Assisted Reproductive Technologies

Quality and Safety

Assisted Reproductive Technologies

Quality and Safety

EDITED BY

Jan Gerris MD PhD
François Olivennes MD PhD
and
Petra De Sutter MD PhD

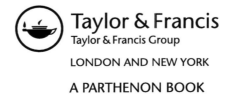

Taylor & Francis
Taylor & Francis Group

LONDON AND NEW YORK

A PARTHENON BOOK

© 2004 Taylor & Francis, an imprint of the Taylor & Francis Group

First published in the United Kingdom in 2004
by Taylor & Francis,
an imprint of the Taylor & Francis Group,
11 New Fetter Lane,
London EC4P 4EE

Tel.:   +44 (0) 20 7583 9855
Fax.:   +44 (0) 20 7842 2298
Website: www.tandf.co.uk

British Library Cataloguing in Publication Data

Data available on application

Library of Congress Cataloging-in-Publication Data

Data available on application

Hardback ISBN 1-84214-231-3
Paperback ISBN 1-84214-313-1

Distributed in North and South America by

Taylor & Francis
2000 NW Corporate Blvd
Boca Raton, FL 33431, USA

Within Continental USA
Tel.: 800 272 7737; Fax.: 800 374 3401
Outside Continental USA
Tel.: 561 994 0555; Fax.: 561 361 6018
E-mail: orders@crcpress.com

Distributed in the rest of the world by
Thomson Publishing Services
Cheriton House
North Way
Andover, Hampshire SP10 5BE, UK
Tel.: +44 (0) 1264 332424
E-mail: salesorder.tandf@thomsonpublishingservices.co.uk

Composition by Parthenon Publishing
Printed and bound by Antony Rowe Ltd., Chippenham, Wiltshire, UK

Contents

List of principal contributors

A. N. Andersen
The Fertility Clinic
Section 4071
Rigshospitalet
Blegsdamvej 9
2100 Copenhagen
Denmark

C. Bergh
Department of Obstetrics and Gynecology
Institute of Children's and Women's Health
Sahlgrenska University Hospital
SE-41345 Göteborg
Sweden

J. Boivin
School of Psychology
Cardiff University
PO Box 901
Cardiff
Wales
CF10 3YG
UK

M. Bonduelle
Centre for Medical Genetics
University Hospital of the Dutch-speaking
  Brussels Free University
Laarbeeklaan 101
1090 Brussels
Belgium

D. Braat
Department of Obstetrics and Gynecology
University Medical Centre Nijmegen
PO Box 9101 nr: GYN 415
6500 HB Nijmegen
The Netherlands

B. Cohlen
Department of Obstetrics and Gynecology
Isala Clinics
Dokter van Heesweg 2
8025 AB Zwolle
The Netherlands

D. De Neubourg
Centre for Reproductive Medicine
Middelheim Hospital
Lindendreef 1
2020 Antwerp
Belgium

P. De Sutter
Centre for Reproductive Medicine
Ghent University Hospital
De Pintelaan 185
9000 Ghent
Belgium

A. Delvigne
Centre for Reproductive Medicine
Hôpital Saint Pierre
Université Libre de Bruxelles
Rue Haute 1
1000 Brussels
Belgium

J. Gerris
Department of Obstetrics, Gynecology and
Fertility
Middelheim Hospital
Lindendreef 1
2020 Antwerp
Belgium

J. Guibert
Sevice de Gynécologie Obstétrique II
Unité de Médecine de la Reproduction
Hôpital Cochin
123 Boulevard de Port-Royal
75014 Paris
France

I. Liebaers
Centre for Medical Genetics
University Hospital of the Dutch-speaking
  Free University of Brussels
Laarbeeklaan 101
1090 Brussels
Belgium

F. Olivennes
Service de Gynécologie Obstétrique II
Unité de Médicine de la Reproduction
Hôpital Cochin
123 Boulevard de Port Royal
75014 Paris
France

G. Pennings
Department of Philosophy
Ghent University
Blandynberg 2
9000 Ghent
Belgium

S. Repping
Center for Reproductive Medicine
Department of Obstetrics and Gynecology
Academic Medical Center
Meibergdreef 9
1105 AZ Amsterdam
The Netherlands

A. Strandell
Reproductive Medicine
Department of Obstetrics and Gynecology
Sahlgrenska University Hospital
SE-41345 Göteborg
Sweden

J. Van der Elst
Infertility Centre
Ghent University Hospital
De Pintelaan 185/2P3
9000 Ghent
Belgium

P. A. van Dop
Department of Obstetrics and Gynecology
Catharina Hospital
PO Box 1350
5602 ZA Eindhoven
The Netherlands

E. Van Royen
Centre for Reproductive Medicine
Department of Obstetrics and Gynecology
Middelheim Hospital
Leindendreef 1
2020 Antwerp
Belgium

A. Van Steirteghem
Centre for Reproductive Medicine
University Hospital of the Dutch-speaking
  Free University of Brussels
Laarbeeklaan 101
1090 Brussels
Belgium

J. P. W. Vermeiden
IVF Laboratory, Division of Reproductive Medicine
Department of Obstetrics and Gynecology
Vrije Universiteit Academic Medical Centre
De Boelelaan 1117
PO Box 7057
1007 MB Amsterdam
The Netherlands

S. Vilska
Infertility Clinic
The Family Federation of Finland
PO Box 849
FIN 00101 Helsinki
Finland

U.-B. Wennerholm
Perinatal Center
Department of Obstetrics and Gynecology
Institute for Women's and Children's Health
Sahlgrenska University Hospital, East
SE-41685 Göteborg
Sweden

Preface

Assisted reproductive technologies (ART) entail a number of risks and complications. These should be minimized, to result in safer treatment; at the same time results should be optimized to generate treatment of high quality. Generally speaking, over the past 20 years, emphasis has been mainly on how to 'improve' results of infertility treatments, not on how to maintain a balance between success, risks and costs. More recently, the need to trade off the efficacy of these treatments against their quality and safety has been introduced by an increasing number of individuals and groups. Worldwide, approximately 500 000 *in vitro* fertilization (IVF) cycles are performed every year, with at least as many ovulation induction or so-called superovulation cycles with or without intrauterine insemination. These treatments and the pregnancies that follow after ART do not come without a price, not only in financial terms but also in terms of medical risks and complications.

The two most frequent and most burdensome complications of ART are twin and high-order multiple pregnancies and the ovarian hyperstimulation syndrome. Other important concerns include uncertainties about the risk for genetic anomalies, congenital malformations and disorders of the reproductive potential of ART offspring, especially after intracytoplasmic sperm injection (ICSI). Also of concern are a possible oncogenic risk, a risk for bleeding at the time of ovum retrieval and for infection both in the patient and in the laboratory, an increased risk for extrauterine pregnancy, a risk for accidental puncture of other organs or pelvic tumors, the risk of inadvertent exposure to gonadotropin releasing hormone (GnRH) agonists, risks related to sedative drugs and a small but existing risk for maternal mortality. There are also relatively minor risks, not strictly medical complications, but which may have a major impact on people's lives, for example, psychological, sexual,

financial, moral, ethical and philosophical dilemmas. All these risks and complications are the focus of concern of this book.

The idea to edit this book arose as a consequence of a 2-day pre-congress course on 'Risks and Complications in ART' organized by a delegation of European Society of Human Reproduction and Embryology (ESHRE) members at the annual American Society for Reproductive Medicine (ASRM) meeting in Seattle, 2002. Clearly, the underlying assumption made by the authors, editors and publishers of this book is the Socratic conviction that humans, being intrinsically good, once knowing what is bad, will naturally try to avoid and prevent it. Both 2400 years of history as well as daily reality seem to indicate that the Socratic axiom – always worth a renewed defense – is at least somewhat less absolute than hoped for, and we may have to settle for a more realistic approach, inspired, for example, by the Kantian principle of never using other humans to reach our own goals, not always less idealistic.

Lack of knowledge of what the risks and complications of a particular medical treatment, e.g. IVF/ICSI with multiple embryo replacement, precisely mean in reality cannot be considered sufficient excuse to continue to cause 'unintended' harm to those who undergo it or who are the result of it. In this context, the word 'knowledge' has a totally different meaning from the media-inflated modernistic concept of 'information'. Many professionals and patients involved in IVF/ICSI are allegedly *informed* about some of the risks the treatment entails, but (more often than not) they do not truly *know* what these risks and complications really mean in terms of time, energy, money and self-questioning guilt. Knowledge is information integrated and settled in the depth of human understanding, characterized by a sense of anticipated experience and creating a sense of accepted responsibility. This book was conceived as an effort to increase knowledge, not only information. Information changes frequently; knowledge deepens slowly.

The major aim of this book is to contribute to ART, to encourage a mature form of alleviation of human suffering due to involuntary childlessness and not only a money-driven businesslike enterprise where major disruptions of fundamental aspects of human reproduction are 'accepted' in order to create pregnancies rather than healthy children. The essence of infertility treatment in general, and of IVF/ICSI in particular, is to provide infertile people with a single healthy baby, with a minimum of complications and at a reasonable cost, so that treatment becomes available to all who have a need for it, endorsed by a competent professional. The end of infertility treatment does not come with a positive pregnancy test but with a liveborn healthy child. It is the professional prerogative as well as the duty of the infertility specialist and the team to guide the patients not only through the *technical* procedure involved, but through the pitfalls that come with it.

This book intends to list and to discuss generally accepted medical risks and complications of ART treatments, their etiology, management and methods of prevention. Although the other risks and complications are not to be underestimated, it will focus heavily on multiple pregnancy (i.e. twin pregnancy and higher-order multiple pregnancy) because these constitute the major risk of ART. The book has been written in the full consciousness that, by the time it is published, the minds and mentalities will have evolved and that not only practitioners but also governments, insurers and patients will have become more aware of their responsibilities. We do not know all we need to know to work perfectly safely, but we know enough to bring our knowledge together under the roof of one unifying concern we share regarding the health of future children.

There is little disagreement as to what is meant by ART: all treatments of infertility in which there is some direct handling of the gametes. Strictly speaking, therefore, induction of ovulation, which by definition solely consists of the administration of drugs to induce follicular maturation and trigger an ovulation in women who otherwise do not ovulate, does not fall within ART. However, given the enormous impact of ovulation induction on the occur-

rence of iatrogenic multiple pregnancies, estimated at about one-third of all multiples, this treatment is also dealt with. The book does not deal with non-ART issues (e.g. reproductive surgery, HIV or other infections), nor does it tackle reproduction in women suffering from particular diseases (e.g. diabetes, lupus) or pre-existing gynecological anomalies (e.g. congenital uterine anomalies). It also does not go into the specific area of certification and accreditation. It deals with the problems specifically caused by ART treatments.

This is a book for all professionals involved in ART: clinicians, embryologists and paramedical personnel working in an IVF/ICSI unit, both newcomers and those established in the field, but also for nurses, laboratory personnel, psychologists and secretarial staff. It takes its inspiration from a wider and holistic view of human reproductive failure. In this sense the book could also appeal to a wider audience consisting of philosophers, ethicists, insurers, politicians involved in health-care management and lawyers. Although it focuses in the first place on facts and data, it also tries to explore the psychological, ethical and moral dimension of our work.

It is also of interest for the potential patient who wants to be well-informed and to understand what the risks and problems related to ART truly are and if and how they can be avoided as far as possible. The responsibility of a treatment that can be applied only through a team effort is also shared by all members of that team, and to a certain degree by the patients as well, since it is, in the end, his or her problem that the team is trying to solve. Through many years of practice, it is my ever-increasing conviction that patients knowing, understanding and correctly anticipating the risks and complications give the best guarantee for a good outcome. We should not underestimate our patients. When the difficulties of the 'average' twin pregnancy are explained to a couple, most will give considerable co-operation to avoid twins. This book can therefore be of great help to those who seek not only treatment but also explanation on a good intellectual level.

The sudden discovery by many around the world of the risks and complications of ART has a somewhat spurious ring, since we have all known for a long time about some of these risks, especially multiple pregnancy. No other medical treatment is accompanied by a complication rate of approximately 50%, which is by and large the proportion of ART children born as part of a set of multiples. As an excuse, the high cost of treatment has been put forward. Again, in the long run, this is more a problem of the medical providers – hence, the politicians – and not one that the children conceived should pay for in terms of quality of life. Another excuse is that patients, women more than men, are ready to accept almost any risk in exchange for a pregnancy. Of course, all mothers love their children, even if they have some minor and even a major disability, so patients can hardly be blamed for a natural wish even if at some risk.

But let there be no misunderstanding: it is from within the profession that both the right questions have been raised and some of the right answers have now started to be given.

For one part of the problem, the answer is easy: single-embryo transfer is not a complex procedure. It is a simple and a logical thing to do. So says the voice of reason. Some scientific, partly academic, questions are still in the open: blastocyst culture, yes or no? If yes, when? Preimplantation aneuploidy screening, yes or no? If yes, when? How to perform optimal embryo selection? How to optimize the increasing importance of our cryopreservation programs? Although topics for further research, in the end, these questions may appear to be irrelevant from the point of view of multiple pregnancy prevention. Even at the price of some loss of ongoing pregnancy rate, single-embryo transfer is a must if certain conditions are met. Patients have to be told that such is the treatment. Less than that is unethical. We can only hope that the embryologists will be well-inspired to agree on efficacious selection characteristics, and not get entangled in sterile discussions. It is quite possible and certainly to be hoped for that, in 20 years from now, a cheap, reliable, simple and universally applicable technique to single out the one genetically perfect embryo with approaching a 100% ongoing implantation rate will be ready to use for all who need it. In the meanwhile, there is no good excuse not to use our simple light microscopic optics in choosing the embryo(s) to transfer to the best of our expertise.

Safety and quality of ART treatments will also depend on both new technology and long-term clinical studies. The latter is the case for the long-term effects on the fertility of ICSI offspring, or for the long-term oncogenic effects of ART treatments on both patients and children. Genetics is certain to play an ever-increasing role in the understanding and the risk assessment of problems of male infertility, and probably in polycystic ovary syndrome and in endometriosis as well. Here further research is needed. The same is true for ovarian hyperstimulation syndrome, where new insights in the molecular pathophysiological mechanisms may open new therapeutic perspectives.

The onus of another part of the problem lies with society as a whole, the politicians and health insurers. Choices will have to be made to allocate limited financial resources. How important for a society is the health of its newborns? Making reproductive medicine accessible for as many persons as truly need it for a reasonable projected cost will become an essential demographic political exercise, especially for the democracies with stable or dwindling populations. Politicians should consider that almost each child born after ART will become a tax payer, reimbursing his or her own coming into existence in a manifold manner, broadening the very social platform that will have to carry the current social costs of society. This is especially so in countries with a long-standing tradition of social security. In other countries, with a more 'liberal', i.e. commercial, view of medicine, things will not be so easy. Physicians will have to be made aware of their moral obligations, possibly through legal initiatives. In the long run, what we need is *multum non multa*, fewer children with an optimal start in life, not many children irrespective of how they start their lives. Patients will have to accept measures that limit the risk for complications, which in itself will become easier if, through financial support, access to treatment if properly indicated has become a right, not a privilege. This may be quite a challenge for politicians who, unfortunately, often have their own hidden electoral agenda. The book is also for them, to see how much more complicated reproductive health issues are than can be solved by pure financial trimming of consumption and cost.

For all of these reasons, the time is ripe for a book reviewing and assessing the medical risks and complications of ART, which constitute the backbone of this book. We did not aim at inducing a negative perception of ART, but rather at creating a positive awareness of how quality care in assisted reproductive medicine can be provided. We strongly believe in the great value of our treatments, in the happiness and fulfilment they cause in large numbers of people. However, if ART is to be a mature form of alleviation of human suffering caused by unwanted childlessness, we have to co-operate worldwide, each one of us in our own practices, in actively convincing patients to accept a wise balance between the chance for a success (a healthy baby) and the risk for complications. We will, therefore, also have to learn to express 'success' other than by just mentioning crude pregnancy rates. The number of singleton children born per started cycle gives a much more quality-related measure. Let us not underestimate our patients by thinking that they will not understand.

These topics of concern have been very much alive within ESHRE. A special task force on risks and complications was created by a number of committed individuals in the year 2000, who initiated a number of educational activities, e.g. an ESHRE Campus Course on 'Prevention of twin pregnancies after ART' in Antwerp in May 2000 and an ESHRE workshop on 'Risks and Complications after ART' in Maastricht in May 2001[1,2]. This resulted in the publication of a campus course report and a summary of guideline proposals, and in the creation of an ESHRE Special Interest Group on Safety and Quality. This SIG-SQART has organized two ASRM pre-congress courses (Seattle, 2002 and San Antonio, 2003) as well as an ESHRE pre-congress course (Madrid, 2003) while planning two others (Berlin, 2004 and Copenhagen, 2005). A structured reflection is taking place on the topic of multiple pregnancy prevention in the Bertarelli Foundation, a think tank uniting the crème de la crème of both American and European reproductive clinicians and embryologists. Many authors of this book are members or active sympathizers of this Special Interest Group. In the future, the SIG will organize other scientific and educational activities and will formulate proposals for minimum quality guidelines to the Executive Committee of ESHRE. It is open to all who want to participate and contribute actively

to its main goal, which is to optimize, not maximize, ART treatments.

Finally, the last chapters of the book should perhaps be read first. As usual, the philosophical and psychological dimensions are almost 'attached files' to the main body of the book. We, clinicians and embryologists, custodians of the so-called 'A' sciences, must learn to think more like those working in the 'B' sciences. In a book on risks I do not mind taking the risk of being considered too moralizing when remembering that philosophy is the mother of all other sciences. The young and frontier-crossing medical adventurers that many of us are (or were) may think our old and wrinkled mother has not so much to say because 'she does not understand' what we are doing. Yet, it is at times stunning with what depth of mind 'old' approaches can give invigorating insights into 'new' problems. For once, these chapters should not just be browsed politely but perhaps be read before all else, to put things in the right human perspective. The present-day result-oriented approach that affects and intoxicates our sphere of action as it does with much other human activity, should be balanced with a personalized approach of sharing experiences.

I heartily thank all authors and contributors to this book, both for their trust in me to edit their work and for the effort they put in. All are persons who are chronically overworked, yet are always prepared to take up a challenge and bring it to good ends. Many of the things that are treated in this book will be dealt with differently in 5 years. In a sense, if that is what happens, it will have served its purpose.

Jan Gerris

REFERENCES

1. Gerris J. ESHRE Campus Course Report. Prevention of twin pregnancies after IVF/ICSI by single embryo transfer. *Hum Reprod* 2001;16:790–800

2. Land JA, Evers JLH. Risks and complications in assisted reproduction techniques: report of an ESHRE consensus meeting. *Hum Reprod* 2003;18:455–7

Assisted reproductive technologies: current achievements and challenges for the future

A. Van Steirteghem

INTRODUCTION

Infertility can be considered as an international health problem. It is one of the most frequently occurring chronic health problems, affecting active young adults. It is time-consuming and costly. It concerns all social classes and races. Infertility has a high prevalence: it affects at least 10% of married or cohabiting women of 18–44 years. A quarter of all married or cohabiting women in that age group are confronted at least once in their lifetime with infertility. The male and female partners in infertile couples represent a substantial part of the population in developed countries.

A survey on the etiology of infertility carried out on publications appearing in the 1960s and 1970s (6814 couples) on the one hand, and reports published in the 1980s and 1990s (9100 couples) on the other, revealed a rather similar prevalence of different diagnostic categories: ovulation disorders in 24 and 28%, semen anomalies in 27 and 23%, tubal infertility in 25 and 20%, idiopathic infertility in 17 and 22% and endometriosis and other causes of infertility in 7 and 7% of couples, respectively.

Over the past four decades, several developments have advanced our knowledge in reproductive science and medicine. Schematically we can say that, in the 1960s we had major developments in reproductive endrocrinology, among other things due to the development of radioimmunoassays, in the 1970s microsurgery was introduced, enabling the repair of a certain number of anomalies in infertile women and men. A major milestone has been *in vitro* fertilization (IVF): Louise Brown was born 25 July 1978 and IVF practice was introduced worldwide in the 1980s[1]. It has proved to be the treatment of choice to alleviate female-factor and idiopathic infertility. A similar solution for treating male-factor infertility was the introduction of intracytoplasmic sperm injection (ICSI)[2]. Since the first birth on 14 January 1992, ICSI has proved to be for male-factor infertility what conventional IVF is for female-factor infertility. The 1990s saw, besides ICSI, the introduction of preimplantation genetic diagnosis (PGD). The question can be asked whether embryonic stem cells will become the new milestone in the current decade.

CURRENT ACHIEVEMENTS OF ASSISTED REPRODUCTIVE TECHNOLOGIES

The *in vitro* fertilization and intracytoplasmic sperm injection procedure

IVF and ICSI treatment cycles can be summarized into the following steps:

(1) Proper patient selection for either IVF or ICSI;

(2) Appropriate patient counseling;

(3) A carefully monitored (ultrasound and hormone assays) controlled ovarian stimulation protocol, mostly a combination of gonadotropin releasing hormone (GnRH) agonists or antagonists in combination with urinary or recombinant gonadotropins and the administration of human chorionic gonadotropin (hCG) at the appropriate moment;

(4) Ultrasound-guided vaginal oocyte retrieval by puncturing of the ovarian follicles;

(5) Search for the cumulus–oocyte complexes in the follicular fluid and incubation of these complexes in adequate culture medium under appropriate physicochemical conditions of pH, O_2, CO_2 and osmolality;

(6) Semen preparation for insemination in IVF or single-sperm microinjection in ICSI;

(7) Assessment of fertilization and embryo cleavage in subsequent days;

(8) Uterine transfer of a limited number of embryos on day 3 or day 5;

(9) Cryopreservation of supernumerary embryos for potential later use[3].

The outcome of these cycles should be carefully followed up until the time of delivery, and the later health of the children born should be fully assessed.

Conventional IVF is applied for different causes of female-factor infertility, including tubal infertility (46%), ovarian or cervical problems (13%), endometriosis (9%) and idiopathic infertility (32%). It became evident that conventional IVF was not very efficient in treating (severe) male-factor infer-

tility: fertilization was much lower when semen parameters were abnormal and up to 50% of all cycles did not result in transfer of at least one embryo[4]. Several assisted fertilization procedures were developed in the late 1980s: first partial zona dissection (PZD), then subzonal insemination (SUZI) and finally ICSI. The first ICSI child was born on 14 January 1992. It became clear that ICSI was consistently better and more efficient than PZD and SUZI for male-factor infertility. ICSI was introduced in many centers worldwide in the mid-1990s[5,6]. It is currently the treatment of choice for male infertility, as IVF is the treatment of choice for female infertility. ICSI can be applied successfully with spermatozoa from the semen in oligo-astheno-teratozoospermia (OAT), with epididymal sperm in obstructive azoospermia and with testicular sperm in obstructive and non-obstructive azoospermia[7].

As indicated in Figures 1 and 2, the results of ICSI are quite similar for the four different types of sperm that can be used in terms of intactness of microinjected oocytes (between 92.1 and 94.1%), normal fertilization (between 60.0 and 75.7% of the injected oocytes) and the percentage of embryos that were transferred or cryopreserved (49.2 and 54.1% of the injected oocytes). In over 90% of ICSI cycles with ejaculated sperm ($n = 2160$), epididy-

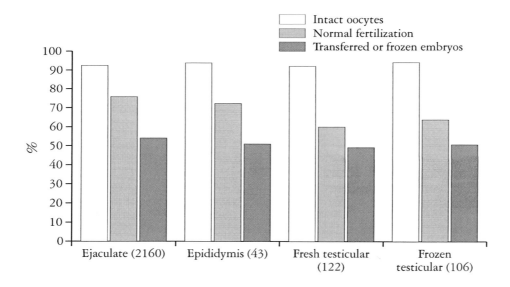

Figure 1 Oocyte intactness, normal fertilization and embryos tranferred or frozen after intracytoplasmic sperm injection with ejaculated, epididymal, fresh or testicular sperm cryopreserved. (Number of treatment cycles in parentheses)

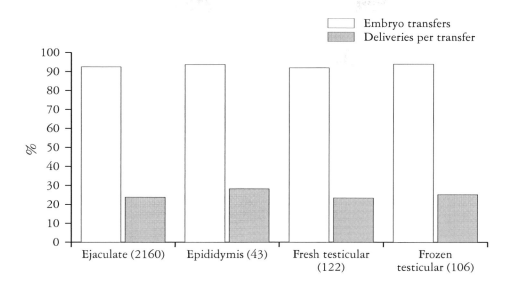

Figure 2 Embryo transfers and delivery rates per transfer after intracytoplasmic sperm injection with four types of sperm. (Number of treatment cycles in parentheses)

mal sperm ($n = 43$), fresh ($n = 122$) and frozen–thawed testicular sperm ($n = 106$), embryo transfer was possible. The percentage of deliveries per transfer in these cycles was 23.8%, 28.2%, 23.4% and 25.3%, respectively[7].

Outcome of *in vitro* fertilization and intracytoplasmic sperm injection

The most important criterion in assessing the outcome of IVF and ICSI procedures has to be the number of treated couples who will end up with a healthy child. As in nature, the preferential outcome is a singleton pregnancy ending in the birth of a healthy child. From the beginning it was clear that the chance of achieving a pregnancy was increased when more embryos were replaced. However, replacing more embryos increases the chance of multiple pregnancy, mostly twins but also triplets and even quadruplets. The occurrence of multiple pregnancies after assisted reproductive technologies (ART), including non-IVF or non-ICSI procedures, has to be considered as the major side-effect of ART. In the later part of this chapter and further in this book, this phenomenon will be discussed, including strategies to avoid multiple ART gestations, including twins.

It is furthermore surprising that, in the first decade of IVF, very few systematic well-designed studies were reported on the outcome, including pregnancy, delivery and health of the children at birth and later in life. When ICSI was introduced at the Vrije Universiteit Brussels (VUB, Free University Brussels) in the early 1990s there was great concern regarding the outcome, because ICSI is an invasive procedure which may damage cellular organelles of the oocyte; ICSI bypasses all steps considered to be involved in the fertilization process; and the sperm used for the microinjection is selected by the embryologist or technician carrying out the ICSI. The sperm used is unable to achieve fertilization *in vivo* or in IVF and this sperm could have more genetic or other abnormalities. Questions were also raised concerning genomic imprinting when non-ejaculated sperm was used; such abnormalities may become evident only later in life. Since in ICSI the whole sperm is introduced into the ooplasm, questions regarding the fate of the paternal mitochondria were also raised.

Since the start of the ART program at the VUB in 1983, a prospective follow-up study was initiated of all pregnancies until delivery as well as the health of all children at birth and later in life. This currently still ongoing study is a joint project between the Center for Reproductive Medicine and the Center for Medical Genetics. This follow-up is carried out with the agreement of the parents. Full information is collected on pregnancy, delivery and, if applicable, prenatal diagnosis. The health of the children is assessed at birth or within 2 months as well as later in life such as at 2, 5 and 8 years of age; the study is planned to continue for as long as possible.

The main observations of this study can be summarized as follows. Genetic counseling is indicated in infertility patients presenting a high risk: i.e. when female age is > 35 years, in situations where one of the partners has an abnormal constitutional karyotype – 5.3% of infertile men – and in situations where there is a higher risk of monogenic disease; an example of the latter is the association of mutations in the *CFTR* gene in male patients with congenital bilateral absence of the vas deferens.

Prenatal karyotypes of 1586 ICSI fetuses obtained after chorionic villus sampling (CVS) or amniocentesis revealed that karyotypes were normal in 97% of the fetuses and that 3.0% of karyotypes were abnormal: 1.4% were inherited chromosome abnormalities – mostly from the infertile father – and 1.6% were *de novo* abnormalities (0.6% sex chromosome aneuploidies and 1.0% autosomal abnormalities, in number as well as in structure)[8]. The mean female age of the patients at the time of prenatal diagnosis was 33.5 years. No such data are available on pregnancies obtained after conventional IVF. This small increase in absolute numbers in *de novo* prenatal chromosome abnormalities after ICSI was correlated with the concentration and motility of the semen used to carry out ICSI. From these data we concluded that it is recommended to counsel ICSI patients to have prenatal diagnosis if sperm concentration is below 5×10^6 per ml and in case of impaired sperm motility.

The results of a cohort study of 2995 IVF and 2889 ICSI children revealed that the percentage of multiple pregnancies was similar after IVF and after ICSI[9]. This high percentage of multiple pregnancies is an important risk factor.

Neonatal data after IVF and ICSI indicate comparable results with regard to birth weight, number of children with low birth weight (< 2500 g), number of perinatal deaths and number of neonatal hospitalizations for medical or surgical treatment. In the studied cohort there was more prematurity in ICSI twins and more very low birth weight (< 1500 g) in IVF twins. When IVF singletons were compared to a reference population IVF had more prematurity, a lower mean birth weight and more babies with low birth weight. A comparison of IVF and ICSI singletons indicated that prematurity, mean birth weight and number of children with low birth weight were similar. When IVF multiples were compared to a reference group of twins, more prematurity was observed, and a mean birth weight that was lower or similar, depending of the study, and more children with a low birth weight. The comparison of IVF and ICSI multiples revealed comparable results regarding prematurity, mean birth weight and number of children with low birth weight. Major congenital anomalies (defined as anomalies leading to death), functional disturbances or requirement for surgery were similar after ICSI (3.4%) and IVF (3.8%). When anomalies detected prenatally or in stillbirths were included, the percentage of anomalies was 4.2% after ICSI and 4.6% after IVF. These percentages are somewhat higher than the anomaly rate reported in national registries, but the methodology used to assess anomalies is different, as will be explained in detail in Chapter 20. Regarding the occurrence of anomalies, there seems to be no influence of the quality or of the origin of the sperm used. Congenital anomalies are more frequent in multiples than in singletons. There was no difference between IVF and ICSI with regard to the organ systems revealing anomalies. In a smaller cohort study of children at the age of 2 years, the two procedures had the same number of anomalies.

The development of ICSI and IVF children was assessed at the age of 2 years using the Bayley test and revealed similar mental scores in the two groups. There was a correlation of this score with the duration of pregnancy, parity and whether the children were singletons or twins. Boys performed somewhat less well than girls, after ICSI and after IVF[10].

Further studies are needed to investigate IVF/ICSI in comparison with spontaneous conceptions regarding liveborn children, fetuses after pregnancy interruption and stillborns. The follow-up of children after ICSI with epididymal or testicular sperm needs to be continued as well as the follow-up of children after replacement of frozen–thawed ICSI embryos. A much longer follow-up of IVF and ICSI children and adults will be needed to assess health, development and fertility.

So far the message to future parents about ICSI should be that multiple pregnancies are a major risk factor, that there is a small increase in the number of inherited and *de novo* chromosomal aberrations, especially in the presence of abnormal sperm, that there is a higher chance of prematurity and lower birth weight even in singletons, that there are probably somewhat more major congenital abnormalities (3.5 instead of 2.5%) which may be related to the age of the female patient and the infertility status, that psychomotor development is normal but neurological development is influenced by neonatal abnormalities and that an increase in rare diseases such as genomic imprinting-related disorders remains a possibility.

PREIMPLANTATION GENETIC DIAGNOSIS

PGD became possible since embryos could be obtained *in vitro* and molecular genetic procedures allowed assessment of abnormalities in single cells such as a blastomere of a preimplantation embryo. PGD is a genetic diagnostic procedure of an embryo prior to transfer into the uterus, i.e. prior to implantation. The first PGD was carried out in the Hammersmith Hospital, London in 1991[11]. It can be considered as an early form of prenatal diagnosis which is performed on an embryo *in vitro*, whereas prenatal diagnosis is performed on a fetus *in vivo*. PGD can be performed in couples with a high recurrence risk for genetic diseases, for example in carriers of a specific genetic disease; carriers of a sex-linked disease; carriers of a chromosomal abnormality. Genetic diagnosis can also be carried out for sporadic chromosomal abnormalities; this approach has been called PGD with aneuploidy screening (PGD-AS; European Society of Human Reproduction and Embryology), preimplantation genetic screening (PGS; UK Human Fertilization and Embryology Authority) and PGD (USA). PGD-AS is practiced to increase the success rate of infertile couples requiring IVF or ICSI in case of: older women, e.g. > 37 years of age; repeated IVF or ICSI failures; recurrent abortions; or severe male factor such as the use of testicular sperm in patients with non-obstructive azoospermia. The role of PGD-AS needs to be assessed by properly conducted controlled studies. In the author's opinions it should at present still be considered as clinical research[12].

PGD *stricto sensu* requires a close collaboration between a center for medical genetics (CMG) and a center for reproductive medicine (CRM). Most couples will be referred to a CMG, where the genetic diagnosis should be firmly established, where the possibility to carry out a robust, reliable and efficient genetic diagnosis on a single cell should be assessed and where proper genetic counseling needs to be done. If the couple accepts PGD they are then referred to a CRM, where a similar approach is applied to that for other ART patients. The clinicians are responsible for the intake, ovarian stimulation and oocyte retrieval; the embryologists will then perform mostly ICSI – to avoid contamination with extraneous DNA – and the embryo biopsy is carried out using acid Tyrode or laser on a day-3 embryo (around the eight-cell stage). In the CMG the genetic diagnosis will then be carried out using fluorescent *in situ* hybridization (FISH) or polymerase chain reaction (PCR) technology. Thereafter, one or two unaffected embryos will be transferred in the CRM. At present, PGD can be performed for several tens of different monogenetic diseases as well as for chromosomal aberrations. As for other active PGD centers, the number of cycles of PGD and PGD-AS in the author's laboratory has increased substantially over the years.

PGD is a novel option for couples with a high recurrence risk of having an affected child. Couples choosing PGD as a prenatal procedure are certainly those requiring ICSI or IVF or those who object to pregnancy termination after amniocentesis or CVS. PGD is possible only when a DNA mutation or chromosomal aberration is known and when a reliable diagnosis on a single cell is possible[13].

CHALLENGES FOR THE FUTURE

Prevention of all assisted reproductive technology multiple pregnancies

It is estimated that, after 25 years of IVF and 12 years of ICSI practice, there have been more than 1 million children born, which can be considered as a positive outcome and a relief for many couples with long-standing infertility. However, about half of these children are not from singleton pregnancies; in other words about 500 000 children are from twin, triplet or higher-order pregnancies. The previously mentioned risks of IVF or ICSI are in terms of prevalence, not important in comparison to the morbidity generated by multiple pregnancies. It is not exceptional that twins after ART are considered as a positive outcome by infertile couples; however, twins have much more problems than singletons: more cases of cerebral palsy, other medical problems and high cost for the community. It is estimated that in the UK the cost of taking care of these children born after multiple IVF or ICSI pregnancies exceeds £50×10^6 per year (about 75×10^6 Euro or $).

The question can be asked why this could occur, since clinicians and other caretakers must have concern for the well-being of infertile patients and their children. Too many embryos are replaced, because the primary goal for many is simply achieving a pregnancy and not achieving a singleton gestation. High pregnancy rates are in many countries part of professional and intellectual competition. Achieving a pregnancy at any price is also influenced by the high cost of ART in many countries such as the USA. In theory the solution to avoid multiple pregnancies including twins is simple, i.e. the replacement of a single embryo. As was stated by Nygren from Sweden: 'You can have as many embryos put back as you like but one at a time'[14]. It is obvious that in the near future the practice of single-embryo transfer is unavoidable. It is already practiced in a number of Scandinavian countries and in Belgium. The following steps are needed to encourage the practice of single-embryo transfer:

(1) Education about the need for single-embryo transfer given to caretakers, patients and health authorities;

(2) Full information given to infertile couples about the important risks related to multiple pregnancies, including twins;

(3) Better methods of choosing the embryo for transfer, having the best chance for implantation;

(4) Better protocols for freezing and thawing of embryos that are not replaced in the initial treatment cycle.

The question can be asked whether PGD-AS may play an additional role to embryo morphology in selecting embryos for transfer. Randomized controlled trials are needed to answer the question of whether single-embryo transfer reduces the chance to fulfil the wish of infertile couples for a child. This aspect will be further developed in greater depth in other chapters.

Human embryonic stem cells

There is currently great interest in stem cells – somatic and embryonic stem cells (ESC) – among other reasons in view of cell transplantation for therapeutic purposes. Using the vast experience with the production of mouse ESC, the derivation of human ESC was reported in 1988. These ESC were derived from the inner cell mass of supernumerary IVF blastocysts which had been donated for research. Isolation and derivation of ESC can be summarized as follows. The first step consists of the isolation of the inner cell mass by immunosurgery. The zona pellucida is removed using pronase. The trophoblast cells are lysed after incubation with anti-2,4-dinitrophenol and guinea-pig complement. What remains is the inner cell mass, which will be plated on a feeder layer of mouse embryonic fibroblasts. After 9–15 days, a central mass is obtained which will be dissociated and plated again. Colonies can be obtained, from which undifferentiated cell colonies can be isolated for further culture. At regular intervals karyotype stability and telomerase activity are monitored. After about ten passages, markers for stem cells are determined: alkaline phosphatase, different cell-surface markers and Oct-4 expression. The potency for differentiation of ESC is determined after formation of embryoid bodies, where the three germ layers are present. The presence of α-fetoprotein is a marker for endoderm, and hCG is a marker for trophoblast differentiation. The capacity of these cells to generate tumors is assessed after injection into SCID mice. Cell lines are cryopreserved after characterization. Before therapeutic use of these cell lines, a number of quality criteria must be fulfilled, such as a proper control of the starting material. Phase I clinical trials must be preceded by a number of preclinical tests[15].

REFERENCES

1. Steptoe PC, Edwards RG, Purdy J. Clinical aspects of pregnancies established with cleaving embryos grown *in vitro*. *Br J Obstet Gynaecol* 1980;87:757–68

2. Palermo G, Joris H, Devroey P, Van Steirteghem AC. Pregnancies after intracytoplasmic injection of single spermatozoon into an oocyte. *Lancet* 1992;340:17–18

3. Van Steirteghem A. Twenty years of *in vitro* fertilization: realization and questions for the future. *Verh K Acad Geneeskd Belg* 2001;63:193–241

4. Tournaye H, Devroey P, Camus M, *et al.* Comparison of *in-vitro* fertilization in male and tubal infertility: a 3 year survey. *Hum Reprod* 1992;7:218–22

5. Van Steirteghem AC, Liu J, Joris H, *et al.* Higher success rate by intracytoplasmic sperm injection than by subzonal insemination. Report of a second series of 300 consecutive treatment cycles. *Hum Reprod* 1993;8:1055–60

6. Van Steirteghem AC, Nagy Z, Joris H, *et al.* High fertilization and implantation rates after intracytoplasmic sperm injection. *Hum Reprod* 1993;8:1061–6

7. De Vos A, Van Steirteghem A. Gamete and embryo micromanipulation. In Strauss J, Barbieri R, eds. *Yen and Jaffe's Reproductive Endocrinology*, 5th edition. Philadelphia: Elsevier Science, 2003:in press

8. Bonduelle M, Van Assche E, Joris H, *et al.* Prenatal testing in ICSI pregnancies: incidence of chromosomal anomalies in 1586 karyotypes and relation to sperm parameters. *Hum Reprod* 2002;17:2600–14

9. Bonduelle M, Liebaers I, Deketelaere V, *et al.* Neonatal data on a cohort of 2889 infants born after ICSI (1991–1999) and of 2995 infants born after IVF (1983–1999). *Hum Reprod* 2002;17:671–94

10. Bonduelle M, Ponjaert I, Van Steirteghem A, *et al.* Developmental outcome at 2 years of age for children born after ICSI compared with children born after IVF. *Hum Reprod* 2003;18:342–50

11. Handyside AH, Kontogianni EH, Hardy K, Winston RML. Pregnancies from biopsied human preimplantation embryos sexed by Y-specific DNA amplification. *Nature (London)* 1990;344:768–70

12. Braude P, Pickering S, Flinter F, Ogilvie CM. Preimplantation genetic diagnosis. *Nature Rev Genet* 2002;3:941–53

13. Geraedts J, Harper J, Braude P, *et al.* Preimplantation genetic diagnosis (PGD), a collaborative activity of clinical genetic departments and IVF centres. *Prenat Diagn* 2001;21:1086–92

14. Templeton A. Avoiding multiple pregnancies in ART. *Hum Reprod* 2000;15:1662

15. Smith AG. Embryo-derived stem cells: of mice and men. *Annu Rev Cell Dev Biol* 2001;17:435–62

2

Epidemiology of multiple pregnancy including natural versus iatrogenic multiple pregnancy

A. Pinborg and A.N. Andersen

INTRODUCTION

The fascination of twins has existed since ancient times. In 1950 the medical literature contained approximately 5000 citations referring to twins[1]. Since then, the number of papers dealing with multiple pregnancies has increased considerably and many countries have established national twin registers to encourage twin surveillance and research. Currently, the high rate of multiple births including twins resulting from assisted reproductive technologies (ART) is a major health issue.

Twin pregnancies are the result of a complex interaction of genetic and environmental determinants. Their frequency has increased considerably over the past two decades, after a decreasing trend lasting 30–40 years. This upward trend has been observed only in dizygotic twinning. The two major contributing factors for the rise in the twin birth rate are the use of ART and the increased age of women at childbirth. An estimation of the factors that have contributed to the increased twinning rate made by Bergh and co-workers revealed that about one-third of the increase is due to increased maternal age, another third is caused by *in vitro* fertilization (IVF) and the remaining third is probably caused by ovarian stimulation[2]. The role of these factors varies in different populations.

Depending on the individual embryo transfer policy and the current practice of replacing two or more embryos into the uterus in most countries, IVF pregnancies carry an increased risk of twin and high-order gestations. It is clear that multiple pregnancies are high-risk pregnancies with risks to both mother and fetuses; hence, they impose a financial burden on maternity and neonatal services. The fetal risks are primarily related to the enormous likelihood of preterm birth in twin and particularly in higher-order multiple pregnancies.

This chapter describes the epidemiology of multiple pregnancies in terms of maternal age, race, populations and zygosity. In addition, spontaneous versus iatrogenic multiple pregnancies and the role of ovarian stimulation and IVF are discussed. Since it has been generally accepted that triplet and higher-order multiple gestations are to be avoided, and many European countries have already recommended the transfer of a maximum of two embryos in ART, the main focus will be on the epidemiology of twin pregnancies.

BIOLOGY (MONOZYGOTIC AND DIZYGOTIC TWINNING)

Twin gestations are divided into two major types: dizygotic (DZ) and monozygotic (MZ). While MZ twins occur sporadically, the DZ twin rate increases with advancing age and parity. The rising gonadotropin levels and the more frequent occurrence of ovulation of more than one mature follicle may explain the higher twin gestation rate seen with advancing maternal age[3]. In some families DZ twinning is apparently inherited[3]. The present increase in the twin birth rate is mainly caused by a rise in the occurrence of DZ twins, whereas the rate of MZ twins remains stable throughout the world. In Caucasians about 30% of twin pregnancies are MZ and about 70% DZ. Zygosity denotes the type of conception, whereas chorionicity refers to the type of placentation. MZ twins result from the splitting of one fertilized ovum during the first 2 weeks of embryogenesis, whereas DZ twins originate from the fertilization of two ova by different spermatozoa[3]. According to the number of layers in the septum between the amniotic sacs, twin placentas are categorized as monochorionic (MC) and dichorionic (DC). DZ twins are always DC, but MZ twins can be either DC or MC. In spontaneously conceived DZ twins the malformation rate per fetus is the same as in singletons, whereas the rate is two- to three-fold higher in MZ twins[4]. Moreover, mortality rates are higher amongst same-sex and MZ twins but only recently has it been shown that this higher rate (in both stillbirths and neonatal deaths) was limited to MC, MZ twins and that there was no significant difference between DZ and DC twin pairs[5]. The proportion of MZ twins among IVF twins (1–2%) is notably lower than in spontaneously conceived twins (30%)[3,6]. Even though the MZ twinning rate is lower in IVF twins, the rate is still more than two-fold over the rate in the general population, where the incidence of MZ twinning has been estimated to be 0.4% in live births[6].

Factors influencing dizygotic twinning rates

DZ twinning has a high heritability. The risk of having twins is roughly doubled in a woman whose mother or sister had DZ twins[7]. Race also plays a major role in DZ twinning rates. Other contributors to DZ twinning rates are maternal age and parity. Maternal age has a considerable effect on DZ twinning rates, which increase more than four-fold from the age of 15 to 37 years, followed by an abrupt decline[7]. Parity has some influence independent of maternal age, with an increase in the twinning rate of 50% from parities of 0 to 10[7]. Surveys on DZ twinning rates suggest an influence of nutrition, since malnutrition in occupied countries during the Second World War caused an acute fall in DZ twinning rates[7]. Obviously, the use of ART plays an important iatrogenic role in the increased DZ twinning rate, as discussed later.

Factors influencing monozygotic twinning rates

It is generally accepted that MZ twinning is a random embryological event, which is not subject to environmental influences and is not genetically determined. While the incidence of MZ twinning is largely independent of race, maternal age, parity and malnutrition, it has been shown that ovarian stimulation more than doubles the incidence of MZ twins[7]. Gonadotropin treatment has been claimed as the major contributing factor for the increased MZ twinning rates in ART, rather than micromanipulation, including intracytoplasmic sperm injection (ICSI), zona drilling and assisted hatching[6]. *In vitro* conditions also play a role, since the incidence of MZ twinning is increased three-fold after blastocyst transfer compared to cleavage-stage transfer[8]. Additionally, it has been shown that a mother who is a MZ twin has a significantly increased risk of herself having MZ twins, indicating that some kind of genetic predisposition to MZ twinning may exist[7].

TIME PATTERNS

Secular changes in dizygotic twinning rates

After a global decline in the DZ twinning rates in developed countries from the beginning of the 1960s to the 1970s, the DZ twinning rate has increased in the USA and in most European countries during the past two decades. Environmental pollutants, the decreasing sperm count or infertility following use of the oral contraceptive pill have been held responsible for the former worldwide decline in the DZ twinning rate, but the exact cause remains unknown[7]. The causes for the increasing DZ twinning rates have previously been discussed.

Secular changes in monozygotic twinning rates

The MZ twinning rate has remained remarkably stable in Italy, Denmark and Israel in recent decades, or increased marginally in a number of countries such as England, Wales, Germany, The Netherlands and Japan. It is generally assumed that the gradual increase is possibly the result of improved obstetric care of mothers carrying twins. The use of ART is negligible, when compared to the great changes in DZ twinning rates[7].

RACIAL FACTORS

The incidence of twin pregnancies is population dependent, the highest rates being reported in Nigeria and the lowest in Japan. As a broad generalization, based on data collected before the advent of ovulation-inducing agents, the DZ twinning rate is about eight per thousand in Caucasians, about twice as large in Blacks and less than half in Mongoloids[9]. The rate of MZ twinning (3.5–4.0 per thousand live births) is fairly constant throughout the world, whereas the differences between racial and ethnic groups are caused mainly by differences in DZ twinning rates. The racial differences in the incidence of DZ twinning have been explained by a number of factors, including genetic predisposition inherited primarily from the mother, undernourishment and possibly rural site of living. The main contributing mechanism, however, has not been identified.

NATIONAL MULTIPLE BIRTH RATES

Imaizumi reported the national changes in twinning and triplet rates from 1972 to 1996 with data originating from vital statistics in 17 countries[10]. The overall twinning and triplet birth rates on a worldwide scale during the period from 1972 to 1996 are listed in Table 1. Apart from the Czech Republic and the Slovak Republic, where the twinning and triplet rates remained fairly constant from 1972 to 1994 followed by a rise in 1995–96, the multiple birth rates in the other 15 countries remained nearly constant or gradually increased until the mid-1980s, with the most rapid increase seen from 1990 to 1996. The range in twin birth rate increases between 1972 and 1996 varied from 1.2-fold observed in Australia to a two-fold increase in Denmark.

For triplets the increase was even more pronounced, from three-fold in Denmark to ten-fold in Norway during the examined period. The same tendency was seen in the USA, where the twinning rate increased 35.8% between 1975 and 1995, and triplet, quadruplet and quintuplet rates increased even more strikingly[1]. The triplet rate in Finland, Norway, Sweden and The Netherlands increased from 1972 until the late 1990s and then decreased[10]. In Switzerland the triplet rate reached a maximum in 1987 and then remained constant. Triplet rates in the remaining countries were rising until 1996. The decreasing triplet rates were due to the recommendation to transfer a maximum of two embryos in the Scandinavian countries. In the 15 countries with rising twinning and triplet rates, the impact of ART has increased from when the first IVF child was born in 1978 to 1996. After the implementation of two-embryo transfer as the standard of good clinical practice in Scandinavia, triplet rates have decreased to a minimum, whereas twinning rates have remained fairly constant and lingered at around 25%. The overall pregnancy rates for IVF patients have not been affected[11]. As previously mentioned, twinning rates were highest in Blacks, intermediate in Caucasians, and lowest in Orientals before treatment with fertility drugs. After the introduction of ART, however, twinning and triplet rates in Singapore, Hong Kong and Japan have exceeded those in the Slovak Republic, indicating that secular changes in multiple birth rates depend on how widespread these techniques are in each country.

This upward trend in multiple pregnancy rates has been particularly remarkable among women aged 30–39 years. In Denmark the national incidence of multiple pregnancies increased 1.7-fold from 1980 to 1994. This increase was almost exclusively observed in women aged ≥ 30 years, for whom the adjusted population-based twinning rates increased 2.7-fold and the triplet rate 9.1-fold. The rise in twinning rates was limited to DZ twinning[12]. This report also yielded a particular impact on infant deaths, in which the proportion of multiple births increased more than two-fold from 11.5% to 26.9% for primiparous women aged ≥ 30 years. The total infant mortality, however, did not increase for this group of women, owing to a significant decrease in the infant mortality rate during the same period among singletons[12].

The secular changes in twinning and triplet rates highlight the substantial effect that the introduction of ART, to a relatively small group of women, has caused on the overall national multiple pregnancy rates. Owing to a concomitant drop in mortality among singletons, the national infant mortality rates have not been affected by the increasing multiple pregnancy rates.

Table 1   National twin and triplet birth rates from 1972 to 1996. From reference 10

Year	Twins (per 1000 births)			Triplets (per 10^6 births)		
	1972	1990	1996	1972	1980–90	1996
Denmark	9.0	11.2	17.8	—	203(1988)	559
Finland	10.4(1975)	11.3(1989)	15.6	122(1975)	229(1987)	545(1992)
Norway	8.9(1974)	—	14.5	50(1974)	133(1986)	507(1991)
Sweden	8.2	9.1(1977)	14.4	77	155(1985)	549(1993)
Austria	8.5	9.4(1987)	11.4	38	—	303
The Czech Republic	8.7	9.6(1994)	11.4	53	181(1994)	320
The Slovak Republic	8.2	—	10.2	30	126(1994)	162
Germany	8.8	9.4(1983)	13.8	70	119(1983)	483
The Netherlands	9.4	10.3(1983)	14.4	79	129(1986)	537(1991)
Switzerland	8.4	—	12.8	55	327(1987)	—
England/Wales	9.5(1974)	10.0(1984)	13.4	94(1974)	125(1984)	402
Canada	9.2	—	11.6	83	187(1990)	320
Australia	—	10.9(1985)	14.1	—	234(1985)	518
Japan	5.8(1974)	—	8.9	58(1974)	109(1988)	275(1994)
Singapore	5.8	7.3	8.4	40	116(1988)	424
Hong Kong	5.5	—	8.7	17	86(1980)	268
Israel	9.4	12.6(1983)	17.4	401(1982)	861(1985)	1297

NATIONAL REGISTRY DATA ON MULTIPLE PREGNANCIES AFTER IVF AND ICSI

The percentages of singleton, twin, triplet and quadruplet deliveries after IVF and ICSI treatments in Europe in 1999 are shown in Table 2. Data originate from the third report of the annual publication of the European Society of Human Reproduction and Embryology (ESHRE) on European data on ART[13]. The distribution of deliveries was: singleton 73.7%, twins 24.0%, triplets 2.2% and quadruplets

0.1%. The incidence of twin deliveries varied from 10.8% in Slovenia to 32.5% in Hungary and the incidence of triplets ranged from 0.3% in Denmark to 7.0% in the Czech Republic. Quadruplets occurred in 0.1% of cases in 1999 with only the Czech Republic exceeding 0.5%.

According to a worldwide collaborative report on ART in 1998, multiple pregnancy rates in Australia and Asia were quite similar to European rates. Twin and triplet rates after IVF in 1998 were 22.0% and 0.7% in Australia; 26.3% and 0% in Hong Kong; 26.6% and 0.9% in Korea; the total

Table 2   Singleton, twin, triplet and quadruplet deliveries after *in vitro* fertilization and intracytoplasmic sperm injection in Europe in 1999. From reference 13

	All deliveries	Singleton deliveries	%	Twin deliveries	%	Triplet deliveries	%	Quadruplet deliveries	%
Belgium	1755	1310	74.6	429	24.4	16	0.9		0.0
Czech Republic	1026	636	62.0	310	30.2	72	7.0	7	0.7
Denmark	1578	1195	75.7	379	24.0	4	0.3	0	0.0
Finland	866	653	75.4	206	23.8	7	0.8	0	0.0
France	7302	5469	74.9	1738	23.8	95	1.3	0	0.0
Germany	7120	5322	74.7	1605	22.5	192	2.7	1	0.0
Greece	1320	979	74.2	332	25.2	9	0.7	0	0.0
Hungary	314	191	60.8	102	32.5	20	6.4	1	0.3
Iceland	111	90	81.1	19	17.1	2	1.8	0	0.0
Ireland	198	144	72.7	47	23.7	7	3.5	0	0.0
Italy	2147	1602	74.6	466	21.7	75	3.5	4	0.2
The Netherlands	NA								
Norway	812	598	73.6	209	25.7	5	0.6	0	0.0
Poland	445	344	77.3	92	20.7	9	2.0	0	0.0
Portugal	271	188	69.4	76	28.0	6	2.2	1	0.4
Russia	604	443	73.3	134	22.2	26	4.3	1	0.2
Slovenia	158	140	88.6	17	10.8	1	0.7	0	0.0
Spain	1843	1236	67.1	513	27.8	91	4.9	3	0.2
Sweden	1670	1259	75.4	405	24.3	6	0.4	0	0.0
Switzerland	300	213	71.0	83	27.7	4	1.3	0	0.0
United Kingdom	NA								
Ukraine	NA								0.0
All	29 840	22 012	73.8	7162	24.0	647	2.2	18	0.1

NA, not available

multiple birth rate in Japan was 22.9%[14]. Data from the American Society for Reproductive Medicine for 1998 gives a similar, albeit worse, picture. Of all IVF deliveries in the USA in 1999, 62.9% were singletons, 32.2% twins, 4.7% triplets and 0.2% quadruplets[15].

With respect to the most important factor – child health – the incidence of multiple deliveries may not be the best outcome measure. Since long-term morbidity, family implications and health economic costs are increased in children of multiple gestations, the number of infants born as multiples should be considered as the preferable outcome measure[16,17]. As listed in Table 3, the distribution of infants born as multiples after IVF and ICSI treatment in several European countries in 1999 varied between 41.6 and 79.0% for singletons, 19.0 and 44.4% for twins, 0.6 and 14.6% for triplets and 0 and 1.9% for quadruplets. In 13 of the 18 countries around 40% of the IVF/ICSI children were born as twins and in 8 European countries nearly 10% of the IVF/ICSI children were born as triplets[13].

Compared with data from the corresponding ESHRE report from 1997, the incidence of multiple deliveries remained fairly unchanged from 1997 to 1999, apart from a marginal decrease in the incidence of triplets and a minor increase in the incidence of singletons and twins. The mean incidence of singleton, twin, triplet and quadruplet deliveries in 1997 was 70.4%, 25.8%, 3.6% and 0.2%, respectively[18]. A reduction in the multiple delivery rates after IVF and ICSI were, however, not observed in Europe from 1998 to 1999[13]. According to the data presented, and to our knowledge regarding the adverse outcome of multiples deliveries, it is clear that the incidence of multiple pregnancies after IVF and ICSI treatment is still much too high.

A change in the embryo transfer policy towards single embryo transfer has been implemented in Finland, resulting in a reduction in the multiple birth rate; in 2001 single embryo transfer constituted one-third of all transfers in Finland and the multiple birth rate was reduced to 17%[19].

MULTIPLE PREGNANCIES AFTER FROZEN EMBRYO REPLACEMENT

The mean percentages of singleton, twin, triplet and quadruplet deliveries after frozen embryo replacement in 17 European countries in 1999 were 84.8%, 14.0%, 0.8% and 0.4%, respectively[13]. Mirroring the lower pregnancy rates after frozen embryo replacement (15.7% pregnancies per transfer) the incidence of multiple pregnancies after frozen embryo replacement was lower than in fresh IVF and ICSI cycles, where the pregnancy rate per transfer in Europe in 1999 was 27.7% and 27.9%, respectively. Multiple pregnancy rates after frozen embryo replacement in Australia and Hong Kong were similar to those reported for Europe, whereas Korea, Singapore and Taiwan revealed substantially higher rates: 27.3–27.8% for twins and 1.1–4.5% for triplets[14]. In the USA, the transfer of cryopreserved embryos resulted in 73.1% singleton, 22.9% twin, 4.0% triplet and < 0.1% more than triplet deliveries[15]. The high multiple pregnancy rates after frozen embryo replacement in the USA and in some Asian and European countries indicate that the numbers of embryos transferred in frozen embryo replacement cycles are high.

NUMBER OF EMBRYOS TRANSFERRED

The number of embryos replaced is of crucial importance in avoiding multiple pregnancies. Table 4 presents data from European registers by ESHRE for the year 1999[13]. The incidence of two-embryo transfers varied from 15 to 84% per country in 1999; transfer of three or four embryos occurred in more than 50% of transfers in 11 of 18 countries, whereas single embryo transfer constituted only 7–23%. Data on the distribution of elective and non-elective single embryo transfer were not available. The European data from 1999 indicate that, while double embryo transfer had become the daily clinical practice in some countries including Scandinavia in 1999, elective single embryo transfer had not yet been introduced. It is clear, when comparing Table 2 and Table 4, that triplet birth rates are high in those countries frequently transferring three to four embryos. Although two-embryo transfer has been implemented in the Scandinavian countries, the twin birth rates in Scandinavia apart from Finland have remained stable. In Finland single embryo transfer constituted 32% of all transfers in 2001, resulting in a multiple birth rate of only 17.4% in 2001 compared with 27.3% in 1992, when only 14.5% of the transfers in Finland were

Table 3   Percentage of infants born as singletons, twins, triplets and quadruplets after *in vitro* fertilization and intracytoplasmic sperm injection in Europe in 1999. From reference 13

	All infants	Singletons	Twins	Triplets	Quadruplets
Belgium	2216	59.1	38.7	2.2	0.0
Czech Republic	1503	62.0	41.3	14.6	1.9
Denmark	1965	60.8	38.6	0.6	0.0
Finland	1086	60.1	37.9	1.9	0.0
France	9230	59.3	37.7	3.1	0.0
Germany	9112	58.4	35.2	6.3	0.0
Greece	1670	58.6	39.8	1.6	0.0
Hungary	459	41.6	44.4	13.1	0.9
Iceland	134	67.2	28.4	4.5	0.0
Ireland	259	55.6	36.3	8.1	0.0
Italy	2775	57.7	33.6	8.1	0.6
The Netherlands	NA				
Norway	1058	59.0	39.5	1.4	0.0
Poland	555	62.0	33.2	4.9	0.0
Portugal	362	51.9	42.0	5.0	1.1
Russia	793	55.9	33.8	9.8	0.5
Slovenia	177	79.0	19.0	1.7	0.0
Spain	2547	48.5	40.3	10.7	0.5
Sweden	2087	60.3	38.8	0.9	0.0
Switzerland	391	42.5	42.5	3.1	0.0
United Kingdom	NA				
Ukraine	NA				
All	36 135	41.6–79.0	19.0–44.4	0.6–14.6	0.0–1.9

NA, not available

Table 4   Number of embryos transferred in *in vitro* fertilization and intracytoplasmic sperm injection in Europe in 1999. From reference 13

	All transfers	One embryo	%	Two embryos	%	Three embryos	%	Four embryos	%
Belgium	8015	852	10.6	3744	46.7	2727	34.0	692	12.7
Czech Republic	5638	577	10.2	1064	18.9	2983	52.9	1014	18.0
Denmark		NA		NA		NA		NA	
Finland	3999	842	21.1	2994	74.9	215	5.4	1	0.6
France	30 459	4200	13.8	12 878	42.3	11 340	37.2	2041	6.7
Germany	41 490	4623	11.1	15 468	37.3	21 399	51.6	0	0.0
Greece	5209	523	10.0	1041	20.0	1677	32.2	1968	37.8
Hungary	1729	134	7.8	293	16.9	823	47.6	479	27.7
Iceland	325	36	11.1	220	67.7	69	21.2	0	0.0
Ireland	972	80	8.2	214	22.0	654	67.3	24	2.5
Italy	10 198	1148	11.3	3167	31.1	4166	40.9	1720	16.3
The Netherlands	NA	NA		NA		NA		NA	
Norway	NA	NA		NA		NA		NA	
Poland	1794	292	16.3	1149	64.0	266	14.8	87	4.9
Portugal	1302	167	12.8	397	30.1	595	45.7	143	11.4
Russia	2819	338	12.0	563	20.0	635	22.5	1283	45.5
Slovenia	1275	287	22.5	795	62.4	193	15.1	0	0.0
Spain	8355	722	8.6	1366	16.3	3809	45.6	2458	29.6
Sweden	6247	699	11.2	5268	84.3	280	4.5	0	0.0
Switzerland	2415	312	12.9	1378	57.1	679	28.1	46	1.9
United Kingdom	NA	NA		NA		NA		NA	
Ukraine	738	49	6.6	114	15.4	136	18.4	439	59.6
All	132 979	15 881	11.9	52 113	39.2	52 646	39.6	12 395	8.6

NA, not available

The sum of all transfers and the sum of transfers with one, two, three or four embryos differ by 56. This is due to unknown number of embryos transferred in some cases single embryo transfers[19]. This clearly illustrates that, in 1999, Finland was the only country where a more-or-less generalized introduction of elective single embryo transfer has been shown to result in a substantial decrease in the number of twins born while maintaining a stable ongoing pregnancy rate.

BLASTOCYST TRANSFER

The ability to select embryos remains an important determinant of the outcome of IVF, despite the limitations of grading the quality of embryos according to morphological criteria, as is done in current clinical practice. Blastocyst transfer has been suggested as a tool in diminishing multiple pregnancies by selecting and transferring the putatively most competent embryo. On the basis of retrospective comparative studies, embryo transfer on day 5 has been claimed to result in higher implantation rates than transfer on day 3. Randomized controlled trials published to date have not supported this convincingly. Another problem is that blastocyst culture seems to entail a higher risk of MZ twinning[20]. There is still a lack of properly designed randomized controlled trials to compare the transfer of one day-3 embryo with one day-5 embryo, which would thereby also address the potential value of single blastocyst transfer in reducing the incidence of multiple pregnancies.

FACTORS PREDICTING MULTIPLE PREGNANCIES

Templeton and Morris studied factors associated with an increased risk of multiple births in 44 236 cycles in 25 240 women in the UK[21]. They concluded that older age, the presence of tubal infertility, four or more previous IVF attempts and long duration of infertility all significantly reduced the odds of a birth as well as the odds of multiple births. A woman having had a previous live birth has increased odds of a birth but not of multiple births. They concluded that the number of embryos available is more important in determining the outcome than the number of embryos actually transferred into the uterus. When more than four eggs had been fertilized, the birth rate was similar whether three or two embryos were transferred. Transfer of more embryos, however, increased the

risk of multiple births. For example, a 30-year-old woman choosing to have two embryos transferred rather than three reduced her risk of multiple birth from 39 to 29% and nearly avoided the risk of triplets[21].

During the 1990s many countries introduced recommendations with respect to the number of embryos to be transferred in ART. In 1997 the Danish National Board of Health recommended the transfer of only two embryos; consequently the triplet rate has been diminished to a minimum, whereas the twinning rate has remained fairly constant. The same pattern was seen in other countries, where double embryo transfer was introduced as daily good clinical practice. In the light of the high twinning rate in ART, elective single embryo transfer is currently a major topic of discussion and has already been introduced in Sweden, Finland and Belgium. In a future perspective, single embryo transfer should be adopted as our daily clinical practice. However, the implementation requires strict patient selection criteria to maintain overall pregnancy rates. One could interpret the dual embryo criteria as an intermediary step towards elective single embryo transfer.

Applying multivariate analysis to a number of variables pertaining to 2107 IVF cycles, Strandell and co-workers found that the number of good-quality embryos transferred, female age, tubal indication and the number of previous IVF cycles were the only independently predictive factors of multiple births. They calculated that the multiple birth rate could be reduced from 26% to 13% in all IVF births, if a single embryo was transferred in selected patients with a high risk of multiple births (50% of all cycles). Concomitantly, they predicted that the total birth rate would decrease from 29% to 25%. The authors claimed that this small decrease could be completely restored by one additional transfer with a single frozen embryo[22]. This goal was almost reached in Finland in 2001 with a multiple birth rate of 17%.

Prospective studies on single embryo transfer have yielded acceptable pregnancy rates of 30–40% in selected patients, provided high-quality embryos are available[23]. One future goal of IVF, seen in the light of the prospective studies on single embryo transfer, is to reduce the multiple pregnancy rate, twins included, to less than 10% without decreasing the overall pregnancy rate.

MULTIPLE PREGNANCIES AFTER OTHER TYPES OF ART

After IVF techniques the incidence of multiple gestations is primarily related to the number of embryos transferred. However, after other types of infertility treatment such as ovulation induction in anovulatory women or superovulation combined with intrauterine insemination (IUI), the key parameter determining the risk of multiple gestations is the number of preovulatory follicles.

The contribution of infertility treatments other than *in vitro* techniques to the increase in multiple deliveries is difficult to assess, as no published national register data are available. In Denmark the Danish Fertility Society has recently made an extension of the national annual data collection of ART by including treatments with IUI. The number of vital pregnancies in relation to singleton, twin and triplet gestations following all types of ART in Denmark in 2002 are presented in Table 5. Data originate from the annual report of the Danish Fertility Society[23]. In Denmark 3176 vital pregnancies were the result of ART in 2002; of these, 742

were twin and 27 triplet pregnancies. IUI accounted for 1311 (33%) of the live gestations, and 2642 (66%) were the result of *in vitro* techniques. In terms of multiple gestations, IUI resulted in 128/742 (17%) of the twin gestations and 13/27 (48%) of the triplet gestations in Denmark in 2002.

In a study combining registration and a questionnaire based on all ART twin deliveries in Denmark in 1997, ART other than *in vitro* techniques accounted for 12.2% of the twin deliveries, whereas 29.4% were the result of *in vitro* methods and 58.4% were spontaneously conceived[17]. In the Dutch-speaking part of Belgium, a survey in 1999 revealed that *in vitro* techniques contributed to 26% of the twin deliveries and that 14% were the result of ovarian stimulation with or without IUI[24]. As previously mentioned, the contribution of ovarian stimulation to the iatrogenic triplet rate in Denmark in 2002 was 48%. Estimation of the contribution of ovarian stimulation to multiple gestations in the USA revealed that approximately 40% of all iatrogenic multiple gestations were caused by ovarian stimulation and 40% by *in vitro* techniques[25].

Table 5 Number of treatments, ongoing vital pregnancies and number of singleton, twin and triplet gestations in 2002 in Denmark following all types of assisted reproduction technology. From Annual Report on National ART data from the Danish Fertility Society[23]

	Number of treatments	Live gestations	Singleton gestations	Twin gestations	Triplet gestations
IVF, ICSI	9630	2411	1817	583	11
FER (thawings)	1543	198	167	28	3
Egg donation	148	33	30	3	0
In vitro techniques (total)	11 321	2642	2014 (76%)	614 (23%)	14 (0.5%)
IUI (husband sperm)	7932	1021	907	103	11
IUI (donor sperm)	1594	290	255	25	2
IUI (total)	9526	1311	1162 (89%)	128 (10%)	13 (1%)
All	20 847	3953	3176 (80%)	742 (19%)	27 (0.7%)

IVF, *in vitro* fertilization; ICSI, intracytoplasmic sperm injection; FER, frozen embryo replacement; IUI, intracytoplasmic insemination

In summary, the proportion of twins born after other types of ART than *in vitro* techniques is not yet evident, owing to a lack of national register data on these treatments. From the existing reports, around 17–35% of the national twin deliveries appear to be due to ovarian stimulation with or without IUI. The rate of higher-order multiple gestations caused by these methods is even higher.

OVULATION INDUCTION IN ANOVULATORY WOMEN

In contrast to other types of ART in which development of multiple preovulatory follicles is the aim of the treatment, the purpose of ovulation induction in anovulatory women is to induce growth and ovulation of a single dominant follicle. Occurrence of multiple gestations is therefore due to lack of control of this process. Even though the concept of low-dose gonadotropin therapy has been widely accepted for ovulation induction, it often remains a difficult clinical task to obtain mono-ovulation. A review by Homburg and Howles showed that the applications of low-dose gonadotropin regimens in clomiphene-resistant women with polycystic ovary syndrome has succeeded in reducing the rate of multiple pregnancies to a minimum of 6%, while mono-ovulation was obtained in 70% of the cycles[26]. Multiple pregnancy rates in clomiphene-stimulated cycles, which are the first choice of treatment for women with polycystic ovary syndrome, are even lower.

INTRAUTERINE INSEMINATION

By far the majority of IUIs combined with ovarian stimulation are performed in women with normal ovulatory cycles. The rationale of this approach is to optimize the chance of conception through ovulation of more than one follicle and through increasing the number of highly motile spermatozoa at the site of fertilization in the distal tube. Consequently, the incidence of multiple gestations following this technique is increased several times when compared with natural cycle conceptions.

In many centers, insemination with donor sperm is also combined with IUI. No ovarian stimulation is required in ovulating women, but in clinical prac-tice ovarian stimulation is frequently performed if conception fails after a number of spontaneous cycles. Therefore, multiple gestation rates in donor sperm insemination programs are also substantially increased.

In a large study of stimulated cycles, multiple regression analysis of 1878 intrauterine pregnancies revealed the following variables as predictors of a high risk of multiple implantations: number of follicles, young age and serum estradiol levels prior to administration of human chorionic gonadotropin[27]. None of the patient characteristics, e.g. duration of infertility, primary versus secondary infertility and body mass index were of predictive value, nor were basal hormone levels, gonadotropin dosage, duration of treatment, or the number of motile spermatozoa.

In addition, a study of 3608 IUI treatments using human menopausal gonadotropin (hMG) or clomiphene citrate (CC) + hMG revealed that the number of follicles, patient age and estradiol levels were correlated with the risk of high-order multiple gestation[28]. Using a regimen of CC combined with hMG in 2473 cycles, Khalil and co-workers showed that, when two mature (> 17 mm) follicles were present, the twinning rate following insemination was 14% and the triplet rate 3.7%. When five mature follicles were present, the twinning and triplet rates were 16.7% and 8.3%, respectively[29].

It is evident that the key variable determining the risk of multiple gestation is the number of observed follicles. Physiologically, only the number of mature follicles should determine this risk. In clinical practice, however, determination of the smallest diameter of a follicle that may give rise to gestation remains difficult to define. Nevertheless, the occurrence of multiple gestations is correlated with the number of follicles of ≥ 12 mm[28]. The number of follicles is closely related to the type of drug used for ovarian stimulation. CC alone gives rise to the development of fewer follicles, a lower pregnancy rate and a lower rate of multiple gestations than CC in combination with gonadotropins or gonadotropins alone[28].

CONCLUSION AND SUMMARY

In 1999 the rates of multiple deliveries after IVF or ICSI in Europe were 24.0% for twin, 2.2% for triplet and 0.1% for quadruplet deliveries. The corresponding numbers from the USA in the same year were 32.2% for twin, 4.7% for triplet and 0.2% for quadruplet deliveries. With up to 4% of all pregnancies being conceived by ART in some developed countries, overall national perinatal statistics are affected by the contribution of ART pregnancies. Although a relatively small proportion of the population uses ART, the introduction of these techniques as well as increasing maternal age has caused worldwide increases in the multiple birth rates from a two-fold increase in the twin birth rate to a ninefold increase in the triplet birth rate in countries with widespread use of ART. In the perspective of the increased risks of multiple pregnancies, the incidence of multiple pregnancies after ART is still too high. The Finnish experience with a reduction of the multiple pregnancy rate to 17% in 2001 has demonstrated that a reduction of the multiple pregnancy rate is possible by national implementation of elective single-embryo transfer.

ACKNOWLEDGEMENTS

We gratefully thank the staff of the European Society of Human Reproduction and Embryology (ESHRE), embryologist K. Erb from the Danish Fertility Society and Dr Y. Imaizumi, National Institute of Population and Social Security Research, Ministry of Health and Welfare, Tokyo, Japan for kindly providing us with the epidemiological data.

REFERENCES

1. Keith LG, Oleszczuk JJ, Keith DM. Multiple gestation: reflections on epidemiology, causes, and consequences. *Int J Fertil* 2000;45:206–14

2. Bergh T, Ericson A, Hillensjö T, *et al.* Deliveries and children born after *in-vitro* fertilisation in Sweden 1982–95: a retrospective cohort study. *Lancet* 1999;354:1579–85

3. Sperling L, Tabor A. Twin pregnancy: the role of ultrasound in management. *Acta Obstet Gynecol Scand* 2001;80:287–99

4. Källen B. Congenital malformations in twins: a population study. *Acta Genet Med Gemellol* 1986;35:167–78

5. Loos R, Derom C, Vlietinck R, *et al.* The East Flanders Prospective Twin Survey (Belgium). *Twin Res* 1998;1:167–75

6. Schachter M, Raziel A, Shevach F, *et al.* Monozygotic twinning after assisted reproductive techniques: a phenomenon independent of micromanipulation. *Hum Reprod* 2001;16: 1264–9

7. Tong S, Short RV. Dizygotic twinning as a measure of human fertility. *Hum Reprod* 1998;13:95–8

8. Milki AA, Sunny HJ, Hinckley MD, *et al.* Incidence of monozygotic twinning with blastocyst transfer compared to cleavage-stage transfer. *Fertil Steril* 2003;79:503–6

9. Bortulus R, Parazzini F, Chatenoud L, *et al.* The epidemiology of multiple births. *Hum Reprod Udate* 1999;5:179–87

10. Imaizumi, Y. A comparative study of twinning and triplet rates in 17 countries, 1972–96. *Acta Genet Med Gemellol* 1998;47:101–14

11. ESHRE Campus Course Report. Prevention of twin pregnancies after IVF/ICSI by single embryo transfer. *Hum Reprod* 2001;16: 790–800

12. Westergaard T, Wohlfahrt J, Aaby P, *et al.* Population based study of rates of multiple pregnancies in Denmark, 1980–94. *Br Med J* 1997;314:775–9

13. Nygren KG, Nyboe Andersen A. Assisted reproductive technology in Europe, 1999. Results generated from European registers by ESHRE. *Hum Reprod* 2002;17:3260–74

14. Healy DL, Kovacs GT, McLachlan R, *et al.* Reproductive Medicine in the twenty-first century. In *Proceedings of the 17th World Congress on Fertility and Sterility, Melbourne, Australia.* London: Parthenon Publishing, 2002;18: 209–19

15. Society for Assisted Reproductive Technology and the American Society for Reproductive Medicine. Assisted reproductive technology in the United States: 1999 results generated from the American Society for Reproductive Medicine/Society for Assisted Reproductive Technology Registry. *Fertil Steril* 2002;78: 918–31

16. Strömberg B, Dahlquist G, Ericson A, *et al.* Neurological sequelae in children born after *in-vitro* fertilisation: a population based study. *Lancet* 2002; 359:461–5

17. Pinborg A, Loft A, Schmidt L, *et al*. Morbidity in a Danish National Cohort of 472 IVF/ICSI twins, 1132 non-IVF/ICSI twins and 634 IVF/ICSI singletons: health-related and social implications for the children and their families. *Hum Reprod* 2003;18:1234–43

18. Nygren KG, Nyboe Andersen A. Assisted reproductive technology in Europe, 1997. Results generated from European registers by ESHRE. *Hum Reprod* 2001;16:384–91

19. http://stakes.info/files/pdf/Tilastotiedotteet/Tt 0703.pdf

20. Kolibianakis EM, Devroey P. Blastocyst culture: facts and fiction. *Reprod Biomed Online* 2002;5:285–93

21. Templeton A, Morris JK. Reducing the risk of multiple births by transfer of two embryos after *in vitro* fertilization. *N Engl J Med* 1998;339:573–7

22. Strandell A, Bergh C, Lundin K. Selection of patients suitable for one-embryo transfer may reduce the rate of multiple births by half without impairment of overall birth rates. *Hum Reprod* 2000;15: 2520–5

23. Danish Fertility Society. Annual Report 2002. www.fertilitetsselskab.dk

24. Dhont M. Single-embryo transfer. *Semin Reprod Biol* 2001;19:251–8

25. Jones H. Multiple births: how are we doing? *Fertil Steril* 2003;79:17–21

26. Homburg R, Howles CM. Low-dose FSH therapy for anovulatory infertility associated with polycystic ovary syndrome: rationale, results, reflections and refinement. *Hum Reprod Update* 1999;5:493–9

27. Tur R, Barri PN, Coroleu B, *et al.* Risk factors for high-order multiple implantation after ovarian stimulation with gonadotrophins: evidence from a series of 1878 consecutive pregnancies in a single centre. *Hum Reprod* 2001;16:2124–9

28. Dickey RP, Taylor S, Lu PY, *et al.* Relationship of follicle numbers and estradiol levels to multiple implantation in 3608 intrauterine insemination cycles. *Fertil Steril* 2001;75: 69–78

29. Khalil MR, Rasmussen PE, Erb K, *et al.* Homologous intrauterine insemination. An evaluation of prognostic factors based on a review of 2473 cycles. *Acta Obstet Gynecol Scand* 2001;80:74–81

3

Obstetric risks and neonatal complications of twin pregnancy and higher-order multiple pregnancy

U.-B. Wennerholm

INTRODUCTION

A dramatic increase in the incidence of multiple pregnancy and delivery has occurred during the past decades, primarily due to a higher childbearing age and the wide availability of assisted reproductive technologies (ART) and non-ART procedures such as intrauterine insemination and ovulation-inducing drugs. Multiple pregnancy (especially twin pregnancy) has been regarded as an almost inevitable but acceptable complication of ART, and many patients consider twins to be a desirable outcome of these procedures. Proponents of this view ignore the serious consequences of multiple pregnancies for the couple, the newborns and the society[1].

Maternal morbidity and mortality are significantly increased in multiple pregnancies, in comparison with singleton pregnancies[2]. Risks to the fetus increase several-fold in multiple pregnancies. The nature and importance of risks vary widely but preterm birth and very preterm birth are the major cause of neonatal mortality and morbidity. Even if the children are healthy, the consequences for the family are severe; among them, long-term stress and depression are well documented, especially in the case of raising triplets. The financial costs per multiple birth are approximately 4-, 11- and 18-fold greater for twins, triplets and higher-order multiple births, respectively, compared with singleton births[3].

This chapter focuses on some of the major maternal and neonatal health consequences of multiple pregnancy.

ZYGOSITY AND PLACENTAL CHORIONICITY

There are two types of twinning: monozygotic (MZ) and dizygotic (DZ). MZ twinning is a result of the splitting of one fertilized ovum during the first 2 weeks of embryogenesis, whereas DZ twins originate from the fertilization of two ova by different spermatozoa. The rate of MZ twinning is believed to be fairly constant around the world and over time (3–4/1000 pregnancies). The incidence of DZ twinning is affected by many factors such as race, heredity, maternal age and ovulation induction and is more variable, ranging from 3 to 40/1000 pregnancies[4]. The highest rates of twin births have been observed in Nigeria, where only 5% were monochorionic (MC) (always MZ) and the lowest in Japan, where more than 60% were MC. In Caucasians, about 30% of twin pregnancies are MZ and about 70% are DZ. The pathogenesis of twinning remains unclear, but increased maternal gonadotropin levels have been implicated.

The overall incidence of twins at delivery is approximately one in 89 births. The incidence of higher-order multiple gestations can be estimated by using a mathematical relationship referred to as Hellin's Law, which dates back to the 19th century. According to this law, if the rate of twins in a population is 1 : 89, then the incidence of triplets is 1 : 89², the incidence of quadruplets 1 : 89³, etc. In reality, a broad range of rates has been described for twinning as well as for higher-order multiple pregnancies and the increasing use of fertility drugs and ART strongly influence current rates.

There are two major types of placenta: MC and dichorionic (DC), depending on the histological composition of the dividing membrane. In MC placentas, the septum consists of two layers of amnion, while DC placental septa consist of two layers of amnion and two layers of chorion. If the dividing membrane is absent, the condition is described as a monoamniotic (MA), MC twin gestation.

DC placentas are found in about 80% of twin gestations and are associated with either DZ or MZ twins. DC placentas may be separate or fused. MC placentation, which may be either MA or diamniotic (DA), accounts for 20% of twin gestations and occurs in only MZ twins.

Placental chorionic status can be determined with ultrasonography aimed at detecting the 'twin peak' or 'lambda' sign, seen only in DC pregnancies. This sign is a triangular projection of placental tissue from the chorionic surface to the area between the two amniotic sacs and accurately identifies chorionicity in 99–100% of twins between 10 and 14 weeks of gestation[5]. Later in pregnancy, it becomes more difficult to visualize; absence of the twin peak sign in the second or third trimester can thus not rule out a DC twin gestation.

Triplet and higher-order multiple conceptions can have a mixture of zygotic patterns, i.e. triplets can be MZ, DZ or trizygotic.

Increased frequency of zygotic splitting has been observed after ovulation-induction alone and after in vitro fertilization (IVF), in the latter case especially when it is associated with zona pellucida manipulation for promoting hatching of blastocysts (assisted hatching)[6,7].

The East Flanders Prospective Twin Survey (EFPTS) is the only population-based register that allows determination of the respective relative frequencies of natural and iatrogenic multiple pregnancies and that includes a description of placentation and zygosity. From 1976 to 1997, the EFPTS registered more than 95% of all multiples born in East Flanders. In the spontaneous twin group ($n = 2731$), about 45% were MZ (30% MC and 15% DC) and in the ART group ($n = 986$), 5% were MZ twins. In the spontaneous triplet group

($n = 23$), 22% were MZ, 52% DZ and 26% trizygotic. In the ART triplet group ($n = 111$), 1%, 12% and 84% were MZ, DZ and trizygotic, respectively[8].

Recent studies have shown that it is chorionicity rather than zygosity that determines outcome in twin gestations, with monochorionic twins being at higher risk than dichorionic twins[9]. In twin studies, variations and type of zygosity in the different populations must thus be taken into consideration.

NATIONAL TRENDS IN MULTIPLE BIRTHS

Since the 1980s, the incidence of multiple pregnancies has risen in developed countries and has reached epidemic proportions, according to some authorities. In France, the incidence of twin deliveries rose from 8.8/1000 to 11.2/1000 and the incidence of triplet deliveries from 0.9/10 000 to 4.4/10 000 between 1972 and 1989[10].

National rates of multiple pregnancies have increased 1.7-fold during the period 1980–94 in Denmark, the rise being most pronounced in recent years[11]. In Sweden, the number of twin deliveries increased from 8.2/1000 to 16.0/1000 between 1973 and 2000[12]. The proportion of triplets and quadruplets is low in Sweden, but has increased slightly during the past 10 years.

A recent report from the USA showed that the twin birth ratio for 2001 continued to climb and that the proportion of all US births that were twins exceeded 3% that year (30.2/1000 total live births)[13]. The twinning rate has increased 33% since 1990 (22.6/1000) and 59% since 1980 (18.9/1000). Twinning rates have risen for all age groups over the past decade, but the largest increases have been among older mothers. Between 1990 and 2001, the twin birth rate for women aged 40–44 years has almost doubled (from 24.7 to 48.1 per 1000), while the rate for women aged 45–49 years has increased more than seven times (from 23.8 to 170.1). In 2001, 17% of all births to women aged 45–49 years were twins. The birth rate for triplets and other higher-order multiples in the USA rose to 185.6 triplets and higher births per 100 000, but the most dramatic surge in triplet births seen between 1990 and 1998 appears to have abated[13].

CONTRIBUTION OF INFERTILITY TREATMENT TO A POPULATION'S MULTIPLE BIRTH RATE

Clomiphene citrate (CC), gonadotropin treatment (without ART) and ART are the infertility treatments most likely to involve multiple births. In a study by Lynch and colleagues, CC, gonadotropins and ART contributed to 14%, 5% and 14% of multiple births, respectively[14]. Natural conceptions, ovulation induction and IVF/intracytoplasmic sperm injection (ICSI) accounted for approximately 20%, 40% and 40%, respectively, of triplets and higher-order multiples in the USA.

In a Boston hospital, IVF treatment accounted for 2% of the singletons, 35% of the twins and 77% of the higher-order multiple births[15]. In Alberta, Canada, IVF treatment accounted for 21% of the twins and all of the triplets born in the province from 1994 to 1996[16].

FREQUENCY OF MULTIPLE GESTATIONS WITH IVF

Recent reports from registries and clinics on the frequency of multiple births in ART programs are shown in Table 1. The fifth world report on the outcome of ART for 1998 showed that multiple births remained at a very high level in several countries, but have started to decline in some countries; this applies especially to the triplet and higher-order multiple rate[17].

Multiple births accounted for 26.3% of IVF-associated live births in Europe[18] and 37% in the USA in 1999[19], resulting in 43% and 55% of the IVF children in Europe and the USA, respectively, being born as multiple birth babies.

The American Society for Reproductive Medicine (ASRM)/Society for Assisted Reproductive Technology (SART) registry reports for the USA from 1992 to 1999 showed that the total multiple births increased from 32% in 1992 to 39% in 1996, falling to 37% in 1999[19]. The decline was mainly attributable to a reduction in triplet deliveries. In Sweden, the proportion of multiple births increased to a maximum of 34% in 1991, after which it declined to 22% in 2000. The decline was primarily due to a decline in triplet births similar to that in the USA; however, there has also been a decrease in twin births in recent years due to the increasing number of elective single-embryo transfers.

In summary, infertility treatments led to a 10- to 20-fold increase in twin birth rates and a 200- to 500-fold increase in triplet rates. Although a relatively small proportion of the population undergoes infertility treatment, the increased risk of multiple pregnancy associated with this treatment has an impact on the national multiple pregnancy rate.

Table 1   Recent multiple birth rates reported in assisted reproductive technology programs

Source	Twins	Triplets	Quadruplets	Triplets and quadruplets	Total
World Report, 1998[17]	27.3			3.4	30.7
Egypt, Serour et al., 1998[77]	19.8	6.0	2.1		27.9
Canada, 1999[78]	29.7			3.6	33.3
USA, ASRM/SART, 1999[19]	32.2	4.7	0.2		37.1
Europe, ESHRE, 1999[18] (mean and range)	24.0 (10.8–32.5)	2.2 (0.3–7.0)	0.1 (0.0–0.7)		26.3 (16.7–39.2)
Sweden, 2000*	21.6	0.4	0		22.0

*P.O. Karlström, personal communication

MATERNAL COMPLICATIONS

Mortality

There is little available information concerning maternal deaths associated with multiple pregnancy in the developed world. As to developing countries, there is an early Nigerian study from 1985 showing that maternal mortality was 1% for singleton, 2% for twin and 6.3% for triplet pregnancies[20].

In 1994, the maternal mortality rate (per 100 000 live births) in France was 10.2 in multiple pregnancies versus 4.4 in singletons. A three-fold increase in maternal mortality was shown (14.9 and 5.2 in multiple and singleton pregnancies, respectively: odds ratio (OR) 2.9, 95% confidence interval (CI) 1.4–6.1) in Europe as a whole[2]. Recently, in a large study from Latin American and Caribbean hospitals, multiple pregnancy was associated with a two-fold increase in mortality, compared with singleton pregnancies, among parous women (adjusted relative risk (RR) 2.1, 95% CI 1.1–3.9)[21]. Maternal death was caused by pulmonary edema following administration of parenteral β-mimetics for tocolysis, by eclampsia or by excessive blood loss.

Morbidity

Maternal morbidity is significantly increased in mothers with multiple pregnancies and seems to be related to the number of fetuses[22]. Risks to the woman include hypertensive disorders, thromboembolism, premature labor and delivery, urinary tract infection, anemia and vaginal–uterine hemorrhage (placental abruption, placenta previa), fluid overload and pulmonary edema in association with parenteral tocolysis. Women with multiple pregnancies are at increased risk of requiring long periods of bed rest, hospitalization, administration of medication to prevent preterm labor and increased risk of surgical procedures (Cesarean section, cerclage). Multiple pregnancies have been shown to be an independent risk factor (OR 2.3) for a woman to be admitted to an intensive care unit[23].

Hypertension

For hypertension, one of the major maternal complications associated with multiple pregnancy, the OR in twins compared to singletons varies from 1.8 to 3.4, according to a recent review[24].

Severe hypertension is 2–3 times more common in twin than in singleton pregnancies, even after adjustment for age and parity[2]. Pre-eclampsia occurs about three times more often in twin than in singleton pregnancies, with an incidence of 10–20%; onset is more often early and the condition of greater severity[2]. In triplet pregnancies the incidence is between 25 and 60% and may be as high as 90% in quadruplet pregnancies[22,25–29].

A six-fold RR of eclampsia in multiple, when compared with singleton, pregnancies was found in a survey in the UK (28.1/10 000 vs. 4.7/10 000 pregnancies, respectively)[30].

To date, no interventions (e.g. low-dose aspirin) have been shown to prevent or reduce the incidence of pre-eclampsia in these high-risk pregnancies.

Preterm labor

The gestational length of a multiple pregnancy is inversely related to the number of fetuses. Although controversial, it has been suggested that uterine overdistention is a cause of preterm labor in multiple gestation. Tocolytic drugs are often indicated to arrest preterm labor, mainly to provide the opportunity for administration of antenatal corticosteroids. However, maternal cardiovascular side-effects of β-mimetics, including pulmonary edema, are more pronounced in multiple than in singleton pregnancies, owing to the increased maternal blood volume and cardiac output.

Anemia

Iron and folate deficiency anemia are more often seen in multiple pregnancies. Abruptio placentae and placenta previa are slightly more common and may cause bleeding. In a study of assisted conception in the UK, 22% of women with multiple pregnancies were admitted to hospital at some time during pregnancy because of bleeding, compared with 17% of mothers with singleton pregnancies[31].

Atony and postpartum hemorrhage due to uterine over-distention occur with a RR of 3.0–4.5[24].

Cesarean section

The much higher frequency of Cesarean section in multiple pregnancies, compared with singleton pregnancies, is mainly due to malpresentation. Cesarean section is associated with more complications than vaginal deliveries. These include infections, hemorrhage and thromboembolic disease. Furthermore, Cesarean section in a multiple pregnancy seems to be associated with an additional risk of endometritis and abdominal wound infections, compared to Cesarean section in a singleton pregnancy, according to a Finnish study[32].

Maternal complications in triplet and quadruplet pregnancies

In a summary of maternal morbidity associated with triplet pregnancies in five published studies comprising a total of 182 triplet pregnancies, preterm labor occurred in 82% (60–92%), pre-eclampsia in 29% (20–39%), preterm premature rupture of membranes (PROM) in 18% (12–20%), anemia in 40% (20–58%), endometritis in 19% (14–24%) and postpartum hemorrhage in 12% (9–15%)[33]. The most recent of these studies showed a 98% risk of antenatal complications (preterm labor 76%, pre-eclampsia 27%, HELLP (hemolysis, elevated liver enzymes, low platelets) syndrome 9%, anemia 27%, preterm PROM 20%, acute fatty liver of pregnancy 7%, gestational diabetes 7%) and a 32% risk of postpartum complications (endometritis 26%, postpartum hemorrhage 9%)[29]. The results from 100 triplet pregnancies were reported recently by the same group[26]. Ninety-six per cent of the pregnancies were afflicted with at least one complication, the most common being preterm labor. No difference in outcome was seen with respect to mode of conception (spontaneous, ovulation induction or IVF).

Few studies have addressed maternal morbidity in quadruplet pregnancies, in connection with which a risk of preterm labor approaching 100% and a 32–90% risk of pregnancy-induced hypertension have been described[27,34].

FETAL AND NEONATAL OUTCOME

Mortality

Following ART, early fetal death in the form of 'vanishing sacs' is a rather common occurrence. In a recent study that summarized several publications, the rate of a 'vanishing twin', when two or three gestational sacs were detected initially, was 33% and 56%, respectively[35]. When two or three embryos were detected initially, the rate was 28.5% and 51.5%, respectively. At our IVF unit, a maximum of two embryos is transferred in the majority of cycles. In an ultrasound study of 230 (221 twins and nine triplets) multiple pregnancies from this unit, Bergh and associates found that spontaneous reduction of at least one gestational sac occurred in 21% (in one case, two sacs disappeared)[36]. Similarly, Manzur and colleagues found a reduction rate of 50% when all implantation sites were considered[37]. It is probable that a similar phenomenon occurs in naturally conceived pregnancies and that the multiple conception rate is much higher than the detected multiple pregnancy rate.

All mortality rates (stillbirths, and early neonatal, late neonatal and infant mortality) are higher in multiple pregnancies compared to singletons and the rates increase with the number of fetuses. Differences in mortality rates, from a population-based registry in England and Wales, are shown in Table 2[38]. This study showed that multiple births make a large contribution to overall mortality rates, despite their relative rarity. In England and Wales, multiple births represented 2.5% of all births but 8% of all stillbirths, 19% of all neonatal deaths and 7% of all post-neonatal deaths in 1991. Disparity related to multiplicity was the greatest when it came to neonatal deaths, the rate of twins being seven times and the rate of triplets and higher-order multiples > 20 times the singleton rate.

A recent article showed that the overall infant mortality rate in the USA fell from 9.5 to 7.0 per 1000 live births between 1989 and 1999[39]. This decline was greater for multiple births than for singletons in all birth weight categories.

The infant mortality rate for singletons and multiples was 6.1 and 31.1 per 1000 live births, respectively, in 2000; this figure can be broken down into 28.9 for twins, 63.2 for triplets and 95.5

Table 2   Mortality and multiplicity of birth in England and Wales, 1991. Adapted from reference 38

	Singletons	Twins	Triplets and higher
Stillbirth rate (late fetal deaths/1000 total births)	4.4	14.2	19.3
Early neonatal mortality (deaths in first 6 days/1000 live births)	2.9	22.8	75.6
Late neonatal mortality (deaths 7–27 days/1000 live births)	0.8	3.9	10.6
Post-neonatal mortality (deaths 28 days to 1 year/1000 live births)	2.4	6.3	15.1
Infant mortality (deaths < 1 year/1000 live births)	6.1	33.0	101.4

for quadruplets. Thus, although infant mortality has declined for both twins and triplets/higher-order multiples, the risk of early death for twins continues to be nearly five times that of singletons and the risk for triplets and higher-order multiples ten times as high.

Not all twins are at similar risk. Several studies have shown that the mortality rate in twins is higher in MZ than in DZ twins and higher in MZ, MC than in DC (DZ or MZ) twins.

In a prospective ultrasound screening study in which chorionicity was determined at 10–14 weeks of gestation, at least one fetal loss occurred before 24 weeks of gestation in 12.7% (13/102) of MC and 2.5% (9/354) of DC pregnancies and there was at least one perinatal loss after 24 weeks in 4.9% (5/102) of MC and 2.8% (10/354) of DC pregnancies[9]. Severe early-onset twin–twin transfusion syndrome (TTTS) in MC twins is considered to be one explanation for this difference in mortality rate between MC and DC twins.

Another study showed that male/female twins born to Caucasian women older than 28 years were at the lowest risk and male/male twins born to young Black women were at the highest risk[40]. In a large population-based study from Sweden (1973–96), in which antenatal death (defined as stillbirth at a minimum of 28 completed gestational weeks) was reported, Rydhström and Heraib showed that the OR for both intrauterine death and intrauterine and infant death combined was 3–4 for

same-sexed twins and 2 for different-sexed twins, compared with singletons[41]. In another large population-based cohort of over one million births in Australia and the USA, of which more than 20 000 were twins, twins were at approximately five-fold increased risk of fetal death and seven-fold increased risk of neonatal death, compared with singletons[42]. Second-born twins, twins from same-sex pairs or growth-discordant pairs and twins whose co-twin died were at increased risk of death.

Gestational age and birth weight

Preterm delivery and low birth weight are the major causes of mortality and morbidity in multiple pregnancy. Gardner and co-workers found that 54% of twins were preterm, compared with 9.6% of singletons, and that birth at < 32 weeks of gestation occurred in 15–17% of twin and 1–2% of singleton pregnancies[43]. As in singleton pregnancies, the causes of preterm twin birth could be divided into three groups: spontaneous preterm labor; preterm PROM; and indicated preterm delivery on maternal or fetal indications. In that study comprising 434 sets of twins, spontaneous labor accounted for 54%, preterm PROM for 22% and indicated delivery for 23% of the preterm deliveries. (The corresponding figures for preterm singleton deliveries were 44%, 31% and 23%, respectively.) The etiology of spontaneous preterm birth may be different in singleton and multiple pregnancies. In a prospective study,

Goldenberg and co-workers found that the usual risk factors for spontaneous preterm birth in singletons (e.g. maternal age, Black race, prior preterm birth, educational level) were not significantly associated with spontaneous preterm birth in twins[44].

Table 3 shows the important differences between singletons, twins and triplets and higher-order multiples in gestational age and birth weight using the latest National Vital Statistics Report for the year 2001 in the USA[13]. This huge resource shows that twins fared substantially worse than singletons and, correspondingly, triplets and higher-order multiples fared substantially worse than twins when it came to both parameters. Generally, gestational age was 3 weeks less for every additional fetus. The average triplet weighed about half of the average singleton at birth.

There is controversy concerning which fetal growth curve should be used in multiple pregnancies. It is well known that the fetal weight of twins is close to that of singletons until 30 weeks, after which it begins to diverge. Some investigators use the 'singleton curve' as a reference, but a special birth weight reference for twins, according to chorionicity, sex and race, has also recently been developed on the basis of longitudinal measurements, and this might serve as an alternative to the singleton reference curve[45].

Median birth weight was significantly lower in MC twins, compared with DC twins, and both babies were small for gestational age (SGA) in significantly more MC twin pairs[9]. No difference was found in the proportion of birth weight discordance (> 25% discordance in birth weight between the twins in each pair) between DC and MC twin sets in that study (11.3% for MC and 12.1% for DC twins). In another study, the frequency of birth weight discordance of > 25% was shown to decrease as a logarithmic function of the total twin birth weight. This would suggest that the better the uterine environment, the fewer discordant twin pairs, and that discordance may represent some form of intrauterine growth restriction. When studying triplets, Mordel and colleagues found that about 25% of the sets had an inter-triplet discordance of > 25%[46], and Vignal and colleagues found a corresponding figure of 34.2[47].

Discordant growth following multifetal pregnancy reduction (MFPR) has been studied by Smith-Levitin and co-workers[48] and Török and co-workers[49]. The rates of birth weight discordance found among twins reduced from triplets were comparable to those among spontaneously reduced triplets and non-reduced twins.

Neonatal morbidity

The vast majority of excess morbidity in multiple births is attributable to low birth weight and preterm delivery. In a study by Gardner and colleagues, twins who constituted only 2.4% of all neonates contributed disproportionately to neonatal morbidity, e.g. low Apgar score at 5 min (7.9%), intraventricular hemorrhage (IVH) grades 3 and 4

Table 3 Gestational age and birth weight characteristics by plurality: USA 2001. Adapted from reference 13

	Singletons	Twins	Triplets	Quadruplets	Quintuplets
Number	3 897 216	121 246	6885	501	85
Per cent < 32 weeks	1.6	11.8	36.7	64.5	78.6
Per cent < 37 weeks	10.4	57.4	92.4	97.8	91.7
Mean GA (weeks) and SD	38.8 (2.5)	35.4 (3.7)	32.0 (4.0)	29.6 (4.1)	29.1 (3.9)
Per cent < 1500 g	1.1	10.2	34.8	68.4	77.4
Per cent < 2500 g	6.0	54.9	94.0	98.4	91.7
Mean BW (g) and SD	3339 (573)	2353 (647)	1678 (574)	1290 (549)	1269 (676)

GA, gestational age; SD, standard deviation; BW, birth weight

(11.4%), sepsis (7.6%), necrotizing enterocolitis (NEC) (9.9%) and respiratory distress syndrome (RDS) (13.8%)[43]. Twin rates of low Apgar scores, RDS, IVH (grade 3–4), sepsis and NEC were significantly higher than singleton rates. Preterm twins had a higher incidence of RDS than preterm singletons, but the difference disappeared after stratification for gestational age.

There are few controlled studies analyzing neonatal morbidity in triplets and higher-order multiples. RDS has been described at different frequencies in different studies: 8.9–43.4% for triplets and 34.8–75% for quadruplets. IVH grade 3–4 has been diagnosed in up to 7.7% of triplets[25] and 8.7% of quadruplets[50]. Kaufman and colleagues compared neonatal morbidity in triplets with that in singletons and twins[28]. Logistic regression analysis, correcting for gestational age, showed a significantly higher incidence of retinopathy of prematurity, patent ductus arteriosus and mild IVH (grade 1–2) in triplets, compared with singletons.

In a recent Israeli population-based study, very low birth weight (VLBW) (< 1500 g) triplets were found to have a higher risk of RDS (RDS was also increased in twins, compared to singletons) as well as death before discharge from hospital than singletons, after consideration of confounding variables and in spite of increased exposure to antenatal steroids[51]. One explanation or theory for this, given by the authors, was a possible diminished efficacy of antenatal steroid treatment in multiples.

As a result of these problems, many multiples require treatment and extended care in neonatal intensive care units (NICUs). According to one study, 15% of singletons, 48% of twins and 78% of triplets and higher-order multiples were admitted to the NICU[15].

Congenital malformations

There are few large population-based studies on the prevalence of congenital malformations in twins and singletons. Such studies are also vulnerable to several methodological pitfalls (i.e. definition and ascertainment biases). In a review, Little and Bryan concluded that there is 'almost certainly' an excess of malformations in twins compared to singletons,

the RR varying between 0.9 and 1.5[52]. MZ twins seem to be more affected than DZ twins, the highest figures being found in monoamniotic twins. Some specific malformations have been found to occur excessively in twins (e.g. cardiac, neural tube and brain defects, facial clefts and gastrointestinal and anterior abdominal wall defects)[53–55].

Recently, a large international registry study ($n = 260\,865$ twins) confirmed the higher risk of malformations in twins, compared with singletons (RR 1.25, 95% CI 1.21–1.28)[56]. However, it was not possible to distinguish between DZ and MZ twins in this study.

Chromosomal abnormalities

The risk of chromosomal abnormalities in twin gestation was analyzed by Rodis and co-workers[57]. Because most twins are dizygotic and each has an *a priori* risk of aneuploidy, the chance that one of the fetuses is affected is greater than would be expected for a singleton. In DZ gestations, any existing chromosomal abnormality will probably involve only one of the twins; in MZ gestations, it will almost always involve both twins. Using the risk estimates for singletons, Rodis and colleagues concluded that a 33-year-old patient with a twin pregnancy has a risk of Down's syndrome in at least one of her twins equivalent to that of a 35-year-old carrying a singleton. However, birth prevalence of Down's syndrome was found to be only marginally increased in twins, compared with singletons[58], an explanation for which might be a higher miscarriage risk in affected pregnancies. Genetic counseling and testing is complex in twin gestations since screening methods are less effective, and amniocentesis or chorionic villus sampling may be associated with a higher risk of miscarriage. If a major non-lethal abnormality is found in only one of the fetuses, selective feticide is an option in subsequent management. The risk of miscarriage and preterm delivery after selective feticide seems to have decreased as clinical experience has increased[59]. However, the ethical dilemmas facing the parents and doctors are complex. It is important to consider chorionicity prior to the procedure, since different techniques should be used in MZ and DC twin pregnancies.

SPECIAL CONSIDERATIONS

Twin–twin transfusion syndrome

The TTTS or fetofetal transfusion syndrome occurs in a multifetal pregnancy in which vascular anastomosis (within the placenta) between two MC fetuses allows shunting of blood from one, the donor, to the other, the recipient, resulting in severe oligohydramnios in the donor and polyhydramnios in the recipient. Usually, TTTS will also cause discordance in size, with the larger twin in the polyhydramniotic sac. It complicates 5–15% of all MC twin pregnancies[60]. Fetal/neonatal mortality is very high, up to 80–100%, without treatment, but it averages 40–60% even with treatment. There is also a high risk of neurological sequelae in surviving fetuses. Hemodynamic imbalance after the death of one twin may cause a fall in blood pressure in the surviving twin, leading to irreversible brain damage.

Recently, staging of TTTS has been proposed, in order to achieve better comparison between centers and more individualized therapy[61]. Ultrasound may be valuable in the prediction of TTTS outcome. Increased nuchal translucency (NT) in weeks 10–14 has been found to be an early sign of TTTS, as has folding of the inter-twin membrane in weeks 15–17[62]. Serial amniocentesis, aimed at relieving polyhydramnios, or fetoscopy with laser coagulation, in order to interrupt the placental vascular anastomoses, are therapeutic options today[63,64].

Monoamniotic twins

In natural conceptions, MA twins comprise about 5% of all MZ twins or 1.7% of all twins; the expected occurrence is 1/5000. An increased rate of MA twins has been reported following zona pellucida manipulation and IVF. In a survey of 143 pregnancies following zona pellucida manipulation, four of the 23 multiple pregnancies (17.4%) were MA, corresponding to a MA twinning rate of 28/1000[65]. MA twins are at increased risk, with a fetal mortality rate of 30–70%. Cord entanglement as well as acute forms of TTTS cause the majority of the fetal losses. Elective preterm Cesarean section at 32 weeks of gestation has been suggested in order to improve survival in MA twins[66].

LONG-TERM OUTCOMES

Multiples may also suffer long-term medical and developmental problems. The major morbidity is neurological impairment and varies from gross clinical neurological impairment to minor and probably subclinical abnormalities.

In one often-quoted study, differential handicap rates in singletons, twins and triplets were analyzed (Table 4)[67]. In this study, it was clearly shown that twins are at considerably higher risk than singletons, especially in the category of severe handicap (twins 1.4 times for all, 1.7 times for severe and 1.3 times for moderate handicap). Triplets fare far worse than singletons in all categories (triplets 2.0 times for all, 2.9 times for severe and 1.7 times for moderate handicap).

Yokoyama and colleagues calculated the risk of handicap in infants from multiple pregnancies born in Japan after 1977[68]. The incidence of handicap was 3.7% in twins, 8.7% in triplets, 11.1% in quadruplets and 10.0% in quintuplets. At least one handicapped infant was born in 7.4% of twin pregnancies, 21.6% of triplet pregnancies and 50% of quadruplet and quintuplet pregnancies.

Table 4   Handicap rates per 1000 post-neonatal survivors (children born in 1988). Adapted from reference 67

	Overall handicap	Severe handicap	Moderate handicap
Singletons	90.4	19.7	70.6
Twins	126.3	34.0	92.3
Triplets	179.1	57.5	121.6

Cerebral palsy

Multiple birth has been recognized as a risk factor for cerebral palsy (CP) for at least a century[69]. A consistent finding in the literature is that the risk of CP increases with plurality. Table 5 presents estimates, from various studies, of the CP prevalence in singleton and multiple births. The risk of CP for twins is approximately five times that for singletons. Triplets had a 17-fold and 20-fold increased risk, compared with singletons, in the two studies using population-based ascertainment.

One of the studies, the Western Australia Study, is particularly instructive, since the rate of CP is also described for singletons, twins and triplets in different categories, e.g. CP per 1000 live births, per 1000 first-year survivors and per 1000 pregnancies[70]. The study design was stringent and the likelihood of ascertainment biases was virtually nil. Table 6 shows the rates of CP for singletons, twins and triplets in each of these categories. When the rates for singletons were standardized to 1, twins were 4.6 times more likely to have CP, compared to singletons, on the basis of 1000 live births or 1000 first-year survivors. Moreover, they were 8.3 times more likely to be afflicted with CP than singletons when this rate was calculated per 1000 pregnancies. The differences are even more pronounced in triplets (17 times and 47 times, respectively).

In the population-based study from Australia and the USA, the CP rate was highest in surviving twins whose co-twins were stillborn, died shortly after birth or had CP[42].

Psychological impact on the family

In addition to the medical risks of multiple pregnancies, there are psychological consequences for the children themselves, their siblings and their parents[71]. Multiple birth children must share parental attention. Some early studies have indicated that multiples begin to speak later than singletons, owing to less individualized attention or because they learn to communicate in another way with each other[72]. Bryan and Read highlighted the special problems caused if one child was disabled, with feelings such as jealousy, anger and depression in the affected child and feelings of guilt and an excessive burden of responsibility in the healthy sibling. The single survivor of a twin set may also

suffer from the loss of his/her companion, the parents' grief or the guilt of having survived[73].

Parents of multiples are also affected socially and psychologically[74]. There are studies indicating that these parents are more likely to be exhausted, depressed, or anxious after birth. An increased rate of depression, extending far beyond the infancy period, has been reported in mothers of twins[75]. The burden of raising multiples may be further increased for the parents if the children are physically or mentally disabled[76]. Social isolation and little time for themselves may place a great deal of stress on the marital relationship and a higher rate of divorces has been reported in families with triplets. Behavioral problems in an older child are more common after the arrival of twins than of a single sibling, as shown in an early study[87].

CONCLUSIONS

The incidence of multiple pregnancy and delivery has increased dramatically over the past decades in many developed countries. Most of the increase in multiple births is iatrogenic, due to fertility-enhancing drugs and ART procedures. Multiple pregnancies remain high-risk pregnancies, entailing more obstetric problems and increased neonatal mortality and morbidity, compared with singleton pregnancies. The risk to the fetuses and infants increase with plurality. Even twins, generally regarded as an acceptable or even desirable outcome of IVF, run an increased risk of death and handicap, compared to singletons. The population-attributable fetal and neonatal risks of twin and triplet gestations are considerable.

In Sweden, there has been a steady decline in the number of multiple births after ART since 1991, due to the decrease in the number of pre-embryos transferred. A maximum of two pre-embryos are generally transferred. This has almost eliminated triplet births; however, twin gestations still account for more than 20% of deliveries after IVF. We have recently advocated a more restrictive embryo transfer policy with single-embryo transfers at least in selected patient groups[88,89] which will, in combination with an optimal freezing program, probably minimally jeopardize the overall probability of a delivery per initiated cycle. However, further research in reproductive medicine is needed to

Table 5 Prevalence of cerebral palsy* and 95% confidence interval in singletons, twins, triplets and quadruplets and higher-order multiples. Adapted from reference 79

Reference	Region and years	Study design	Singletons	Twins	Triplets	Quadruplets and higher
Grether et al. (1993)[80]	California (1983–85)	population-based	1.1 (0.97–1.3)	6.7 (4.2–11)		
King and Johnsson (1995)[81]	Oxford, UK (1984–91)	population-based	2.3 (2.1–2.4)	7.4 (5.3–9.5)		
Nelson and Ellenberg (1995)[82]	USA (1959–66)	population-based	3.8 (3.2–4.3)	10.5 (4.0–17.0)		
Petterson et al. (1993)[70]	Western Australia (1980–89)	population-based	1.6 (1.4–1.8)	7.4 (5.2–10.0)	27.9 (11.0–63.0)	
Pharoah and Cooke (1996)[83]	Mersey, UK (1982–89)	population-based	2.3 (2.1–2.5)	12.6 (9.7–16.1)	44.8 (16.6–95)	
Williams et al. (1996)[84]	London, UK (1985–86)	population-based	1.0 (0.8–1.2)	7.4 (4.3–11.9)		
Yokoyama et al. (1995)[68]	Japan	survey		8.5 (4.4–14.8)	31.4 (14.4–58.7)	111.1 (23.5–291.6)
McFarlane et al. (1990)[85]	UK	survey			17.4 (7.4–34.0)[†]	
Liu et al. (2000)[86]	China	prevalence in 0–7 year olds	1.5 (1.4–1.7)	9.7 (6.5–14.0)[‡]		

*Rates per 1000 1-year survivors except Grether (rate per 1000 3-year survivors) and King and Johnsson (rate per 1000 live births); † triplets and higher-order multiples; ‡ multiples

Table 6   Cerebral palsy in Western Australia during the period 1980–89. Adapted from reference 79

	Singletons		Twins		Triplets	
		Standardized		Standardized		Standardized
Per 1000 live births	1.60	1	7.40	4.6	26.7	16.6
Per 1000 first-year survivors	1.60	1	7.32	4.6	27.9	17.4
Per 1000 pregnancies	1.59	1	13.24	8.3	75.95	47

develop effective elective single-embryo transfer regimens and to improve the selection of one good-quality embryo. For all those concerned with perinatal medicine, the management of multiple pregnancies represents a true challenge. Many controversial clinical dilemmas remain to be solved in multiple pregnancies in order to improve outcome. For example, these include the definition of 'term' in multiples, discordant fetal conditions, the controversies regarding the mode of delivery, management of TTTS and multifetal pregnancy reduction.

REFERENCES

1. Elster N. Less is more: the risks of multiple births. The Institute for Science, Law, and Technology Working Group on Reproductive Technology. *Fertil Steril* 2000;74:617–23

2. Senat MV, Ancel PY, Bouvier-Colle MH, Breart G. How does multiple pregnancy affect maternal mortality and morbidity? *Clin Obstet Gynecol* 1998;41:78–83

3. Multiple gestation pregnancy. The ESHRE Capri Workshop Group. *Hum Reprod* 2000;15:1856–64

4. Derom R, Orlebeke J, Eriksson A, Thiery M. The epidemiology of multiple births in Europe. In Keith LG, Papiernik E, Keith DM, Luke B, eds. *Multiple Pregnancy, Epidemiology, Gestation and Perinatal Care*. Carnforth, UK: Parthenon Publishing, 1995:145–62

5. Finberg HJ. The 'twin peak' sign: reliable evidence of dichorionic twinning. *J Ultrasound Med* 1992;11:571–7

6. Edwards RG, Mettler L, Walters DE. Identical twins and *in vitro* fertilization. *J In Vitro Fertil Embryo Transf* 1986;3:114–17

7. Wenstrom KD, Syrop CH, Hammitt DG, Van Voorhis BJ. Increased risk of monochorionic twinning associated with assisted reproduction. *Fertil Steril* 1993;60:510–14

8. Derom R, Derom C, Vlietinck R. The risk of monozygotic twinning. In Blickstein I, Keith LG, eds. *Iatrogenic Multiple Pregnancies*. London, UK: Parthenon Publishing, 2001: 9–20

9. Sebire NJ, Snijders RJ, Hughes K, Sepulveda W, Nicolaides KH. The hidden mortality of monochorionic twin pregnancies. *Br J Obstet Gynaecol* 1997;104:1203–7

10. Tuppin P, Blondel B, Kaminski M. Trends in multiple deliveries and infertility treatments in France. *Br J Obstet Gynaecol* 1993;100:383–5

11. Westergaard T, Wohlfahrt J, Aaby P, Melbye M. Population based study of rates of multiple pregnancies in Denmark, 1980–94. *Br Med J* 1997;314:775–9

12. Odlind V, Haglund B, Pakkanen M, Olausson PO. Deliveries, mothers and newborn infants in Sweden, 1973–2000. *Acta Obstet Gynecol Scand* 2003;82:516–28

13. Martin JA, Hamilton BE, Ventura SJ, Menacker F, Park MM, Sutton PD. Births: final data for 2001. *Natl Vital Stat Rep* 2002;51:1–102

14. Lynch A, McDuffie R, Murphy J, Faber K, Leff M, Orleans M. Assisted reproductive interventions and multiple birth(1). *Obstet Gynecol* 2001;97:195–200

15. Callahan TL, Hall JE, Ettner SL, Christiansen CL, Greene MF, Crowley WF Jr. The economic impact of multiple-gestation pregnancies and the contribution of assisted-reproduction techniques to their incidence. *N Engl J Med* 1994;331:244–9

16. Tough SC, Greene CA, Svenson LW, Belik J. Effects of *in vitro* fertilization on low birth weight, preterm delivery, and multiple birth. *J Pediatr* 2000;136:618–22

17. Adamson D, Lancaster P, de Mouzon J, Nygren KG, Zegers-Hochschild F. World collaborative report on assisted reproductive technology, 1998. In Healy DL, Kovacs GT, McLachlan R, Rodriguez-Armas O, eds. *Reproductive Medicine in the Twenty-First Century*. London: Parthenon Publishing, 2002:209–19

18. Nygren KG, Andersen AN. Assisted reproductive technology in Europe, 1999. Results generated from European registers by ESHRE. *Hum Reprod* 2002;17:3260–74

19. American Society for Reproductive Medicine/Society for Assisted Reproductive Technology. Assisted reproductive technology in the United States: 1999 results generated from the American Society for Reproductive Medicine/Society for Assisted Reproductive Technology Registry. *Fertil Steril* 2002;78:918–31

20. Harrison KA. Child-bearing, health and social priorities: a survey of 22 774 consecutive hospital births in Zaria, Northern Nigeria. *Br J Obstet Gynaecol* 1985;92 (Suppl 5):1–119

21. Conde-Agudelo A, Belizan JM, Lindmark G. Maternal morbidity and mortality associated with multiple gestations. *Obstet Gynecol* 2000;95:899–904

22. Sebire NJ, Jolly M, Harris J, Nicolaides KH. Risks of obstetric complications in multiple pregnancies: an analysis of more than 400 000 pregnancies in the UK. *Prenat Neonat Med* 2001;6:89–94

23. Bouvier-Colle MH, Varnoux N, Salanave B, Ancel PY, Breart G. Case–control study of risk factors for obstetric patients' admission to intensive care units. *Eur J Obstet Gynecol Reprod Biol* 1997;74:173–7

24. Santema JG, Koppelaar I, Wallenburg HC. Hypertensive disorders in twin pregnancy. *Eur J Obstet Gynecol Reprod Biol* 1995;58:9–13

25. Albrecht JL, Tomich PG. The maternal and neonatal outcome of triplet gestations. *Am J Obstet Gynecol* 1996;174:1551–6

26. Devine PC, Malone FD, Athanassiou A, Harvey-Wilkes K, D'Alton ME. Maternal and neonatal outcome of 100 consecutive triplet pregnancies. *Am J Perinatol* 2001;18:225–35

27. Elliott JP, Radin TG. Quadruplet pregnancy: contemporary management and outcome. *Obstet Gynecol* 1992;80:421–4

28. Kaufman GE, Malone FD, Harvey-Wilkes KB, Chelmow D, Penzias AS, D'Alton ME. Neonatal morbidity and mortality associated with triplet pregnancy. *Obstet Gynecol* 1998;91:342–8

29. Malone FD, Kaufman GE, Chelmow D, Athanassiou A, Nores JA, D'Alton ME. Maternal morbidity associated with triplet pregnancy. *Am J Perinatol* 1998;15:73–7

30. Douglas KA, Redman CW. Eclampsia in the United Kingdom. *Br Med J* 1994;309:1395–400

31. Beral V, Doyle P, Tan SL, Mason BA, Campbell S. Outcome of pregnancies resulting from assisted conception. *Br Med Bull* 1990;46: 753–68

32. Suonio S, Huttunen M. Puerperal endometritis after abdominal twin delivery. *Acta Obstet Gynecol Scand* 1994;73:313–15

33. Malone F, D'Alton M. Multiple gestation: clinical characteristics and management. In Creasy R, Resnik R, eds. *Maternal-Fetal Medicine* vol 4. Philadelphia: WB Saunders, 1999:598–615

34. Collins MS, Bleyl JA. Seventy-one quadruplet pregnancies: management and outcome. *Am J Obstet Gynecol* 1990; 162:1384–91; discussion 1391–2

35. Landy HJ, Keith LG. The vanishing twin: a review. *Hum Reprod Update* 1998;4:177–83

36. Bergh C, Strandell A, Lundin K. 'Vanishing twin' in spontaneous and induced pregnancies. *Reprod Technol* 2000;10:158–61

37. Manzur A, Goldsman MP, Stone SC, Frederick JL, Balmaceda JP, Asch RH. Outcome of triplet pregnancies after assisted reproductive techniques: how frequent are the vanishing embryos? *Fertil Steril* 1995;63:252–7

38. Doyle P. The outcome of multiple pregnancy. *Hum Reprod* 1996;11(Suppl 4):110–7; discussion 118–20

39. Russell RB, Petrini JR, Damus K, Mattison DR, Schwarz RH. The changing epidemiology of multiple births in the United States. *Obstet Gynecol* 2003;101:129–35

40. Powers WF, Wampler NS. Further defining the risks confronting twins. *Am J Obstet Gynecol* 1996;175:1522–8

41. Rydhström H, Heraib F. Gestational duration, and foetal and infant mortality for twins vs singletons. *Twin Res* 2001;4:227–31

42. Scher AI, Petterson B, Blair E, *et al.* The risk of mortality or cerebral palsy in twins: a collaborative population-based study. *Pediatr Res* 2002;52:671–81

43. Gardner MO, Goldenberg RL, Cliver SP, Tucker JM, Nelson KG, Copper RL. The origin and outcome of preterm twin pregnancies. *Obstet Gynecol* 1995;85:553–7

44. Goldenberg RL, Iams JD, Miodovnik M, *et al.* The preterm prediction study: risk factors in twin gestations. National Institute of Child Health and Human Development Maternal–Fetal Medicine Units Network. *Am J Obstet Gynecol* 1996;175:1047–53

45. Min SJ, Luke B, Gillespie B, *et al.* Birth weight references for twins. *Am J Obstet Gynecol* 2000;182:1250–7

46. Mordel N, Benshushan A, Zajicek G, Laufer N, Schenker JG, Sadovsky E. Discordancy in triplets. *Am J Perinatol* 1993;10:224–5

47. Vignal J, Daures JP, Vergnes C, Giacalone PL, Boulot P. Assessment of triplet fetal growth by using cross-sectional analysis of the birth weight. *Fetal Diagn Ther* 1999;14:31–4

48. Smith-Levitin M, Kowalik A, Birnholz J, *et al.* Selective reduction of multifetal pregnancies to twins improves outcome over nonreduced triplet gestations. *Am J Obstet Gynecol* 1996;175:878–82

49. Török O, Lapinski R, Salafia CM, Bernasko J, Berkowitz RL. Multifetal pregnancy reduction is not associated with an increased risk of intrauterine growth restriction, except for very-high-order multiples. *Am J Obstet Gynecol* 1998;179:221–5

50. Lipitz S, Frenkel Y, Watts C, Ben-Rafael Z, Barkai G, Reichman B. High-order multifetal

gestation – management and outcome. *Obstet Gynecol* 1990;76:215–18

51. Shinwell ES, Blickstein I, Lusky A, Reichman B. Excess risk of mortality in very low birth-weight triplets: a national, population based study. *Arch Dis Child Fetal Neonat Ed* 2003;88:F36–40

52. Little J, Bryan E. Congenital anomalies in twins. *Semin Perinatol* 1986;10:50–64

53. Doyle PE, Beral V, Botting B, Wale CJ. Congenital malformations in twins in England and Wales. *J Epidemiol Community Health* 1991;45:43–8

54. Kallen B. Congenital malformations in twins: a population study. *Acta Genet Med Gemellol (Roma)* 1986;35:167–78

55. Kato K, Fujiki K. Multiple births and congenital anomalies in Tokyo Metropolitan Hospitals, 1979–1990. *Acta Genet Med Gemellol (Roma)* 1992;41:253–9

56. Mastroiacovo P, Castilla EE, Arpino C, et al. Congenital malformations in twins: an international study. *Am J Med Genet* 1999;83:117–24

57. Rodis JF, Egan JF, Craffey A, Ciarleglio L, Greenstein RM, Scorza WE. Calculated risk of chromosomal abnormalities in twin gestations. *Obstet Gynecol* 1990;76:1037–41

58. Cuckle H. Down's syndrome screening in twins. *J Med Screen* 1998;5:3–4

59. Berkowitz RL, Stone JL, Eddleman KA. One hundred consecutive cases of selective termination of an abnormal fetus in a multifoetal gestation. *Obstet Gynecol* 1997;90:606–10

60. Wee LY, Fisk NM. The twin–twin transfusion syndrome. *Semin Neonatol* 2002;7:187–202

61. Quintero RA, Dickinson JE, Morales WJ, et al. Stage-based treatment of twin–twin transfusion syndrome. *Am J Obstet Gynecol* 2003;188:1333–40

62. Sebire NJ, Souka A, Skentou H, Geerts L, Nicolaides KH. Early prediction of severe twin-to-twin transfusion syndrome. *Hum Reprod* 2000;15:2008–10

63. Odibo AO, Macones GA. Management of twin–twin transfusion syndrome: laying the foundation for future interventional studies. *Twin Res* 2002;5:515–20

64. Ropacka M, Markwitz W, Blickstein I. Treatment options for the twin–twin transfusion syndrome: a review. *Twin Res* 2002;5:507–14

65. Slotnick RN, Ortega JE. Monoamniotic twinning and zona manipulation: a survey of U.S. IVF centers correlating zona manipulation procedures and high-risk twinning frequency. *J Assist Reprod Genet* 1996;13:381–5

66. Su LL. Monoamniotic twins: diagnosis and management. *Acta Obstet Gynecol Scand* 2002;81:995–1000

67. Luke B, Keith LG. The contribution of singletons, twins and triplets to low birth weight, infant mortality and handicap in the United States. *J Reprod Med* 1992;37:661–6

68. Yokoyama Y, Shimizu T, Hayakawa K. Prevalence of cerebral palsy in twins, triplets and quadruplets. *Int J Epidemiol* 1995;24:943–8

69. Blickstein I. Cerebral palsy in multifetal pregnancies. *Dev Med Child Neurol* 2002;44:352–5

70. Petterson B, Nelson KB, Watson L, Stanley F. Twins, triplets, and cerebral palsy in births in Western Australia in the 1980s. *Br Med J* 1993;307:1239–43

71. Bryan E. Educating families, before, during and after a multiple birth. *Semin Neonatol* 2002;7:241–6

72. Allen MC. Factors affecting developmental outcome. In Keith LG, Papiernik E, Keith DM, Luke B, eds. *Multiple Pregnancy, Epidemiology, Gestation and Perinatal Outcome.* Carnforth, UK: Parthenon Publishing, 1995:599–612

73. Bryan E, Read B. Guidance after twin and singleton death. *Arch Dis Child Fetal Neonat Ed* 1995;73:F123

74. Garel M, Salobir C, Blondel B. Psychological consequences of having triplets: a 4-year follow-up study. *Fertil Steril* 1997;67:1162–5

75. Thorpe K, Golding J, MacGillivray I, Greenwood R. Comparison of prevalence of depression in mothers of twins and mothers of singletons. *Br Med J* 1991;302:875–8

76. Joesch JM, Smith KR. Children's health and their mothers' risk of divorce or separation. *Soc Biol* 1997;44:159–69

77. Serour GI, Aboulghar M, Mansour R, Sattar MA, Amin Y, Aboulghar H. Complications of medically assisted conception in 3,500 cycles. *Fertil Steril* 1998;70:638–42

78. Collins JA, Bustillo M, Visscher RD, Lawrence LD. An estimate of the cost of *in vitro* fertilization services in the United States in 1995. *Fertil Steril* 1995;64:538–45

79. Petterson B, Watson L, Kurinczuk J. Cerebral palsy in triplets. In Keith LG, Blickstein I, eds. *Triplet Pregnancies and their Consequences.* London, UK: Parthenon Publishing, 2002: 321–32

80. Grether JK, Nelson KB, Cummins SK. Twinning and cerebral palsy: experience in four northern California counties, births 1983 through 1985. *Pediatrics* 1993;92:854–8

81. King R, Johnson A. *Oxford Register of Early Childhood Impairments: Annual Report 1995.* Oxford: Women's Centre, Oxford Radcliffe Hospital, 1995

82. Nelson KB, Ellenberg JH. Childhood neurological disorders in twins. *Paediatr Perinat Epidemiol* 1995;9:135–45

83. Pharoah PO, Cooke T. Cerebral palsy and multiple births. *Arch Dis Child Fetal Neonat Ed* 1996;75:F174–7

84. Williams K, Hennessy E, Alberman E. Cerebral palsy: effects of twinning, birth-weight, and gestational age. *Arch Dis Child Fetal Neonat Ed* 1996;75:F178–82

85. MacFarlane AJ, Johnson A, Bower P. Disabilities and health problems in childhood. In Botting BJ, MacFarlane AJ, eds. *Three, Four or More.* London: HMSO, 1990

86. Liu J, Li Z, Lin Q, *et al.* Cerebral palsy and multiple births in China. *Int J Epidemiol* 2000;29:292–9

87. Hay DA, McIndoe R, O'Brien PJ. The older sibling of twins. *Aus J Early Child* 1987;13:25–8

88. Bergh T, Ericson A, Hillensjö T, Nygren K-G, Wennerholm UB. Deliveries and children born after *in vitro* fertilization in Sweden 1982–1995: a retrospective cohort study. *Lancet* 1999;354:1579–85

89. Strömberg B, Dahlquist G, Ericson A, Finnström O, Köster M, Stjernqvist K. Neurological sequelae in children born after *in vitro* fertilization: a population-based study. *Lancet* 2002;359:461–5

4

Prevention of multiple pregnancies after non-*in vitro* fertilization treatment

B. Cohlen and P. A. van Dop

INTRODUCTION

The aim of any infertility treatment should be a healthy, singleton baby born after an uncomplicated pregnancy. For many years fertility specialists have been focusing on achieving pregnancy as the main goal without realizing the consequences of multiple pregnancies on patients, obstetric care and society. The costs of a multiple pregnancy for the health service and community as well as the family will be 100–200 times greater than the costs of a singleton[1]. In *in vitro* fertilization (IVF)/intracytoplasmic sperm injection (ICSI) the number of transferred embryos can be controlled and therefore the chance of achieving a multiple pregnancy minimized. In many countries, only two embryos are replaced and the discussion of single-embryo transfer is ongoing.

The number of twins and high-order multiple pregnancies (HOMP) after infertility treatment is nevertheless still too high. This is also due to treatments other than IVF/ICSI. In this chapter we focus on prevention of multiple pregnancies after assisted reproduction technologies (ART) other than IVF or similar invasive treatments. In daily practice ovulation induction and controlled ovarian hyperstimulation (COH) with or without intrauterine insemination (IUI) are by far the most widely applied non-IVF infertility treatments. In reproductive medicine there is a distinction between ovulation induction and COH. Whereas ovulation induction is indicated for patients with amenorrhea or oligomenorrhea causing subfertility, COH is applied in patients with usually regular menstrual cycles. Although both groups of patients share subfertility as a common characteristic, from an endocrinological point of view they are quite different. In patients

with oligo/amenorrhea, monofollicular development should be the main goal, while with COH most physicians strive towards multifollicular development to enhance the probability of conception. COH with or without IUI is therefore a treatment modality with a potentially high risk for multiple pregnancies.

One could indeed argue about whether the word 'controlled' in COH is appropriate. In fact, the individual reaction of a particular patient's ovaries after the administration of a fixed dose of follicle stimulating hormone (FSH) is unpredictable, let alone controlled. We claim to apply COH in the sense of a 'controlled' quantitative steering of the number of follicles. However, at present we are not able to manage the number of follicles in an efficient way.

Since the prevention of multiple pregnancies is the main theme of this chapter, we first have to consider the natural factors influencing multiple pregnancies.

NATURAL DETERMINANTS OF MULTIPLE PREGNANCY

Under natural circumstances the multiple pregnancy rate is mainly influenced by race, age and hereditary factors. Dizygotic multiple pregnancies are a result of multiple follicular growth[2]. As is the case in ovulation induction and COH, under spontaneous circumstances this is due to an increase in FSH levels[3] and influenced by the ovarian reserve[4]. In many cultures women are of a significantly older age when they start their procreation. This delay in timing of pregnancy results in an increase in the spontaneous multiple pregnancy rate.

CONTROLLED OVARIAN STIMULATION WITH OR WITHOUT IUI

Because COH is the main risk factor for achieving multiples, it should only be applied in daily practise after being proven effective in randomized trials. Ovarian hyperstimulation is often followed by IUI, but in some cases IUI could be as effective when applied in natural cycles. IUI has therefore been the subject of many randomized trials[5–7]. It has been compared with timed intercourse, and natural cycles have been compared with COH cycles (Figure 1). Meta-analyses combining all evidence per indication have shown IUI in natural cycles to be effective in couples with male subfertility and cervical hostility[5,8]. IUI in natural cycles is ineffective in couples with unexplained or mild male subfertility[8]. Hughes published a robust meta-analysis on the efficiency of IUI and COH in the treatment of pertinent infertility[9]. He concluded that both IUI and FSH independently improved the probability of conception. Across all diagnostic groups (5214 cycles) the likelihood of conception was about two-fold higher with FSH and about three-fold higher with IUI.

In summary, the combination of COH followed by IUI has been proven effective in couples with unexplained and mild male subfertility only and should therefore be restricted to these specific indications.

CONTROLLED OVARIAN HYPERSTIMULATION WITH IUI AND MULTIPLE PREGNANCIES

The literature regarding prevention of multiples after COH/IUI is extensive, but most trials have a retrospective cohort design. Such trials can identify prognostic variables after multivariate analysis, but can never result in as robust conclusions as prospective (randomized) trials[10]. Various indications for subfertility treatment are often combined and the power of most retrospective trials is insufficient to detect statistically significant predicting parameters. Furthermore, the American literature focuses on preventing HOMP while twins are often hardly considered a problem. Several large (retrospective) studies searching for parameters to predict multiple pregnancies after COH/IUI have been published[11–14] and will be discussed later.

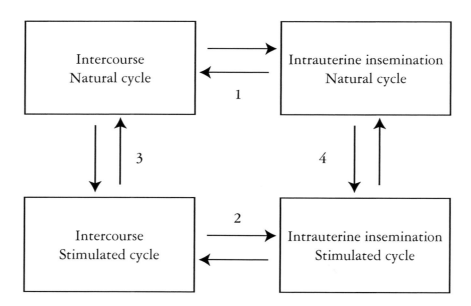

Figure 1   The four comparisons that have to be made in randomized trials to (dis)prove the efficacy of intrauterine insemination and/or controlled ovarian hyperstimulation

MULTIPLE PREGNANCIES AFTER IUI: SHOULD WE USE CLOMIPHENE CITRATE INSTEAD OF GONADOTROPINS?

Since COH turns out to be a major risk factor for multiple pregnancies in IUI and since both clomiphene citrate (CC) and gonadotropins are used in combination with IUI, it is mandatory to see whether the risks (and efficacy) are comparable.

Several small randomized controlled trials (RCTs) combining various indications have compared the efficacy of CC with gonadotropins, both in combination with IUI[15–18]. Regrettably the results of these trials are contradictory. Whereas Balasch and colleagues[15] and Matorras and colleagues[16] concluded that low-dose FSH was superior to CC, Ecochard and co-workers[17] concluded both treatment modalities to be at least as effective with a trend favouring CC. A fourth randomized trial with a factorial design with eight different treatment alternatives concluded that COH with human menopausal gonadotropin (hMG) was more effective than CC in insemination cycles, but insemination as such seemed to have no beneficial effect on the pregnancy rate in stimulated cycles for treatment of unexplained infertility[18].

Do these four randomized trials say anything about the risk of multiple pregnancies after CC stimulation compared with gonadotropins? Ecochard and associates did not mention the number of multiples at all, whereas Balasch and colleagues (using only 75 IU FSH every other day) achieved singleton pregnancies only. Increasing the dose of gonadotropins to 150 IU daily results in a higher multiple pregnancy rate, becoming as high as 46% in the trial by Karlstrom and associates[18]. It is beyond doubt that increasing the daily dose of gonadotropins results in higher pregnancy rates (Table 1)[19]. However, the price that has to be paid in terms of an increased proportion of multiple pregnancies is too high.

Both Hughes and Cohlen and colleagues discussed the use of CC in IUI cycles in their systematic reviews and concluded that CC seemed less effective[9,20]. However, large RCTs with sufficient power to detect clinically relevant differences in cost-effectiveness between CC and gonadotropins in IUI cycles are still lacking. Large retrospective studies found multiple pregnancy rates of approximately 10% with the use of CC[21].

In conclusion, it seems that CC is less potent when compared to gonadotropins, resulting probably in a lower pregnancy rate but also in a lower proportion of multiple pregnancies. Large RCTs comparing CC with gonadotropins should focus not only on efficacy but also on side-effects such as multiple pregnancies. Cost-effectiveness should also include the costs of multiples, to be able to reach conclusions about the treatment modality that should be the first choice.

Table 1 Results of intrauterine insemination with more or less aggressive stimulation protocols from 17 studies carried out between 1986 and 1993

Reference numbers	Type of stimulation	Number of cycles	Monthly fecundity rate	% Multiple pregnancies	% Triplets
35–37	CC/hMG	593	0.09	5	0.0
18, 36, 38–42	150 IU hMG	1528	0.12	19	3.2
43–48	150–225 IU hMG	1500	0.18	21	4.5
45, 47, 49, 50	analog/hMG	259	0.20	31	8.5

CC, clomiphene citrate; hMG, human menopausal gonadotropin

MONITORING CONTROLLED OVARIAN HYPERSTIMULATION/IUI CYCLES: CAN WE PREDICT AND/OR PREVENT MULTIPLES?

Cycles with ovarian hyperstimulation are usually monitored by frequent ultrasound assessment of follicular number and size and/or serum estradiol measurements. The value of cycle monitoring in COH/IUI cycles has recently been the subject of a discussion in *Fertility and Sterility*[22]. Several large retrospective trials have been published on this subject[11–14]. However, these trials used different study populations, different stimulation protocols, different cancellation criteria (if any), and different statistical methods. It is therefore not surprising that these trials found different predicting parameters and came to different conclusions. Overall the probability of achieving a multiple pregnancy seemed to be related to the age of the woman, the total number of follicles and/or the number of follicles larger than 11 mm at the time of human chorionic gonadotropin (hCG) administration. The parameters found in these retrospective trials should be checked in large prospective trials using receiver-operating characteristic (ROC) curves to determine optimal cut-off values. Finally, these parameters should be the subject of internal and external validation before they are used in daily practice.

Several randomized trials on COH/IUI have been published using low-dose step-up protocols, with intensive monitoring and strict cancellation criteria. Did these protocols result in low multiple pregnancy rates? As mentioned before, Balasch and colleagues[15] used 75 IU FSH every other day, resulting in singleton pregnancies only (pregnancy rate/cycle: 13%). Goverde and associates[6] used 75 IU FSH daily in a step-up protocol and cancelled cycles when more than three follicles of ≥ 18 mm or more than six follicles of ≥ 14 mm were present. This resulted in a multiple pregnancy rate of 29%, with twins only, for a pregnancy rate/cycle of 8.7%. Cohlen and co-workers[5] used the same dosage of FSH and cancelled the insemination when more than three follicles of ≥ 18 mm were seen or when serum estradiol levels exceeded 6000 pmol/l. They found a multiple pregnancy rate of 9.5%, with twins only (pregnancy rate/cycle: 13.7%). Gregoriou and co-workers[23] published a randomized trial using a low-dose step-up protocol starting with 75 IU hMG/day with strict cancellation criteria of more than four follicles ≥ 16 mm and serum estradiol levels not exceeding 1500 pmol/l. In couples with unexplained subfertility this resulted in a multiple pregnancy rate of 9.1% (pregnancy rate/cycle: 25.7%). When we compare the results of these trials with the results of the largest randomized trial published on COH/IUI, by Guzick and co-workers[7], who used a higher fixed-dose regimen of 150 IU FSH/day and cancelled cycles only when serum estradiol levels exceeded 11 010 pmol/l, the differences are striking. The combination of COH and IUI yielded a multiple pregnancy rate of over 25% with two quadruplet and three triplet pregnancies (pregnancy rate/cycle: 9%).

Therefore, besides the parameters found in retrospective trials, it seems reasonable to assume that the probability of achieving a multiple pregnancy is correlated with the aggressiveness of the stimulation protocol and the applied cancellation criteria. Table 1 illustrates these conclusions. Randomized trials comparing different stimulation protocols for IUI (for instance 50 IU FSH/day versus 75 IU FSH/day) in a well-defined subfertile population using strict cancellation criteria should first be conducted to define the optimal stimulation protocol: acceptable pregnancy rates with only very few or even no multiple pregnancies.

GONADOTROPIN RELEASING HORMONE AGONISTS AND IUI

Does the addition of a gonadotropin releasing hormone (GnRH) agonist prevent multiple pregnancies in IUI cycles? Three randomized trials have been published that investigated the efficacy of GnRH agonists in COH/IUI programs[24–26]. All trials concluded that GnRH agonists are not cost-effective. Two trials mentioned the number of multiple pregnancies and these rates varied between 22 and 55%. It can be concluded that there is no role for GnRH agonists in COH/IUI programs. It is not cost-effective, nor does it prevent multiples. No data are at present available on GnRH antagonists and IUI.

PREOVULATORY SUPERNUMERARY FOLLICLE REDUCTION BY ASPIRATION IN IUI

De Geyter and colleagues[27,28] published two retrospective studies on prevention of multiple pregnancies by aspiration of supernumerary follicles just before ovulation. In their first paper they reported similar pregnancy rates between cycles with aspiration (when more than three follicles of > 14 mm were present) and cycles where aspiration was not necessary (24.4% vs. 21.9%). However, the multiple pregnancy rates were still too high: 10.4%, including triplets. In a second paper[28] based on more patients they reported a significant reduction in the multiple pregnancy rate in their program (from 19.6% to 9.4%) and no hospital admission for ovarian hyperstimulation syndrome (OHSS), while stable pregnancy rates were achieved. However, still five triplets, one quadruplet and one quintuplet were diagnosed, necessitating selective fetal reduction. Albano and co-workers[29] studied the effects of follicular aspiration when more than three follicles of ≥ 15 mm were present in 26 cycles, resulting in seven singleton pregnancies only.

From the point of view of reducing multiple pregnancy rates in COH/IUI programs, follicular reduction by aspiration may be a useful method that needs further investigation in large prospective randomized trials. Whether this method can be safely applied in centers not carrying out IVF and lacking procedures for routine follicle aspiration and oocyte identification in the aspirate needs to be investigated.

CONVERSION OF IUI TO IVF

Owing to excessive follicular development, Nisker and co-workers[30] converted 25 COH/IUI cycles to IVF/embryo transfer (ET). This resulted in 13 pregnancies (52%) including two twins and one triplet (multiple pregnancy rate: 23%). Moreover, four patients developed severe OHSS, including two cases requiring paracentesis. One might wonder whether this treatment prevents multiple pregnancies. It seems that this aggressive kind of ovarian hyperstimulation (GnRH agonist with high dosage of hMG) in IUI programs is out of place. Furthermore, conversion to IVF might suddenly surprise unprepared, non-informed couples and make treatment more expensive and invasive. Therefore, it is our strong opinion that conversion to IVF/ET should be discouraged.

CONCLUSIONS AND RECOMMENDATIONS

Two review papers[31,32] on the use of ovarian hyperstimulation make it unmistakably clear that multiple pregnancies are unavoidable using gonadotropins. Multiple pregnancies are high-risk pregnancies not only for the mother, but even more so for the unborn and the newborn. When multiple pregnancies cannot be avoided, should we abandon ovarian hyperstimulation with or without IUI from the pool of our therapeutic options, although effectiveness has been proven? Should we instead start treating subfertile couples with IVF/ET or ICSI immediately?

Not many trials have been published that compared the cost-effectiveness and safety of COH/IUI compared with IVF/ET. However, the investigators who performed this comparison all concluded that COH/IUI was more cost-effective[6,33]. Furthermore, subfertile couples prefer less invasive and stressful treatments, such as COH/IUI[6]. Future randomized trials will have to focus on the role of natural-cycle IVF and whether this 'new' treatment modality can replace COH/IUI, being not only safer with regard to multiple pregnancies, but also cost-effective and more appreciated by couples.

In the meantime, it is our duty to develop COH/IUI programs that minimize the risks without compromising the results. Figure 2 shows a proposed strategy that can be applied to minimize the risk for multiples.

When COH/IUI is applied it should be offered to couples with mild male subfertility (average total motile sperm count > 10 million) or unexplained subfertility only. Low-dose step-up protocols should be used with close ultrasound monitoring and strict cancellation criteria (maximum two or three follicles of ≥ 15 mm or four to five follicles of ≥ 11 mm). No GnRH agonists should be used. When the cancellation criteria are exceeded, cycles should be cancelled and couples should be advised to abstain from unprotected intercourse. Alternatively, aspiration of supernumerary follicles can be proposed. The center should have experience in performing follicle aspirations and in detecting oocytes in the aspirate. Only two follicles should be left over. Conversion to IVF/ET can be proposed in IVF centers when couples are informed beforehand, but high-quality randomized trials investigating the cost-effectiveness of this escape route have not been performed. Furthermore, most couples will not be informed and

prepared beforehand, costs will rise tremendously and risks of invasive treatments will be introduced.

It is of paramount importance that, before starting treatment, couples are well informed of all risks, including those of multiple pregnancies. Many couples do not object to becoming pregnant with twins, because they do not understand the consequences. It is our duty to explain these conse-

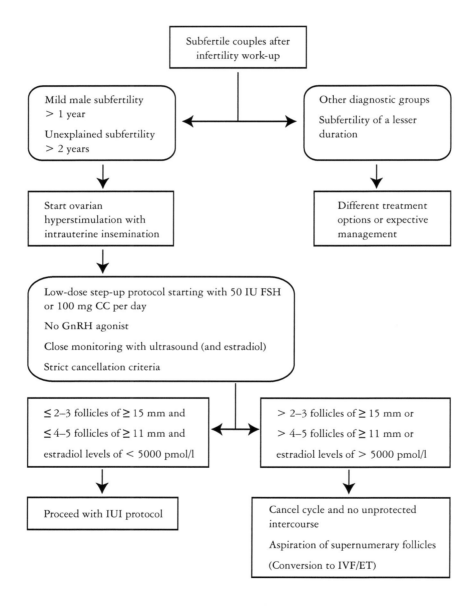

Figure 2 Proposed strategy to prevent multiple pregnancies in ovarian stimulation programs in combination with intrauterine insemination (IUI). FSH, follicle stimulating hormone; CC, clomiphene citrate; GnRH, gonadotropin releasing hormone; IVF, *in vitro* fertilization; ET, embryo transfer

quences, based on reliable literature and the data of our own centers.

The study of Guzick and co-workers[7] is regarded as the gold standard in IUI studies. In an invitational editorial in the same issue of the *New England Journal of Medicine*, te Velde and Cohlen[34] raise the question: 'How should we guide these couples in a manner that maximizes the chances of conception while minimizing the risks and complications?' They emphasized the 'overlooked' importance in subfertility of the likelihood of spontaneous conceptions if infertility had been ruled out. The authors underlined the importance of spontaneous pregnancies during the non-insemination cycles (3%) during the trial. The observed pregnancy rate in non-treatment cycles of 3% corresponds to a yearly fecundity rate of 31%. Another concern raised in the editorial was the multiple pregnancy rate in this prospective multicenter study of 30%, with a rate of triplet and quadruplet pregnancies of almost 9%, matching those reported in IVF/ET. Te Velde and Cohlen come to the conclusion that the same pregnancy rate in six months obtained during the trial of Guzick and colleagues could also have been reached when treatment had been postponed for 12 months. They ended their editorial with 'Most important, the fertility and infertility information given to individual couples should fundamentally change. The marketing of assisted reproductive technology should include realistic perspectives instead of hyperstimulated illusions'.

REFERENCES

1. FIGO Committee Report. Ethical guidelines in the prevention of iatrogenic multiple pregnancy. *Int J Gynecol Obstet* 2000;71:293–4

2. Gilfillan CP, Robertson DM, Burger HG, *et al.* The control of ovulation in mothers of dizygotic twins. *J Clin Endocrinol Metab* 1996;81:1557–62

3. Lambalk CB, Boomsma DI, De Boer L, *et al.* Increased levels and pulsatility of follicle-stimulating hormone in mothers of hereditary dizygotic twins. *J Clin Endocrinol Metab* 1998;83:481–6

4. Oosterhuis GJ, Vermes I, Michgelsen HW, *et al.* Follicle stimulating hormone measured in unextracted urine throughout the menstrual cycle correlates with age and ovarian reserve. *Hum Reprod* 2002;17:641–6

5. Cohlen BJ, te Velde ER, van Kooij RJ, *et al.* Controlled ovarian hyperstimulation and intrauterine insemination for treating male subfertility: a controlled study. *Hum Reprod* 1998;13:1553–8

6. Goverde AJ, McDonnell J, Vermeiden JP, *et al.* Intrauterine insemination or *in-vitro* fertilisation in idiopathic subfertility and male subfertility: a randomized trial and cost-effectiveness analysis. *Lancet* 2000;355:13–18

7. Guzick DS, Carson SA, Coutifaris C, *et al.* Efficacy of superovulation and intrauterine insemination in the treatment of infertility. National Cooperative Reproductive Medicine Network. *N Engl J Med* 1999;340:177–83

8. Cohlen BJ, te Velde ER. Mild ovarian hyperstimulation for intrauterine insemination. In Tarlatzis B, ed. *Ovulation Induction*. Paris: Elsevier, 2002:53–64

9. Hughes EG. The effectiveness of ovulation induction and intrauterine insemination in the treatment of persistent infertility: a meta-analysis. *Hum Reprod* 1997;12:1865–72

10. Daya S. Inappropriate use of cohort studies to formulate treatment guidelines. *Fertil Steril* 2003;79:27

11. Dickey RP, Taylor SN, Lu PY, *et al.* Relationship of follicle numbers and estradiol levels to multiple implantation in 3,608 intrauterine insemination cycles. *Fertil Steril* 2001;75:69–78

12. Tur R, Barri PN, Coroleu B, *et al.* Risk factors for high-order multiple implantation after ovarian stimulation with gonadotrophins: evidence from a large series of 1878 consecu-

tive pregnancies in a single centre. *Hum Reprod* 2001;16:2124–9

13. Kaplan PF, Patel M, Austin DJ, Freund R. Assessing the risk of multiple gestation in gonadotropin intrauterine insemination cycles. *Am J Obstet Gynecol* 2002;186:1244–9

14. Gleicher N, Oleske DM, Tur-Kaspa I, *et al.* Reducing the risk of high-order multiple pregnancy after ovarian stimulation with gonadotropins. *N Engl J Med* 2000;343:2–7

15. Balasch J, Ballesca JL, Pimentel C, *et al.* Late low-dose pure follicle stimulating hormone for ovarian stimulation in intra-uterine insemination cycles. *Hum Reprod* 1994;9:1863–6

16. Matorras R, Diaz T, Corostegui B, *et al.* Ovarian stimulation in intrauterine insemination with donor sperm: a randomized study comparing clomiphene citrate in fixed protocol versus highly purified urinary FSH. *Hum Reprod* 2002;17:2107–11

17. Ecochard R, Mathieu C, Royere D, *et al.* A randomized prospective study comparing pregnancy rates after clomiphene citrate and human menopausal gonadotropin before intrauterine insemination. *Fertil Steril* 2000; 73:90–3

18. Karlstrom PO, Bergh T, Lundkvist O. A prospective randomized trial of artificial insemination versus intercourse in cycles stimulated with human menopausal gonadotropin or clomiphene citrate. *Fertil Steril* 1993;59: 554–9

19. Nan PM, Cohlen BJ, te Velde ER, *et al.* Intrauterine insemination or timed intercourse after ovarian stimulation for male subfertility? A controlled study. *Hum Reprod* 1994;9: 2022–6

20. Cohlen BJ, Vandekerckhove P, te Velde ER, Habbema JD. Timed intercourse versus intra-uterine insemination with or without ovarian hyperstimulation for subfertility in men.

Cochrane Database Syst Rev 2000;(2): CD000360

21. Dickey RP, Holtkamp DE. Development, pharmacology and clinical experience with clomiphene citrate. *Hum Reprod Update* 1996;2:483–506

22. Dickey RP. A year of inaction on high-order multiple pregnancies due to ovulation induction. *Fertil Steril* 2003;79:14–16

23. Gregoriou O, Vitoratos N, Papadias C, *et al.* Controlled ovarian hyperstimulation with or without intrauterine insemination for the treatment of unexplained infertility. *Int J Gynecol Obstet* 1995;48:55–9

24. Dodson WC, Olive DL, Hughes CL, Haney AF. The prognostic value of serum concentrations of progesterone, estradiol, and luteinizing hormone during superovulation with and without adjunctive leuprolide therapy. *Fertil Steril* 1993;59:1174–8

25. Sengoku K, Tamate K, Takaoka Y, Morishita N, Oshikawa M. A randomized prospective study of gonadotrophin with or without gonadotrophin-releasing hormone agonist for treatment of unexplained infertility. *Hum Reprod* 1994;9:1043–7

26. Karlstrom PO, Bergh T, Lundkvist O. Addition of gonadotrophin-releasing hormone agonist and/or two inseminations with husband's sperm do not improve the pregnancy rate in superovulated cycles. *Acta Obstet Gynecol Scand* 2000;79:37–42

27. De Geyter C, De Geyter M, Castro E, *et al.* Experience with transvaginal ultrasound-guided aspiration of supernumerary follicles for the prevention of multiple pregnancies after ovulation induction and intrauterine insemination. *Fertil Steril* 1996;65:1163–8

28. De Geyter C, De Geyter M, Nieschlag E. Low multiple pregnancy rates and reduced frequency of cancellation after ovulation

induction with gonadotropins, if eventual supernumerary follicles are aspirated to prevent polyovulation. *J Assist Reprod Genet* 1998;15:111–16

29. Albano C, Platteau P, Nogueira D, *et al.* Avoidance of multiple pregnancies after ovulation induction by supernumerary preovulatory follicular reduction. *Fertil Steril* 2001;76: 820–2

30. Nisker J, Tummon I, Daniel S, *et al.* Conversion of cycles involving ovarian hyperstimulation with intra-uterine insemination to *in-vitro* fertilization. *Hum Reprod* 1994;9: 406–8

31. Dickey RP, Olar TT. Hormone treatment for infertility. Restrictions won't prevent multiple pregnancies. *Br Med J* 1993;307:1281–2

32. Child TJ, Barlow DH. Strategies to prevent multiple pregnancies in assisted conception programmes. *Baillières Clin Obstet Gynaecol* 1998;12:131–46

33. Peterson CM, Hatasaka HH, Jones KP, *et al.* Ovulation induction with gonadotropins and intrauterine insemination compared with *in vitro* fertilization and no therapy: a prospective, nonrandomized, cohort study and meta-analysis. *Fertil Steril* 1994;62:535–44

34. te Velde ER, Cohlen BJ. The management of infertility. *N Engl J Med* 1999;340:224-6

35. Horvath PM, Bohrer M, Sheldon RM, Kemmann E. The relationship of sperm parameters to cycle fecundity in superovulated women undergoing intrauterine insemination. *Fertil Steril* 1989;52:288–94

36. Kemmann E, Bohrer M, Sheldon R, Fiasconaro G, Beardsley L. Active ovulation management increases the monthly probability of pregnancy occurrence in ovulatory women who receive intrauterine insemination. *Fertil Steril* 1987;48:916–20

37. Sunde A, Kahn J, Molne K. Intrauterine insemination. *Hum Reprod* 1988;3:97–9

38. Cruz RI, Kemmann E, Brandeis VT, *et al.* A prospective study of intrauterine insemination of processed sperm from men with oligoasthenospermia in superovulated women. *Fertil Steril* 1986;46:673–7

39. Dickey RP, Olar TT, Taylor SN, Curole DN, Rye PH, Matulich EM. Relationship of follicle number, serum estradiol, and other factors to birth rate and multiparity in human menopausal gonadotropin-induced intrauterine insemination cycles. *Fertil Steril* 1991;56:89–92

40. Ho PC, So WK, Chan YF, Yeung WS. Intrauterine insemination after ovarian stimulation as a treatment for subfertility because of subnormal semen: a prospective randomized controlled trial. *Fertil Steril* 1992;58:995–9

41. Hurst BS, Tjaden BL, Kimball A, Schlaff WD, Damewood MD, Rock JA. Superovulation with or without intrauterine insemination for the treatment of infertility. *J Reprod Med* 1992;37:237–41

42. Remohi J, Gastaldi C, Patrizio P, *et al.* Intrauterine insemination and controlled ovarian hyperstimulation in cycles before GIFT. *Hum Reprod* 1989;4:918–20

43. Chaffkin LM, Nulsen JC, Luciano AA, Metzger DA. A comparative analysis of the cycle fecundity rates associated with combined human menopausal gonadotropin (hMG) and intrauterine insemination (IUI) verus either hMG or IUI alone. *Fertil Steril* 1991;55:252–7

44. Dodson WC, Whitesides DB, Hughes CL Jr, Easley HA III, Haney AF. Superovulation with intrauterine insemination in the treatment of infertility: a possible alternative to gamete intrafallopian transfer and *in vitro* fertilization. *Fertil Steril* 1987;48:441–5

45. Dodson WC, Walmer DK, Hughes CL Jr, Yancy SE, Haney AF. Adjunctive leuprolide therapy does not improve cycle fecundity in controlled ovarian hyperstimulation and intrauterine insemination of subfertile women. *Obstet Gynecol* 1991;78:187–90

46. Dodson WC, Haney AF. Controlled ovarian hyperstimulation and intrauterine insemination for treatment of infertility. *Fertil Steril* 1991;55:457–67

47. Gagliardi CL, Emmi AM, Weiss G, Schmidt CL. Gonadotropin-releasing hormone agonist improves the efficiency of controlled ovarian hyperstimulation/intrauterine insemination. *Fertil Steril* 1991;55:939–44

48. Serhal PF, Katz M, Little V, Woronowski H. Unexplained infertility – the value of Pergonal superovulation combined with intrauterine insemination. *Fertil Steril* 1988;49:602–6

49. Allegra A, Volpes A, Coffaro F, Guida S, Francofonte R. Superovulation with buserelin and gonadotropin dramatically improves the success rate of intrauterine insemination with husband's washed semen. *Acta Eur Fertil* 1990;21:191–5

50. Zikopoulos K, West CP, Thong PW, Kacser EM, Morrison J, Wu FC. Homologous intra-uterine insemination has no advantage over timed natural intercourse when used in combination with ovulation induction for the treatment of unexplained infertility. *Hum Reprod* 1993;8:563–7

5

Patient selection for single-embryo transfer

A. Strandell

BACKGROUND

Children born after *in vitro* fertilization (IVF) constitute at least 2% of all newborn babies in many industrialized countries. Parallel to the increasing success of IVF, the rate of multiple births has increased and is commonly 25–35% among IVF births and in some countries even more than 40%. The increase is mainly due to the occurrence of twins, but the incidence of higher-order multiple births has increased as well. There is no disagreement concerning triplets and higher-order multiple births: they cause major medical, social and financial consequences. Whether the high rate of twins is a major health issue is being debated, and is not completely accepted by all physicians or by their patients. However, the follow-up of children born after IVF has shown that giving birth after IVF is associated with a greater risk of prematurity and with a lower birth weight, resulting in a somewhat increased risk of perinatal death, mainly attributed to twins[1]. The risk of cerebral palsy is evidently increased in triplets and higher-order multiples but it is also significantly increased in twins when compared with singletons, ranging from two- to ten-fold in different reports[2]. There has been an obvious change in patient attitude as this information has spread, resulting in a demand for single-embryo transfer, which was previously an uncommon practice.

The negative outcome in IVF children is mainly due to the increased risk of multiple pregnancy and the associated risk of prematurity, and it is urgent to decrease the rate of multiple birth after IVF, at the same time aiming at preventing the pregnancy rate from falling. The most important factor influencing the rate of multiple birth is the number of embryos transferred, which has gradually decreased but still shows a wide range worldwide. Several reports aiming at reducing the multiple birth rate by transferring two instead of three embryos, published during the 1990s, showed that the pregnancy rate was unaffected while the rate of multiple pregnancy decreased. In one of the largest studies, using the national British IVF database[3], it was demonstrated within different age groups that only the multiple birth rate and not the overall birth rate increased when three instead of two embryos were transferred, if more than four eggs had been fertilized. In Sweden, as well as in the other Nordic countries, transfer of a maximum of two embryos has become the norm, resulting in a pregnancy rate of 35–40% and a live birth rate of approximately 25% per transfer. This routine was introduced in 1993 and resulted in the maintenance of a stable pregnancy rate, while triplets almost disappeared, but the twin rate remained unchanged at around 25%. Twin pregnancies are still associated with an increased risk of prematurity and there is an obvious need further to reduce the rate of multiple births.

STRATEGIES TO REDUCE THE MULTIPLE PREGNANCY BIRTH RATE

There are four obvious strategies to reduce the rate of multiple birth. The simplest method is to perform single-embryo transfer as a routine in all cases, which certainly would result almost exclusively in singletons, but pregnancy and birth rates would probably decrease substantially, which would be unlikely to be accepted by the infertile patients and their physicians, both of whom are motivated to maximize the outcome in each cycle.

The second method — elective single-embryo transfer to a selected group of patients — is advocated by an increasing number of centers and physicians, either on a voluntary basis or through health authority regulations. This chapter focuses on the issue of how to select patients for single-embryo transfer.

A third option to reduce the multiple birth rate would be to perform blastocyst culture, which theoretically would enable a better and more secure selection of viable embryos. The method still needs to be further evaluated in a large randomized controlled trial and compared with transfer of cleavage-stage embryos. In the first randomized study[4], including 200 patients, pregnancy rates were the same whether day-3 or day-5 embryos were transferred (39%) and implantation rates were 21% and 24%, respectively. The second randomized study[5] was somewhat smaller ($n = 162$) and showed similar pregnancy rates in day-3 (29%) and blastocyst (35%) transfer. However, significantly more embryos were transferred at the cleavage stage (3.5 vs. 2.0), resulting in a lower implantation rate (13% vs. 26%) and a higher rate of high-order multiple gestation (19% vs. 4%). The use of blastocyst transfer still needs to prove its value in the transfer of a single blastocyst as compared to a single cleavage-stage embryo.

These three methods are aimed at reducing multiple birth rate by preventing multiple conceptions and implantations, as opposed to the fourth method, embryo reduction. A policy to transfer an excess of embryos with the intention of reducing a high-order multiple gestation is not acceptable from an ethical point of view, nor from a medical point of view, considering the risk of side-effects associated with high-order multiple gestation and with additional unnecessary invasive procedures. However, the reduction method has its place when a high-order multiple pregnancy has occurred despite all precautions.

ELECTIVE SINGLE-EMBRYO TRANSFER

An alternative to consistent single-embryo transfer would be an individualized embryo transfer policy, discussed by Coetsier and Dhont[6], who developed a theoretical model in which multiple pregnancies were predicted to be reduced from 28% to 15% and pregnancy rates from 30% to 26% if single-embryo transfer were applied in selected patients. A Finnish study[7] was the first to demonstrate satisfactory pregnancy rates (29.7%) after single-embryo transfers in selected groups of patients. In a follow-up study[8] of 127 elective single-embryo transfers, the results of subsequent cycles with frozen–thawed embryos were analyzed. Both single and double transfers were performed, resulting in a cumulative delivery rate per oocyte retrieval of 52.8% and a twin rate of 7.6%. The decision of single-embryo transfer in these studies was based on medical reasons (diabetes mellitus, risk of ovarian hyperstimulation syndrome, uterine malformation, etc.), on the wish to avoid multiple pregnancy or on the desire of the patient to receive only one embryo. The first randomized study[9] in this area focused on embryo quality and demonstrated a significantly higher twin rate if both embryos transferred, as opposed to one of two, were of top quality (57% vs. 21%).

Several reports had identified prognostic factors for pregnancy and multiple pregnancy and their influence when the number of embryos transferred was reduced from three to two, but there was a lack of knowledge about whether these were applicable also in the discussion of single-embryo transfer. We analyzed a large dataset from our IVF center at the Sahlgrenska University Hospital where two-embryo transfer had been a routine for the entire study period, with the intention of describing risk factors for multiple pregnancy and birth.

SWEDISH PREDICTION MODEL FOR ELECTIVE SINGLE-EMBRYO TRANSFER

We performed a retrospective study[10] covering 1995 to 1997 and including 1441 women undergoing 2107 IVF cycles in which two embryos were transferred. Factors with a possible correlation with pregnancy, multiple pregnancy, birth and multiple birth were studied in a multivariate analysis. The factors included background data (female age, previous pregnancies and births, previous IVF cycles, indication for IVF) and IVF cycle characteristics such as need for follicle stimulating hormone (FSH), number of retrieved and fertilized oocytes, fertilization method, day of transfer and number of good-quality embryos available for selection, number transferred and number suitable for freezing.

A primary logistic regression analysis with adjustment for previous cycles identified several factors correlating with pregnancy outcome, as presented in Table 1. Factors of significance were included in a secondary multivariate regression analysis identifying independent predictors (Table 2). In the final model, the following factors were independently predictive of multiple birth after accounting for the contribution of women with more than one cycle. Female age expressed a negative correlation, while number of good-quality embryos transferred (one vs. two) was positively correlated. The same factors (female age and absence of good-quality embryos transferred) and number of previous cycles (> 2) were independently negatively predictive of birth. All three FSH variables were positively correlated with age and the total dose of FSH showed the highest predictive capacity. Total dose of FSH was considered as an impractical clinical variable to work with and was thus omitted from the final model, which resulted in female age being included instead. One may conclude from the model in which FSH dosage was included that low ovarian reserve, expressed as high total dose of FSH, is independently correlated with a decreased risk of both live birth and multiple birth (data not shown). Possibly, poor responders to gonadotropins, regardless of age, would thus not be candidates for single-embryo transfer, although the number and quality of embryos have to be considered.

Birth is the most important outcome variable, but pregnancy is often reported instead. The dataset was also analyzed regarding predictors of pregnancy and multiple pregnancy, where pregnancy was defined as a viable pregnancy with heartbeat detected by transvaginal ultrasound. Similar results were obtained for predictors of pregnancy and multiple pregnancy as for birth and multiple birth (Table 1). Female age, FSH dose, numbers of good-quality embryos available, transferred and suitable for freezing were predictive of both pregnancy and multiple pregnancy when adjustment for rank of cycle was included. In addition, the number of oocytes retrieved and fertilized was positively predictive of pregnancy, whereas a tubal indication for IVF was negatively predictive of multiple pregnancy. In the multivariate analysis after adjustment for all other variables and after recalculation of variance, considering that several cycles per women were included, only rank of cycle > 2 and absence of good-quality embryos at transfer were negatively predictive of pregnancy, while female age and tubal infertility were both independently negatively predictive of multiple pregnancy. These results are further presented in Table 2 as odds ratios and 95% confidence intervals for each level of the variables that were independently predictive of birth, multiple birth, pregnancy and multiple pregnancy.

Obviously, to a large extent, the same factors are predictive of both pregnancy and multiple pregnancy as of birth and multiple birth. Inevitably, the reduction of multiple pregnancies by the introduction of single-embryo transfer will also reduce the chance of pregnancy. However, by using the presented data in a theoretical model, setting the aim for reduction of multiple births together with an acceptable reduction in birth rates, a population at risk for multiple birth may be defined.

We aimed at reducing the rate of multiple births by half from 26% to 13% by applying single-embryo transfer to a high-risk population defined by age, cycle number and the number of good-quality embryos available. Good-quality embryos were defined by the number of blastomeres (3–4 on day 2, or 6–8 on day 3) and degree of fragmentation ($< 20\%$). According to the theoretical calculation, the total birth rate will decrease from 29% to 25% but may be completely restored by performing one additional transfer of a single frozen/thawed embryo in high-risk patients who do not achieve a term pregnancy. This hypothesis is currently being tested in a Scandinavian multicenter randomized study, in which the enrollment has recently been completed and the results are awaited. This theoretical model is graphically illustrated in Figure 1, which expresses the calculated birth rates at different ages if one or two embryos of good quality are transferred to the defined population at high risk for multiple birth, considering rank of cycle and presence of tubal infertility.

Instead of defining the desired reduction in multiple birth rate and subsequently calculating age limits, the data can also be used to explore at what levels the impact of female age becomes more important. Three different methods were used:

Table 1 Factors analyzed for possible correlation with birth, multiple birth, pregnancy and multiple pregnancy, adjusted for number of previous *in vitro* fertilization (IVF) cycles

	Birth		Multiple birth		Pregnancy		Multiple pregnancy	
Variable	Odds ratio	p Value	Odds ratio	p Value	Odds ratio	p Value	Odds ratio	p Value
Background factors								
Female age (per year)	0.96 (0.93, 0.99)	0.02*	0.90 (0.85, 0.95)	0.0002*	0.97 (0.94, 0.99)	0.03*	0.92 (0.88, 0.96)	0.0007*
Previous pregnancy	0.84	0.8	1.3	0.3	0.97	0.9	1.2	0.5
Previous childbirth	1.2	0.5	1.1	0.8	1.2	0.6	1.1	0.9
IVF indication								
Tubal infertility	0.76 (0.59, 0.99)	0.04*	0.63 (0.38, 1.02)	0.06	0.78 (0.60, 1.0)	0.06	0.59 (0.37, 0.95)	0.03*
Endometriosis	1.1	0.7	0.9	0.8	1.0	0.9	1.1	0.7
Male factor	1.1	0.5	1.3	0.2	1.1	0.5	1.3	0.2
Unexplained	1.2	0.3	1.0	0.9	1.2	0.4	1.0	0.9
Hormonal	1.5	0.3	1.1	0.9	1.4	0.4	1.3	0.7
IVF performance								
FSH initial daily dose (per ampule, 75 IU)	0.71 (0.61, 0.82)	0.00001*	0.62 (0.50, 0.79)	0.0001*	0.995 (0.993, 0.997)	0.0000*	0.994 (0.990, 0.997)	0.0004*
Duration of ovarian stimulation (per day)	0.97 (0.92, 1.0)	0.14	0.98	0.6	0.96 (0.91, 0.99)	0.047*	0.97	0.4
FSH total dose (per ampule, 75 IU)	0.98 (0.97, 0.99)	0.00001*	0.97 (0.95, 0.98)	0.0002*	0.9996 (0.9995, 0.9998)	0.0000*	0.9996 (0.9993, 0.9998)	0.0004*
Number of retrieved oocytes	1.02 (1.0, 1.04)	0.1	1.0	0.9	1.02 (1.001, 1.04)	0.03*	1.0	0.6
Fertilization method	1.0	1.0	1.2	0.2	0.97	0.7	1.2	0.4
Number of fertilized oocytes	1.02 (1.0, 1.05)	0.09	1.0	0.3	1.03 (1.01, 1.06)	0.02*	1.03	0.1

continued

Table 1 Continued

Variable	Birth		Multiple birth		Pregnancy		Multiple pregnancy	
	Odds ratio	p Value	Odds ratio	p Value	Odds ratio	p Value	Odds ratio	p Value
Proportion of fertilized oocytes	1.16	0.6	1.78	0.2	1.3	0.3	2.02	0.1
Day of transfer (day 2 vs. 3)	0.8	0.1	0.7	0.2	0.77 (0.58, 1.01)	0.05	0.68	0.1
Number of good-quality embryos available	1.04 (1.00, 1.08)	0.03*	1.05	0.08	1.05 (1.01, 1.08)	0.01*	1.07 (1.01, 1.13)	0.02*
Number of good-quality embryos transferred	1.49 (1.18, 2.0)	0.005*	2.18 (1.3, 3.8)	0.006*	1.61 (1.21, 2.15)	0.001*	2.28 (1.98, 4.36)	0.01*
Number of embryos suitable for freezing	1.04 (1.01, 1.08)	0.03*	1.05 (0.99, 1.10)	0.08	1.05 (1.01, 1.09)	0.01*	1.07 (1.01, 1.13)	0.02*

95% confidence interval (CI) is shown in parentheses when the corresponding p value is < 0.1; * $p < 0.05$
95% CI and p values have been adjusted, accounting for the individuals undergoing more than one cycle
FSH, follicle stimulating hormone

Table 2 Variables independently predictive of birth, multiple birth, pregnancy and multiple pregnancy, adjusted for all other variables

Variable	Birth		Multiple birth		Pregnancy		Multiple pregnancy	
	Odds ratio	p Value	Odds ratio	p Value	Odds ratio	p Value	Odds ratio	p Value
Background factors								
Female age (per additional year)	0.97 (0.94, 0.999)	0.02*	0.91 (0.86, 0.96)	0.0005*	0.97 (0.94, 1.00)	0.06	0.93 (0.88, 0.97)	0.003*
Tubal infertility (vs. non-tubal)	0.78 (0.59, 1.01)	0.063	0.68 (0.42, 1.12)	0.13	0.78 (0.60, 1.02)	0.07	0.60 (0.37, 0.98)	0.04*
Previous IVF cycles (vs. none)								
1–2	0.90 (0.71, 1.14)	0.40	0.89 (0.59, 1.35)	0.59	0.88 (0.70, 1.1)	0.28	0.98 (0.67, 1.44)	0.91
>2	0.47 (0.24, 0.90)	0.02*	0.72 (0.23, 2.22)	0.56	0.46 (0.24, 0.87)	0.02*	0.61 (0.20, 1.89)	0.39
IVF performance								
Day of transfer (vs. 2)								
Day 3					0.77 (0.59, 1.02)	0.07		
No. of good-quality embryos available (vs.2)								
3–4							1.31 (0.75, 2.30)	0.34
>4							1.52 (0.98, 2.36)	0.06
No. of good-quality embryos transferred (vs. 2)								
1	0.78 (0.53, 1.16)	0.22	0.38 (0.15, 0.97)	0.04*	0.71 (0.48, 1.06)	0.09	0.46 (0.19, 1.38)	0.09
None	0.32 (0.14, 0.75)	0.008*	0.31 (0.06, 1.75)	0.19	0.30 (0.13, 0.70)	0.005*	0.32 (0.06, 1.80)	0.20

95% confidence interval (CI) is shown in parenthese when the corresponding *p* value is < 0.1; * *p* < 0.05
IVF, *in vitro* fertilization

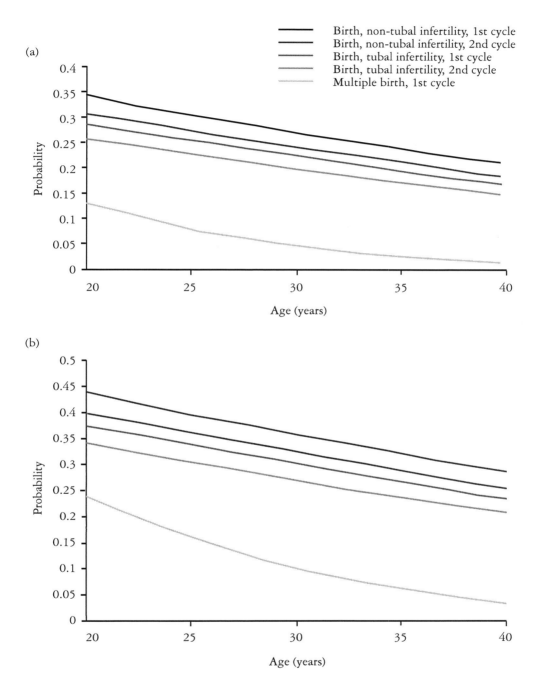

Figure 1   Probability of birth and multiple birth in relation to female age, number of previous transfer cycles and presence of tubal infertility if one (a) or two (b) good-quality embryos are transferred to a specified group of patients with high risk for multiple birth. The probability estimations refer to the total population including patients without high risk for multiple births, receiving two embryos

(1) Compare slope coefficients in the logistic regression equation between different age groups;

(2) Analyze the effect on birth and multiple birth when moving between two adjacent age groups;

(3) Compare age intervals with a young standard.

The first method revealed that the chance of a birth declined steeper at female age ≥ 36 years, whereas the concurrent risk of a multiple birth declined steeper 1 year earlier (≥ 35 years). The comparison of adjacent age interval of 2 or 4 years did not show any statistically significant difference when the outcome was birth, but for multiple birth any comparison to the next group of higher age resulted in a significantly decreased risk of multiple birth. If the young standard in the third method was set to < 33 years, the chance of birth decreased significantly in patients ≥ 37 years. Using the same standard, the risk reduction for multiple birth was 50% in women of 35–36 years, and 70% in patients of ≥ 37 years.

To summarize the Swedish data, patients at high risk for multiple birth were women under 35 years of age with at least two good-quality embryos available for transfer. Since the obvious decline in birth rate occurred 1 year later, 36 years can be recommended as an age limit for single-embryo transfer. Only first and second transfer cycles were suitable for single-embryo transfer, since the chance of a birth declined in the third cycle. Patients with tubal factor infertility had a reduced risk of multiple pregnancy.

EUROPEAN PREDICTION MODELS

A second retrospective analysis of predictors of birth and multiple birth, from a large dataset of 7700 cycles in 4417 patients, was published from the UK in 2001[11], confirming the results of the Swedish study. Younger age (< 35 years), diagnosis other than tubal infertility, fewer than three previous unsuccessful cycles, previous IVF live birth and a large number of embryos created were identified as risk factors for an increased chance of birth and multiple birth (Table 3). It was clearly shown that,

given these factors, increasing the number of embryos transferred (ranging from 2 to ≥ 4) did not increase the chance of a birth, but only the chance of a multiple birth. The study supported our own finding that tubal infertility can be regarded as indicating a poor prognosis compared with other indications.

A third prediction model for selecting patients for elective single-embryo transfer was presented in 2002[12]. The study included 642 patients and their first IVF cycle in which no more than two embryos were transferred. The outcome was pregnancy and multiple pregnancy instead of birth and multiple birth. The primary univariate analysis identified several variables associated with pregnancy and multiple pregnancy, but only the embryo morphology score reached significant statistical independent power to predict pregnancy, but not multiple pregnancy, in the multivariate analysis (Table 3). Female age was not independently predictive of either pregnancy or multiple pregnancy and the explanation might be found in the smaller sample size, which gives a wider confidence interval and/or a strong association between age and morphology score. The association between female age and oocyte/embryo quality was clearly demonstrated in another study analyzing almost 7000 cycles using donor oocytes[13]. In donor cycles, higher maternal age did not decrease multiple birth risk, whereas in non-donor cycles, a significantly decreased chance of both live birth delivery and multiple live birth was evident.

Embryo quality is certainly one of the most important variables, and prediction models for selecting the single best embryo have been developed. This issue is further explored in Chapter 6. A summary of the three prediction studies on patient selection is displayed in Table 3. Note that no embryo quality measure was included in the study by Engmann and co-workers[11], and that cycles with replacement of ≥ 4 embryos were included, as opposed to the two other studies with a maximum of two embryos[12] or two embryos in all cycles[10].

IS THERE A NEED FOR RANDOMIZED STUDIES?

During the past decade there has been an intense debate on the issue of how many embryos to transfer, trading off the risk of high-order multiple birth against the reduced chance of pregnancy. Reducing the recommended number of embryos from three to two was preceded by several prediction studies showing that, given certain conditions of embryo quality and female age, the transfer of two embryos as opposed to three did not decrease the chance of pregnancy but only the risk of multiple birth. No randomized controlled trials were needed and two-embryo transfers were gradually introduced as a routine in many countries. Now, when the discussion concerns the move from two to one embryo, the arguments are very similar. Is there a need for randomized studies to show that pregnancy rates will not be too impaired, or will the accumulating data from cohort studies suffice? Is the fear of losing in terms of pregnancy rate greater when moving towards single-embryo transfer so that the professional community is more difficult to convince? If the answer is 'yes' to these questions, randomized studies are certainly warranted, since they are less likely to be biased than cohort studies.

There are few randomized studies on the topic of single-embryo transfer. The largest randomized study published to date included 144 patients undergoing their first or second cycle, resulting in at least four available embryos of good quality[14]. Pregnancy rates were 32% and 47% (NS) in the two groups who received one or two embryos, respectively. The twin rate in the double-embryo group was 39% but twinning was not completely avoided in the single-embryo group, owing to one monozygotic pair of twins. The results supported the option of changing embryo transfer policy towards single-embryo transfer without any remarkable decrease in success rate.

A smaller randomized trial from Belgium looking at embryo quality analyzed pregnancy outcome in women under 34 years of age, undergoing their first IVF cycle, randomized to receive one or two embryos if at least two top-quality embryos were available[15]. Among 26 patients who received one embryo, the implantation rate was 42.3% and the ongoing pregnancy rate was 38.5%. In 27 patients who received two embryos, the corresponding results were 48.1% and 74%. It was concluded that, by applying strict embryo criteria and single-embryo transfer, an ongoing pregnancy rate similar to that in normal fertile couples could be achieved, whereas the rate of twin pregnancy was diminished.

The same center in Belgium has published the largest dataset of almost 400 single-embryo transfer cycles in a retrospective cohort study[16]. The pregnancy rates in single or double transfers were similar (32.6% vs. 36.2%). The inclusion of patients comprised not only patients with a good prognosis but also those older than 38 years and without top-quality embryos. A prospective cohort study from the same center, including patients aged < 38 years in their first IVF cycle yielding at least one top-quality embryo[17], demonstrated an ongoing pregnancy rate of 40% even if a top-quality embryo was not available.

A summary of retrospective and prospective studies is presented in Table 4. The results from hitherto published studies seem to be reassuring with respect to the maintenance of the pregnancy rate after single-embryo transfer, although the impact of bias from patient selection is obvious. Some may regard the published data to be sufficient to change transfer policy, whereas others do not. The largest study, which has not yet been published, will hopefully supply us with a sufficient amount of data for future policy decisions. The study is a Scandinavian multicenter randomized controlled trial, designed on the basis of the results of the retrospective cohort study[10] and aimed at demonstrating a reduction by 50% of the multiple birth rate while maintaining the same birth rate, if single-embryo transfer is performed in a selected group of patients. Patients who are randomized to single-embryo transfer, but do not conceive in the fresh cycle, receive one frozen–thawed embryo at a second transfer. Thus, the result after receiving two embryos on one occasion is compared with the result after receiving one embryo on two different occasions. The recruitment of 660 patients will give sufficient statistical power to the study, aiming at demonstrating that there is no difference in birth rates between the groups. The enrollment of patients has recently been completed and the results will be available in the near future. As this is the largest randomized study on this topic, the results are likely to have a great impact on transfer policies, from the point of view of both the physicians and the health authorities.

Table 3 Summary of three studies using logistic regression to identify independently predictive factors of birth and multiple birth (or pregnancy and multiple pregnancy)

	Strandell et al. (2000)[10]	Engman et al. (2001)[11]	Hunault et al. 2002[12]
Years	1995–97	1984–97	1993–98
Cycles/women	2107/1441	7700/4417	642/642
No. of embryos transferred	2	1 to ≥ 4	1–2
Pregnancy rate %	38	25	26
Multiple pregnancy rate (%)	28	—	35
Birth rate (%)	29	16	—
Multiple birth rate (%)	26	28	—
Outcome	birth/multiple birth	birth/multiple birth	pregnancy/multiple pregnancy

Univariate analysis of positive and negative predictors of **birth** (pregnancy in the Hunault study)

+ no. of good-quality embryos available		+ total no. of spermatozoa cells
+ quality of embryos transferred		+ no. of retrieved oocytes
+ no. of embryos suitable for freezing		+ no. of embryos suitable for transfer
− female age		+ stage of development of 1st and 2nd best embryo
− tubal infertility		+ morphology score of 1st and 2nd best embryo
− > 2 previous unsuccessful IVF cycles		− female age
− FSH dose		

Univariate analysis of positive and negative predictors of **multiple birth** (pregnancy in the Hunault study)

+ quality of embryos transferred		+ no. of embryos suitable for transfer
− female age		+ stage of development of 1st and 2nd best embryo
− FSH dose		+ morphology score of 1st and 2nd best embryo
		− female age

continued

Table 3 *continued*

	Strandell et al. (2000)[10]	Engman et al. (2001)[11]	Hunault et al. 2002[12]
Multivariate analysis of positive and negative predictors of **birth** (pregnancy in the Hunault study)	+ quality of embryos transferred − female age − > 2 previous unsuccessful IVF cycles	+ previous IVF live birth + large number of embryos created − female age ≥ 35 years − tubal infertility − >2 previous unsuccessful IVF cycles	+ morphology score of the best embryo
Multivariate analysis of positive and negative predictors of **multiple birth** (pregnancy in the Hunault study)	+ quality of embryos transferred − female age	+ previous IVF live birth − female age ≥ 40 years − > 3 previous unsuccessful IVF cycles	no significant predictors

IVF, *in vitro* fertilization; FSH, follicle stimulating hormone

Table 4   Summary of studies comparing elective single-embryo transfer (SET) with double-embryo transfer (DET) in fresh cycles

Authors	Type of study	Inclusion criteria	Cycles (n)		Pregnancy rate (%)		Twin rate (%)	
			SET	DET	SET	DET	SET	DET
Vilska et al. (1999)[7]	retrospective cohort	subject's wish; risk of OHSS; medical reasons	74	742	29.7	29.4	0	23.9
Gerris et al. (1999)[15]	randomized controlled trial	first cycle; < 34 years; 2 top-quality embryos	26	27	53.8	77.8	7.1	28.6
Tiitinen et al. (2001)[8]	retrospective cohort	subject's wish; medical reasons	127	517	38.6	40.0	2.9*	26.2
Martikainen et al. (2001)[14]	randomized controlled trial	< 36 years; ≥ 4 good-quality embryos	74	76	32.4	47.1	4.2*	33.3
De Neubourg et al. (2002)[17]	prospective cohort	first cycle; < 38 years	127	116	42.5	40.5	0	23.4
Gerris et al. (2002)[16]	retrospective cohort	patient's wish; inclusion in other studies	385	852	32.2	36.2	0.8*	35.3[†]

OHSS, ovarian hyperstimulation syndrome; * one monozygotic twin in each of the studies; [†] including three sets of triplets

CONCLUSION

Generally in IVF treatments, the number of embryos transferred has decreased, but even in countries with two-embryo transfer as a routine, multiple birth and its associated problems still constitute an important impact on medical, economic and social needs. Several countries have taken steps towards single-embryo transfer, but there is also a suspicion that too radical a policy might impair pregnancy rates unacceptably. Important factors when selecting patients for single-embryo transfer are:

(1) Female age (< 35–37 years);

(2) IVF cycle number (1st or 2nd);

(3) Number of good-quality embryos available (≥ 2);

(4) Absence of severe tubal disease.

Since patient populations differ between countries and even centers, it is recommended that each center explore its own data to retrieve accurate limits for the above-mentioned risk factors, resulting in recommendations for that specific population. Introducing 'deliveries of singletons at term' or 'birth per embryo transferred' as outcome measures should give a more appropriate definition of IVF success than merely recording pregnancy and birth rates, and may constitute an incentive to make efforts to reduce the rate of multiple births.

REFERENCES

1. Bergh T, Ericson A, Hillensjö T, Nygren K, Wennerholm U. Deliveries and children born after *in-vitro* fertilisation in Sweden 1982–95 – a retrospective cohort study. *Lancet* 1999;354:1579–85

2. Olivennes F. Double trouble: yes a twin pregnancy is an adverse outcome. *Hum Reprod* 2000;15:1663–5

3. Templeton A, Morris JK. Reducing the risk of multiple birth by transfer of two embryos after *in vitro* fertilization. *N Engl J Med* 1998;339:573–7

4. Coskun S, Hollanders J, Al-Hassan S, Al-Sufyan H, Al-Mayman H, Jaroudi K. Day 5 versus day 3 embryo transfer: a controlled randomized trial. *Hum Reprod* 2000;15:1947–52

5. Karaki RZ, Samarraie SS, Younis NA, Lahloub TM, Ibrahim MH. Blastocyst culture and transfer: a step toward improved *in vitro* fertilization outcome. *Fertil Steril* 2002;77:114–18

6. Coetsier T, Dhont M. Avoiding multiple pregnancies in *in-vitro* fertilization: who's afraid of single embryo transfer? *Hum Reprod* 1998;13:2663–4

7. Vilska S, Tiitinen A, Hydén-Granskog C. Elective transfer of one embryo results in an acceptable pregnancy rate and eliminates the risk of multiple births. *Hum Reprod* 1999;14:2392–5

8. Tiitinen A, Halttunen M, Härkki P, Vuoristo P, Hydén-Granskog C. Elective single embryo transfer: the value of cryopreservation. *Hum Reprod* 2001;16:1140–4

9. Van Royen E, Mangelschots K, De Neubourg D, *et al.* Characterization of a top quality embryo, a step towards single-embryo transfer. *Hum Reprod* 1999;14:2345–9

10. Strandell A, Bergh B, Lundin K. Selection of patients suitable for one-embryo transfer may reduce the rate of multiple births by half without impairment of overall birth rates. *Hum Reprod* 2000;15:2520–5

11. Engmann L, Maconochie N, Tan SL, Bekir J. Trends in the incidence of births and multiple births and the factors that determine the probability of multiple birth after IVF treatment. *Hum Reprod* 2001;16:2598–605

12. Hunault CC, Eijkemans MJ, Pieters MH, *et al.* A prediction model for selecting patients undergoing *in vitro* fertilization for elective single embryo transfer. *Fertil Steril* 2002;77:725–32

13. Reynolds MA, Schieve LA, Jeng G, Peterson HB, Wilcox LS. Risk of multiple birth associated with *in vitro* fertilization using donor eggs. *Am J Epidemiol* 2001;154:1043–50

14. Martikainen H, Tiitinen A, Tomás C, *et al.* One versus two embryo transfer after IVF and ICSI: a randomized study. *Hum Reprod* 2001; 16:1900–3

15. Gerris J, De Neubourg D, Mangelschots K, Van Royen E, Van de Meerssche M, Valkenburg M. Prevention of twin pregnancy after *in-vitro* fertilization or intracytoplasmic sperm injection based on strict embryo criteria: a prospective randomized clinical trial. *Hum Reprod* 1999;14:2581–7

16. Gerris J, De Neubourg D, Mangelschots K, *et al.* Elective single day 3 embryo transfer halves the twinning rate without decrease in the ongoing pregnancy rate of an IVF/ICSI programme. *Hum Reprod* 2002;17:2626–31

17. De Neubourg DD, Mangelschots K, Van Royen E, *et al.* Impact of patients' choice for single embryo transfer of a top quality embryo versus double embryo transfer in the first IVF/ICSI cycle. *Hum Reprod* 2002;17:2621–5

6

Embryo selection for elective single-embryo transfer

E. Van Royen

INTRODUCTION

To make single-embryo transfer an acceptable treatment, the advantages should outweigh the disadvantages. The arguments in favor are obvious: no multiple pregnancies and consequently fewer complications for mother and child(ren). This means less mortality, less morbidity and fewer disabled children. Arguments against single-embryo transfer seem very strong, however. If we compare the few papers that have been published on the implementation of single-embryo transfer with the overwhelming majority of papers in which two, three or more embryos are transferred, we must conclude that only a few centers are convinced of the feasibility of single-embryo transfer. The arguments against single-embryo transfer are mainly economic. The only way to refute these arguments is to optimize single-embryo transfer to such an extent that it becomes at least a competitive and eventually the most cost-effective treatment. This chapter focuses on optimization of the laboratory procedures and of the transfer procedure as prerequisites for single-embryo transfer in an assisted reproduction technologies (ART) program with a stable high implantation rate. Reduction of the number of embryos transferred is required to establish a one-to-one link between embryo and outcome. In these conditions an evidence-based selection system can be developed that relies exclusively on embryos with a documented outcome.

The goal of embryo selection should not only be to select the 'putative high-competence' embryo. Often, there will be no putative high-competence embryo available within the cohort of embryos resulting from a stimulation cycle. The goal should be more ambitious. It is to make an evidence-based estimate of the implantation potential of different types of embryos – not just the best – and to provide a qualitative and a quantitative ranking. This will not only allow the selection of the putative high-competence embryo (when present), but will also offer a solid basis to outweigh the risk and benefit of transferring two embryos of moderate or low quality.

Embryo quality is an intrinsic property of the embryo. It can be preserved as much as possible but it cannot be improved by extended culture. This intrinsic quality that enables some embryos to develop into blastocysts was already present at the zygote stage. The aim of any selection strategy for a high-quality embryo is to detect it as soon as possible. Embryo culture beyond the pronuclear stage has no other purpose than embryo selection. During culture, in order to fully express its intrinsic quality, each embryo should be subjected to only optimal laboratory procedures.

EMBRYO QUALITY MARKERS AND EMBRYO SELECTION IN THE LITERATURE

Many different quality-related parameters have been described in the literature and some of these have been proven to allow a statistically significant discrimination between embryos with a high and with a low implantation rate. We attempt to discuss them in the sequence in which they appear during embryo development.

Quality markers of the gametes

Embryo quality starts with the quality of the gametes. For evaluating oocyte quality several quality-related factors have been proposed: cumulus–coronal morphology, oocyte morphology (darkness or excessive granularity of the cytoplasm, the presence of vacuoles or other cytoplasmic inclusions, the perivitelline space, smooth endoplasmic reticulum clustering and refractile bodies) and first polar body morphology. Each of these factors has been shown to have an impact on implantation[1–5]. ATP content of oocytes and the dissolved oxygen content of follicular fluid have been suggested as epigenetic influences on oocyte development[6–8]. Poor sperm morphology is a major obstacle for fertilization in *in vitro* fertilization (IVF). Intracytoplasmic sperm injection (ICSI) seems to bypass this obstacle completely. Sperm morphology was thought to have no further impact on fertilization, embryo development and implantation. However, it was recently demonstrated that sperm quality has an impact on the development of the early cleaving embryo[9]. Moreover, poor sperm morphology has been associated with an increased spontaneous abortion rate[10,11]. Recently it was demonstrated that progressive motility and sperm morphology were significantly correlated with diminished blastocyst development and quality[12].

Quality markers of zygotes

Polarity

The concept of oocyte polarity and cell determination in the early embryo was elegantly developed by Edwards and Beard[13]. They offered some features that were tested for their relationship with embryo quality; only the orientation of the pronuclei relative to the polar bodies proved to be related to embryo quality[14]. However, the identification and assessment of pronuclear structures requires some awkward micromanipulation for positioning and measurement of angles.

Nucleolar precursor bodies

Observation of pronuclei and nuclear precursor bodies requires rotation of embryos to observe both pronuclei side by side in the same focal plane.

Because nucleolar precursor bodies move about, different scores may be attributed to the same embryo when observed at different moments.

The halo effect

The 'halo effect', i.e. the appearance of a cytoplasmic halo, has been related to embryo morphology. Embryos derived from halo-positive zygotes had significantly better morphology (60.9%) than embryos derived from halo-negative zygotes (52.2%) ($p < 0.05$), but in terms of pregnancy rates no difference was found[15]. Others found that cycles with halo-positive oocytes showed a significantly higher pregnancy rate (44.0% vs. 31.1%; $p < 0.05$)[16].

Zygote score

Using time-lapse video cinematography, a definite course of events after normal fertilization leading to particular morphological phenomena was observed: organelles contracting from the cortex towards the center of the oocyte (causing the halo effect) and a significant decrease in diameter (by 6 μm) of the oocytes[17]. These authors also demonstrated that the female pronucleus was smaller in diameter than the male pronucleus and that it contained on average fewer nucleoli (4.2 and 7.0, respectively). These findings paved the way for studies using a single static observation of zygotes. A scoring system was designed and refined based on the size and relative positioning of pronuclei, the distribution and alignment of nucleoli, the appearance of a halo in the cytoplasm and the time of first cleavage[18,19]. A significant predictive power was demonstrated of this scoring system with respect to implantation and pregnancy rates. Distinct patterns of pronuclear organization were proposed and later related to embryos with an increased implantation potential[20,21]. Only cycles in which all embryos transferred were characterized as good-quality embryos (by fragmentation, size and number of blastomeres and appearance of the cytoplasm) were included in this study, and zygote parameters were not used as the criterion for embryo selection. Transfers of embryos that developed exclusively from oocytes showing this optimal pronuclear pattern gave significantly higher pregnancy and implantation rates compared with transfers where no such embryos were involved. These findings were later confirmed, although the authors failed to demonstrate that a higher proportion of these oocytes with the optimal pronuclear pattern developed into good-morphology embryos on day 2[22].

The German embryo protection law does not allow culture beyond the pronuclear stage of more embryos than are to be transferred. Supernumerary zygotes have to be frozen. The importance of a pronuclear scoring system under these conditions is obvious. These are the ideal circumstances for a prospective randomized study on the impact of zygote scoring on embryo selection. A German prospective multicenter study revealed that both pattern 0B and pattern 3, as proposed by Tesarik and Greco[20], yielded significantly higher pregnancy and implantation rates of 37.9% and 20.5%, respectively, for pattern 0B and 36.4% and 23.4%, respectively, for pattern 3 zygotes. Pattern 0B and pattern 3 are both patterns with a symmetrical and polarized distribution of nucleolar precursor bodies[20,23]. The scoring system described by Scott and Smith was also used for prospective evaluation and selection of the three best pronuclear-stage zygotes[18,24]. These zygotes were kept in culture for another 24 h before transfer. The clinical pregnancy rate (when transferring a mean of 2.9 embryos per transfer) was 15%. No implantation rates were provided. Despite the very low number (11 pregnancies) reported, these authors also found a relation between the mean pronuclear score and the percentage of pregnancies, a lower score leading to a lower pregnancy rate.

The predictive value of pronuclear morphology of zygotes has also been evaluated by means of a series of exclusively single-embryo transfers[25]. This approach allows a one-to-one link between score and outcome. Results indicated no significant impact of embryo quality on implantation or pregnancy rates using zygote patterns as proposed by Tesarik and Greco[20].

In conclusion, several authors have demonstrated a relationship between pronuclear characteristics and embryo quality. In the situation where the decision on which embryos to cultivate further has to be made at the zygote stage it has been proved to be advantageous to use zygote scoring. If the selection can be delayed to day 2 or 3 after fertilization the benefit is less obvious, because other selection parameters are available at that time. Most of the studies involved use double- or triple-embryo transfers and this makes it difficult to establish clear relationships. The only series of single-embryo transfers offering an indisputable link between pronuclear embryo characteristics and outcome, from a Finnish group, failed to demonstrate any impact on implantation rates[25]. A comparison between the maximum implantation rates obtained by different authors using different selection methods is shown. Methods including zygote scoring achieve no higher maximum implantation rates than methods without. We think there may be some pronuclear parameters that might contribute to embryo selection, but they need better specification and verification by unequivocal studies.

Quality markers of cleavage-stage embryos

Quality features at the cleaving embryo stage that have been used are:

(1)   Number of blastomeres;

(2)   Fragmentation;

(3)   Multinucleation;

(4)   Relative size of blastomeres;

(5)   Early cleavage.

Prolonging culture to the cleavage stage allows for a number of parameters related to embryo quality to be studied and used. The degree of fragmentation and the number of blastomeres have been used for many years by most centers to select embryos to transfer. Different individual or cumulative embryo scores have been designed, relying on observations of transfers with embryos of mixed quality[26–30]. Two papers have described a direct link between score, observed quality criteria and outcome: one paper considering exclusively transfers of embryos showing homogeneous quality characteristics and the other making a retrospective analysis of exclusively compulsory single-embryo transfers[31,32]. Multinucleation is also an important quality-related criterion[33]. This observation was confirmed by others[34–36]. Multinucleation proved to be useful in combination with fragmentation and cleavage rate for embryo scoring[37]. By means of single- as well as double-embryo transfers with exclusively multinucleated embryos, we have recently demonstrated that these embryos have a significantly decreased implantation rate (4.3% and 5.7%, respectively)[38]. Embryos with unevenly sized blastomeres were reported to have lower pregnancy and implantation rates, and the same paper showed some evidence that this phenomenon was often associated with multinucleation[39]. Early cleavage was found to be strongly correlated with increased implantation, and recently this was unequivocally confirmed in a study using exclusively single-embryo transfers[40,41].

An approach including several morphological criteria was recently reported, but resulted in a maximum implantation rate of only 18%[42]. It must indeed be difficult to make a link between embryo quality and outcome while transferring a mean of 3.4 embryos per transfer.

The ultimate test for embryo selection is single-embryo transfer. In the first paper on the subject, a 29.7% pregnancy rate was achieved after elective single-embryo transfer of either day-2 or day-3 cleavage embryos[43]. In a subsequent study the same group obtained a clinical pregnancy rate of 32.4% after single-embryo transfer and demonstrated the beneficial effect of cryopreservation[44]. Our group has reported high ongoing implantation rates of 49% in a retrospective analysis of double-embryo transfers in women younger than 38 years of age ($n = 37$) and of 38.5% in a prospective study of single-embryo transfers in women younger than 34 years of age[45]. Later, an ongoing pregnancy rate after single-embryo transfer of 43% was reached in a prospective study in women younger than 38 years of age[46]. Recently, an implantation rate of as high as 50% after single-embryo transfer for early cleaving embryos transferred on day 2 was reported by a Finnish group[41].

Quality markers of day-5 blastocysts

As early as 1994 it was demonstrated that extended culture to the blastocyst stage was possible[47]. The development of sequential culture media has largely contributed to the increasing interest in extended culture. At first, not much attention was paid to differences in blastocyst quality; the development to this stage seemed proof enough of quality. High implantation rates of 43% with exclusively expanded blastocysts and of 47% have been reported[48,49]. Recently it was shown that the introduction of quality-related parameters allowed char-

acterization of blastocysts with a superior implantation potential[50]. Blastocysts with the blastocele completely filling the embryo, with an expanded volume larger than the early cleaving embryo, hatching or completely hatched in combination with a tightly packed inner cell mass consisting of many cells and a trophectoderm also consisting of many cells forming a cohesive epithelium resulted in an 87% clinical pregnancy rate and a 70% implantation rate after homogenous double-embryo transfers. A survey of these different selection strategies is provided in Table 1.

PRACTICAL MODALITIES FOR EMBRYO SELECTION

The optimal day for transfer

In the literature two contrasting approaches have been described for selecting the best embryos. The first method tries, as soon as possible, to identify the optimal embryos by means of a selection strategy. The second proposes to culture the embryos for as long as possible to enable the embryos to select themselves[19,20,51]. Between these two opposite poles, several intermediate paths have been followed. Owing to religious or legal obligations, selection sometimes has to be made at the zygote stage. From a scientific point of view this situation is not optimal[23,24]. The longer the culture period the more selection parameters become available. Selection will improve only if proper use is made of the opportunities offered by these parameters. During culture, some embryos will have arrested growth while others will develop to blastocysts. These blastocysts have been claimed to possess superior implantation potential[49]. Until now only a few papers have compared day-3 transfers with blastocyst transfers in a population that had been prospectively randomized before stimulation and where comparable numbers of embryos were transferred in both groups. These papers have failed to demonstrate the superiority of blastocyst transfer[52–55]. Day-5 culture seems to provide no better outcome, and it has been associated in several reports with an increased monozygotic twinning rate[56–58]. Recently, Blake and colleagues, after a meta-analysis, concluded: 'Overall this review of the

Table 1 Embryo selection methods from the literature, stratified according to the day of selection. For each day methods are ranked according to the maximum implantation rate obtained

Reference	Selection	Pregnancy rate (%)	Embryos/ transfers	Implantation rate (%)
Wittemer et al., 2000[22]	day 3 + zygote	39.3	1.78	26
Scott et al., 2000[19]	day 3 + zygote	57	3.2	31
Rienzi et al., 2002[53]	day 3	56	2	35
Gerris et al., 1999[45]	day 3	42.3	1	42
De Neubourg et al., 2002[46]	day 3		1	43
Bungum et al., 2003[55]	day 3	61	2	44
Van Royen et al., 1999[37]	day 3	63	2	49
Huisman et al., 2000[63]	day 5	27.8	1.9	26
Rijnders and Jansen, 1998[64]	day 5	53	2.25	30
Coskun et al., 2000[52]	day 5	39	2	24
Bungum et al., 2003[55]	day 5	51	2	37
Rienzi et al., 2002[53]	day 5	58	2	38
Shapiro et al., 2000[48]	day 5	63	2.73	43
Milki et al., 2000[49]	day 5	68	2.4	47
Gardner et al., 2000[50]	day 5	87	2	70

best available evidence based on data from randomized controlled trials, suggests that to date little difference in the major outcome parameters has been demonstrated between early embryo transfer and blastocyst culture. Collectively, the increase in cancellation and the possible decrease in cryopreservation rates suggest that the routine practice of blastocyst culture should be offered to patients with caution. The subgroup of trials employing sequential media did however demonstrate a substantial improvement in implantation rates and similar pregnancy rates, despite the transfer of less embryos. Whether this trend will culminate in convincingly higher live birth rates per woman has yet to be validated'[59]. In their review, Kolibianakis and Devroey decided that, in the absence of convincing evidence of the superiority of extended culture, there was no reason to switch to a culture method that takes more time and is more expensive in terms of personnel, media and laboratory resources[60]. These arguments seemed sufficiently convincing for us to maintain our policy of transferring on day 3.

Selection methods

Selection should have no (negative) impact on the embryo quality. In order to make a selection we need selection methods that should preferably be non-invasive, to distinguish embryos with a low and a high implantation potential. Invasive methods should be considered only secondary, after optimal non-invasive selection, and if they have been proved to offer a substantial benefit. In the near future, methods based on the analysis of embryo metabolites might provide new selection options. Optical methods allow fast and low-cost assessment of several selection parameters and therefore they are most often used. Today they require far less effort than methods based on embryo metabolism and offer data without delay and without extra cost for additional chemical analysis. The required equipment is limited – an inverted microscope with suitable optics, an instrument that is available in most IVF laboratories.

Observations on oocytes and embryos

Oocytes and embryos should be individually traceable. This enables follow-up of early embryo development during culture. Later, it provides information on their individual outcome. Oocytes and embryos can be cultivated in groups in order to improve culture conditions, but for the sake of selection they should be individually traceable as soon as markers of different qualities can be attributed to them.

Timing

From the moment the oocytes have been inseminated or injected, the continuous process of embryo development starts. Because this is a dynamic process it is essential that observations be made systematically after the same time intervals from fertilization onwards. These observations should be made within narrow time intervals. This is a prerequisite if these observations are to be used to compare results from different IVF/ICSI procedures in comparative studies, and if reference values are to be established.

Optics

In order to see small structures such as nuclear precursor bodies it is essential to use high magnification. Modulation contrast is preferable to other contrasts, because it allows good visualization of nuclei in blastomeres. An inverted microscope with 400 × magnification and modulation contrast is adequate. In order to preserve its optical quality this microscope should receive regular maintenance. Consequences of different magnification factors and poor microscope maintenance have to be taken into account.

Selection criteria

Quality (or lack of it) needs to be expressed in the embryo by means of detectable quality-related parameters. This sets the limits on every optical selection strategy: genetic defects that have no visible impact on embryo development will not be detected. Selection parameters are quality-related parameters with a high power of discrimination between embryos with a high and a low implantation potential. Observations made at each developmental stage of the embryo can serve as selection criteria. As we have shown earlier, several parameters have been described in the literature. To make them useful tools in embryo selection they should be tested for their relevance at each developmental stage. The longer the culture lasts, the more selection criteria will become available. The problem is to learn which are meaningful at each stage of development and which will have lost their impact, because other more discriminative parameters have become available. Consequently, a decisive factor for the selection parameters to be used will be the developmental stage at the moment of selection and/or transfer.

Data management

Recording observations separately

It is important to keep observation of variables simple without combining them. As an example: it seems logical to keep records separately of length and weight of a person and not combine both into a body mass index (BMI). Although BMI is a useful tool for some purposes, it provides less information than length and weight separately. Two people with the same BMI may be very different in posture; this is why the police will never use BMI in a person's description. They always will use length and weight as separate characteristics. The same goes for embryos: combining the number of blastomeres and the degree of fragmentation into a single score does not provide the same information as the two individual variables. It will create a less precise image of the embryo and cause loss of information. Combining different parameters (such as fragmentation and cleavage pattern) into one score implies the introduction of a certain weighting to each of these parameters and this will be purely arbitrary. In other words: do both factors (fragmentation and number of blastomeres) have the same impact on embryo quality? This is obviously not so and can be clearly demonstrated. Higher fragmentation is associated with lower implantation, but maximum implantation on day 2 coincides with four blastomeres. Both lower and higher cleavage rates are associated with lower implantation rates.

The need for a computer database

Looking at nature we see that evolution has elected monofollicular ovulation and consequently singleton pregnancy as the optimum method of human procreation despite a rather poor success rate of 25% per cycle in the fertile population. In order to have monofollicular ovulation a subtle but highly efficient feedback mechanism is in operation regulating the hypothalamic–pituitary–gonadal axis.

If we want to move to single-embryo transfer we will have to implement a similar feedback mechanism in order to optimize laboratory results first, transfer policy later and finally doctor and patient information. Essential for this feedback are specific and meaningful messages and specific receptors. In order to create a meaningful message we have to gather information that is relevant. This information has to be stored, organized and analyzed and that is exactly what a computer database is meant for. If the information thus obtained proves to be reliable, doctors will gain confidence in it and eventually will become receptive to it. Once they are convinced of the feasibility of single-embryo transfer themselves, they will convince their patients. Thus the feedback system will have been established. We would strongly advocate the addition of a new topic in the next version of the guidelines of the European Society of Human Reproduction and Embryology (ESHRE) advising the use of such a database with a user-friendly system, because information retrieval and analysis are useful only if they are easily available without too much effort.

The results of this analysis would be useful for evaluating the performance of an ART program and would stimulate its optimization. It would allow detection of flaws in the system or below-standard performances and would help provide guidance for the improvement of the continuous training of the team. A database is also a highly efficient tool in ordinary quality control, e.g. for keeping track of batches of media and materials.

Some examples of where results of an IVF/ICSI database could be of use are:

(1) Fertilization rate per operator performing ICSI;

(2) Number of oocytes retrieved per operator performing oocyte pick-up;

(3) Implantation rate per provider of embryo transfer;

(4) Implantation rate per operator performing embryo selection;

(5) Fertilization rate according to the duration of stimulation;

(6) Outcome results according to stimulation protocol;

(7) Regular checks of fertilization and pregnancy rates.

All of this is possible without a database, but the effort required is so much greater that it will be realised only on exceptional occasions.

Ideally this database should be a relational database with at least three levels with a one-to-many relationship: the top level should contain the patient data, the second level the cycle data (stimulation, sperm parameters, culture data, materials used, transfer, outcome) and the bottom level the oocyte–embryo data (maturity, injection, fertilization, quality parameters, destination). This structure would allow analysis of data as they are required to set up a quality control and optimization system and that can provide the necessary feedback as described above.

Selection strategies

Should we be satisfied with the characterization of top-quality embryos or should we try to calculate and predict the implantation potential of different types of embryos? Selecting the best embryo is imperative if we want to move to single-embryo transfer. However, the best embryo in a treatment cycle sometimes may be of poorer quality than was hoped for. This implies that it is desirable to have a reliable estimate of the implantation potential of all embryos in order to adapt transfer policy. Thus, the chance of success (a singleton pregnancy) could be mathematically weighted against the risk of producing a multiple pregnancy if more than one embryo is to be transferred.

We have designed and applied two distinct selection strategies, which are both based on the same combination of different quality markers. As a comparison, in the detection of Down's syndrome, for which there is no single efficaciously predicting parameter, attempts have been made to improve the screening by means of a combination of several (three in the triple test) variables[61]. In ART we have sought the benefit of a similar approach by combining several quality parameters. In both our models, apart from the woman's age, we have used four such parameters: fragmentation, multinucleation and the number of blastomeres on day 2 and on day 3 after fertilization.

The aim of the first selection strategy was the characterization of a top-quality embryo[37]. It was developed to allow the selection of embryos with a high implantation potential and was useful in reducing the number of embryos transferred and in allowing the progressive introduction of single-embryo transfer. Although this selection method falls short in optimizing the selection between different top-quality embryos or between non-top-quality embryos, it offers a simple tool for optimizing the implantation rate of the program. The aim of the second method is the calculation of the implantation potential of individual embryos[62]. It offers a far more refined selection method because it allows the calculation of a quantitative measure for the ongoing implantation for each type of embryo, characterized by its number of blastomeres, its fragmentation and its absence of observed multinucleation on days 2 and 3. This means that a ranking of the ongoing implantation potential can be made for all types of embryos exclusively based on facts, not assumptions. This can be achieved by relying exclusively on transfers where all embryos evolved either into ongoing implantations or into no implantations at all. It is no coincidence that these two different selection strategies were designed in this order. The first needs only a limited number of transfers with 100% implantation, whereas the second requires a far greater number of observations in order to make it a useful tool. The first approach sets the conditions to start with elective single-embryo transfer and gradually to accumulate data from both single-embryo transfer and double-embryo transfer. When sufficient data are available a switch can be made to the second, more refined, selection method.

Characterization of top-quality embryos

The gold standard for the quality or competence of an embryo is its ongoing implantation potential. Retrospective analysis of the characteristics of embryos that had all implanted allowed us to establish reference values for the quality-related parameters of such a top-quality embryo. The procedure used is common for establishing reference values of any biochemical marker. Between 1 January 1996 and 19 May 1997, 23 double-embryo transfers resulted in 23 ongoing dizygotic twin pregnancies[37]. These 46 embryos with proven quality (because they all resulted in healthy babies) had been analyzed on both day-2 and day-3 quality-related parameters. All embryos showed 20% or less fragmentation on both day 2 and day 3 and none of them showed multinucleation either on day 2 or on day 3. Except for three embryos, all others showed four or five blastomeres on day 2 and at least seven on day 3. These observations have led to the characterization of a top-quality embryo as an embryo with a count of four or five blastomeres on days 2 and 7 or more on day 3, in which fragmentation does not exceed 20% and no multinucleation is present either on day 2 or on day 3.

Retrospective evaluation and validation of the implantation potential of top-quality embryos

Between 20 May 1997 and 31 July 1998, 400 consecutive cycles led to 221 double transfers in women < 38 years of age. This was the standard transfer procedure in this age category for the first two cycles. These 221 transfers of two embryos were divided into three groups according to the number of top-quality embryos as defined earlier: two, one or zero. Results are shown in Table 2. Mean age (29.9, 29.3 and 29.6 years, respectively) was not different in the three groups consisting of 104, 65 and 52 transfers. Ongoing pregnancy rates are 65 (63%), 38 (58%) and 12 (23%).

Pregnancy rates were not different between the first two groups (OR 1.18; 95% CI 0.63–2.23), i.e. between the groups that contained either one or two top-quality embryos. Pregnancy rates were significantly different between the group with two top-quality embryos and the group without a top-quality embryo (OR 5.56; 99% CI 2.60–11.85) as well as between the group with only one top-quality

Table 2 Ongoing pregnancy and implantation rates in 221 two-embryo transfers as a function of the number of top-quality (TQ) embryos per transfer

	Two TQ embryos	One TQ and one non-TQ embryo	Two non-TQ embryos
Number of transfers	104	65	52
Ongoing pregnancy	65 (63%)	38 (58%)	12 (23%)
Singleton	28 (43%)	30 (79%)	12 (100%)
Twin	37 (57%)	8 (21%)	0
Ongoing implantation	102/208 (49%)	46/130 (35%)	12/104 (12%)

embryo and the group without a top-quality embryo (OR 4.69; 99% CI 2.08–10.57). Twinning rates were significantly different between groups: 37 twins in 65 pregnancies (57%) in the first group versus eight twins in 38 pregnancies (21%) in the second group (OR 4.96; 99% CI 1.97–12.45). In the third group there were no twins in 12 pregnancies. Ongoing implantation rates of 102/208 (49%) versus 46/130 (35%) were significantly different between both groups with top-quality embryos (OR 1.76; 95% CI 1.12–2.76). There was a significant difference between the groups that contained either two or one top-quality embryo versus the group that contained none and that had an ongoing implantation rate of only 12/104 (12%) (OR 7.28; 99% CI 3.81–14.28 and OR 4.20; 99% CI 2.08–8.46, respectively).

This high ongoing implantation rate of 49% led to a pregnancy rate of 63% and a twinning rate of 57% in double-embryo transfers of only top-quality embryos in women younger than 38 years of age. It convinced us of the feasibility of and the need for single-embryo transfer in this age category whenever a top-quality embryo is available.

Calculating the implantation potential of individual embryos

Principles The characterization of a top-quality embryo allows the selection of a group of embryos with superior implantation potential. It is clear that, on the one hand not all the different types of top-

quality embryos will have the same implantation potential and that, on the other hand not all non-top-quality embryos will have the same decreased chance of implantation. A ranking of the implantation potential allows the optimal selection of embryos.

It is possible to calculate, for each type of embryo characterized by its cleavage pattern, its fragmentation and its multinucleation, a measure (the implanted fraction) for the ongoing implantation rate. This requires embryos with documented implantation, i.e. embryos from transfers where either all or none of the embryos implanted. For this kind of transfers we can calculate for each type of embryo the ratio of the number implanting over the number transferred. The data provided here represent an updating from data that have been published previously[62]. Between 20 May 1997 and 31 July 2002, there were 1765 oocyte retrievals leading to 1669 (94.6%) transfers in women younger than 38 years of age. Of these, there were 160 single-embryo transfers leading to 158 ongoing singleton and two ongoing monozygotic twin pregnancies, 134 double-embryo transfers leading to 130 ongoing twins and four dizygotic triplet pregnancies and five triple transfers leading to five ongoing triplet pregnancies (Table 3). In total there were 443 embryos with proven (or 100%) ongoing implantation. The number that did certainly not implant is to be found in the transfers followed by a negative human chorionic gonadotropin (hCG) value.

Sample of embryos used for the calculation Between 20 May 1997 and 31 July 2002, 3108 embryos were transferred in women younger than 38 years of age. Of these, 443 certainly did implant and 1579 certainly did not (Table 4). Thus, there were 443 + 1579 = 2022 embryos with documented implantation and these represent 2022/3108 (65.1%) of all transferred embryos. As can be seen in Table 4 only 17/443 (3.8%) embryos with 100% implantation showed more than 20% fragmentation. Of the remaining 426 embryos only six showed multinucleation. If we assume that these embryos with 100% implantation are a representative sample of all implanting embryos, we can conclude that 420/443 (94.8%) of all implanting embryos have a fragmentation of ≤ 20% and show

Table 3 The number of transfers resulting in ongoing implantations stratified according to the number of embryos replaced and outcome. Embryos with 100% implantation are printed in bold type

Embryos transferred	Singleton	Twin	Triplet
1	158	2	
2	256	130	4
3	28	15	5
4	6	2	1
5	4		
6	1		
7	1		1
9			1

Table 4 The number of transferred embryos categorized according to six different types of implantation and three levels of fragmentation. The number of embryos of each category showing multinucleation on day 2 and/or on day 3 is shown in parentheses. Embryos with 0% and 100% implantation are printed in bold type

	Fragmentation			
Outcome	F_1	F_2	F_{3-5}	Total
Zero implantation	728 (78)	522 (81)	329 (67)	1579 (226)
Biochemical pregnancy	121 (11)	81 (7)	21 (3)	223 (21)
Clinical abortion	87 (3)	40 (7)	7 (2)	134 (12)
Ectopic pregnancy	20 (1)	7 (0)	1 (0)	28 (1)
< 100% ongoing implantation	354 (16)	258 (22)	89 (11)	701 (49)
100% ongoing implantation	300 (5)	126 (1)	17 (1)	443 (7)
Total	1610 (114)	1034 (118)	464 (84)	3108 (316)

F_1, < 10% fragmentation; F_2, < 20% fragmentation; F_{3-5}, ≥ 20–< 50% fragmentation

no observed multinucleation in any stage of their development. This sample of embryos with 100% implantation represents 433/778 (55.7%) of all ongoing implantations. We can conclude that our sample of embryos with documented implantation covers a substantial part of more than 55% of all ongoing implantations and, if we exclude all embryos with multinucleation or with a fragmentation higher than 20%, it allows for calculations concerning 95% of all ongoing implantations.

Because only embryos with < 10% and < 20% fragmentation have to be considered, calculations can be summarized (Tables 5 and 6). Implanted fractions can be calculated from Table 5 for fragmentation < 10% (F1) and from Table 6 for fragmentation between 10 and 20% (F2), where, for each cleavage pattern, we can find the ratio between the number with certain implantation over the number of documented implantation.

Ranking of embryos From these two tables we can extract a ranking of implanted fractions for different morphological types of embryo. Table 7 was constructed using the ratios of those types of embryo of which at least ten embryos with documented implantation were available and after having sorted them in descending order of implanted fraction. The ranking obtained offers a qualitative and a quantitative instrument for optimum embryo selection. The efficiency of this selection with respect to pregnancy rate and prevention of multiple pregnancies is demonstrated in the following paragraph.

APPLICATION OF THESE SELECTION METHODS IN DAILY ROUTINE

The results of our two preliminary studies were such that it was decided in our center to change our

Table 5 Transferred embryos with fragmentation F_1 categorized according to the number of blastomeres on day 2 and day 3: number with 100% implantation/number with documented implantation. The implanted fraction is shown in parentheses

			Blastomeres on day 2				
	2	3	4	5	6	7	8
Blastomeres on day 3							
3	0/1 (0)						
4	2/33(6)	0/5 (0)	0/18 (0)				
5	1/10 (10)	2/10 (20)	2/20 (10)	0/4 (0)			
6	3/13 (23)	2/9 (22)	3/36 (8)	1/4 (25)	0/1 (0)		
7	4/13 (31)	1/9 (11)	19/83 (23)	3/20 (15)			
8	6/20 (30)	2/16 (13)	187/429 (44)	10/31 (32)	1/6 (17)	0/2 (0)	
9		1/4 (25)	12/30 (40)	13/38 (34)	0/2 (0)		
10			3/21(14)	5/19 (26)	3/11 (27)	0/1 (0)	
11			4/5 (80)	1/3 (33)	0/1 (0)	0/1 (0)	
12			1/3 (33)	1/2 (50)			
13			1/1 (100)	0/1 (0)			
14			1/2 (50)				
15				0/3 (0)			0/1 (0)

Table 6 Transferred embryos with fragmentation F_2 categorized according to the number of blastomeres on day 2 and day 3: number with 100% implantation/number with documented implantation. The implanted fraction is shown in parentheses

| | Blastomeres on day 2 | | | | | | |
Blastomeres on day 3	2	3	4	5	6	7	8
2	0/1 (0)						
3	0/3 (0)	0/2 (0)					
4	5/34 (15)	0/7 (0)	2/18 (11)	0/1 (0)			
5	1/9 (11)	1/12 (8)	3/21 (14)	0/4 (0)			
6	2/14 (14)	1/16 (6)	7/43 (16)	1/8 (13)			
7	0/3 (0)	1/8 (13)	10/45 (22)	4/20 (20)	0/3 (0)		
8	1/8 (13)	3/8 (38)	50/129 (39)	5/20 (25)	0/7 (0)		
9			8/20 (40)	10/38 (26)	0/4 (0)		
10			3/6 (50)	3/11 (27)	0/6 (0)	1/2 (50)	
11				2/5 (40)			
12				0/3 (0)			
13				1/1 (100)			
14							
15			0/1 (0)				0/1 (0)

transfer policy[45,46]. From 1 January 2002 all patients younger than 38 years of age having their first IVF/ICSI cycle, or after a delivery, would receive only one embryo for transfer if a top-quality embryo was available and two if there was no such embryo. As much as possible, patients were also counseled to accept single-embryo transfer if an embryo with a good prognosis was available in the second and third cycles. As before, we only discuss patients younger than 38 years of age. There were 386 oocyte retrievals leading to 360 (93%) transfers. Of the patients having transfer, 183 (51%) received a single embryo, 163 (45%) two embryos, 13 (4%) three embryos and one four embryos. Single-embryo transfers resulted in 71 ongoing singleton and two monozygotic twin pregnancies, double transfers in 39 ongoing singletons and 14 twins, triple transfers in three singletons and one twin pregnancy. The total ongoing pregnancy rate was 130/360 (36%) per transfer with a twinning rate of 17/130 (13%). There were no triplets.

CONCLUSION

The introduction of an evidence-based quantitative selection method has paved the way for a transfer policy that can be adapted to the 'risk' of implantation. It has enabled the combination of a high pregnancy rate with a low twinning rate. It has largely contributed to the acceptance of single-embryo transfer as the treatment of choice in the appropriate cycles by both doctors and patients. Even in second and third treatment cycles, patients themselves have become motivated and prefer the transfer policy of single-embryo transfer if a top-quality embryo is available, and double-embryo transfer if there is no such embryo. The selection strategy can still be improved by the introduction of other highly

Table 7 Ranking in descending order of implanted fraction of different types of embryos characterized by fragmentation, number of cells on day 2, number of cells on day 3 and absence of multi-nucleation. Types of which less than 10 embryos have been transferred have not been listed

Fragmentation	Cells on day 2	Cells on day 3	100% Implantation	0% + 100% Implantation	Implanted fraction (%)
1	4	8	187	429	43.6
1	4	9	12	30	40.0
2	4	9	8	20	40.0
2	4	8	50	129	38.8
1	5	9	13	38	34.2
1	5	8	10	31	32.3
1	2	7	4	13	30.8
1	2	8	6	20	30.0
2	5	10	3	11	27.3
1	6	10	3	11	27.3
2	5	9	10	38	26.3
1	5	10	5	19	26.3
2	5	8	5	20	25.0
1	2	6	3	13	23.1
1	4	7	19	83	22.9
2	4	7	10	45	22.2
2	5	7	4	20	20.0
1	3	5	2	10	20.0
2	4	6	7	43	16.3
1	5	7	3	20	15.0
2	2	4	5	34	14.7
2	4	5	3	21	14.3
1	4	10	3	21	14.3
2	2	6	2	14	14.3
1	3	8	2	16	12.5
2	4	4	2	18	11.1
1	4	5	2	20	10.0
1	2	5	1	10	10.0
1	4	6	3	36	8.3
2	3	5	1	12	8.3
2	3	6	1	16	6.3
1	2	4	2	33	6.1
1	4	4	0	18	0.0

discriminative quality parameters such as early cleavage[40,41]. Cryopreservation will also be of major importance in the general acceptance of single-embryo transfer; the better the survival and implantation of frozen/thawed embryos, the stronger the arguments in favor of single-embryo transfer. Finally, it should be stressed that, in this chapter, exclusively 'low tech' methods have been discussed. However, these have been proved to be sufficient to allow the selection of a single embryo for transfer.

REFERENCES

1. Ng ST, Chang TH, Wu TC. Prediction of the rates of fertilization, cleavage, and pregnancy success by cumulus–coronal morphology in an *in vitro* fertilization program. *Fertil Steril* 1999;72:412–17

2. Loutradis D, Drakakis P, Kallianidis K, *et al*. Oocyte morphology correlates with embryo quality and pregnancy rate after intracytoplasmic sperm injection. *Fertil Steril* 1999;72:240–4

3. Xia P. Intracytoplasmic sperm injection: correlation of oocyte grade based on polar body, perivitelline space and cytoplasmic inclusions with fertilization rate and embryo quality. *Hum Reprod* 1997;12:1750–5

4. Serhal PF, Ranieri DM, Kinis A, *et al*. Oocyte morphology predicts outcome of intracytoplasmic sperm injection. *Hum Reprod* 1997;12:1267–70

5. Ebner T, Moser M, Yaman C, *et al*. Elective transfer of embryos selected on the basis of first polar body morphology is associated with increased rates of implantation and pregnancy. *Fertil Steril* 1999;72:599–603

6. Van Blerkom J, Davis PW, Lee J. ATP content of human oocytes and developmental potential and outcome after *in-vitro* fertilization and embryo transfer. *Hum Reprod* 1995;10:415–24

7. Van Blerkom J, Antczak J, Schrader R. The developmental potential of the human oocyte is related to the dissolved oxygen content of follicular fluid: association with vascular endothelial growth factor levels and perifollicular blood flow characteristics. *Hum Reprod* 1997;12:1047–55

8. Van Blerkom J. Epigenetic influences on oocyte developmental competence: perifollicular vascularity and intrafollicular oxygen. *J Assist Reprod Genet* 1998;15:226–34

9. Tesarik J, Mendoza C, Greco E. Paternal effects acting during the first cell cycle of human preimplantation development after ICSI. *Hum Reprod* 2002;17:184–9

10. Kiefer D, Check JH, Katsoff D. Evidence that oligoasthenozoospermia may be an etiologic factor for spontaneous abortion after *in vitro* fertilization–embryo transfer. *Fertil Steril* 1997;68:545–8

11. Lundin K, Soderlund B, Hamberger L. The relationship between sperm morphology and rates of fertilization, pregnancy and spontaneous abortion in an *in-vitro* fertilization/ intracytoplasmic sperm injection program. *Hum Reprod* 1997;12:2676–81

12. Miller JE, Smith TT. The effect of intracytoplasmic sperm injection and semen parameters on blastocyst development *in vitro*. *Hum Reprod* 2001;16:918–24

13. Edwards RG, Beard HK. Oocyte polarity and cell determination in early mammalian embryos. *Mol Hum Reprod* 1997;3:863–905

14. Garello C, Baker H, Rai J, *et al*. Pronuclear orientation, polar body placement, and embryo quality after intracytoplasmic sperm injection and *in-vitro* fertilization: further evidence for polarity in human oocytes? *Hum Reprod* 1999;14:2588–95

15. Salumets A, Hydèn-Granskog C, Suikkari A-M, *et al*. The predictive value of pronuclear

morphology of zygotes in the assessment of human embryo quality. *Hum Reprod* 2001; 16:2177–81

16. Stalf T, Herrero J, Mehnert C, *et al.* Influence of polarization effects in ooplasma and pronuclei on embryo quality and implantation in an IVF program. *J Assist Reprod Genet* 2002;19:355–62

17. Payne D, Flaherty SP, Barry MF, *et al.* Preliminary observations on polar body extrusion and pronuclear formation in human oocytes using time-lapse video cinematography. *Hum Reprod* 1997;12:532–41

18. Scott LA, Smith S. The successful use of pronuclear embryo transfers the day following oocyte retrieval. *Hum Reprod* 1998;13:1003–13

19. Scott L, Alvero R, Leondires M, *et al.* The morphology of human pronuclear embryos is positively related to blastocyst development and implantation. *Hum Reprod* 2000;15:2394–403

20. Tesarik J, Greco E. The probability of abnormal preimplantation development can be predicted by a single static observation on pronuclear stage morphology. *Hum Reprod* 1999; 14:1318–23

21. Tesarik J, Junca AM, Hazout A, *et al.* Embryos with high implantation potential after intracytoplasmic sperm injection can be recognized by a simple, non-invasive examination of pronuclear morphology. *Hum Reprod* 2000;15:1396–9

22. Wittemer K, Bettahar-Lebugle J, Ohl C, *et al.* Zygote evaluation: an efficient tool for embryo selection. *Hum Reprod* 2000;15:2591–7

23. Montag M, van der Ven H. Evaluation of pronuclear morphology as the only selection criterion for further embryo culture and transfer: results of a prospective multicentre study. *Hum Reprod* 2001;16:2384–9

24. Ludwig M, Schöpper B, Al-Hasani S, *et al.* Clinical use of a pronuclear stage score following intracytoplasmic sperm injection: impact on pregnancy rates under the conditions of the German embryo protection law. *Hum Reprod* 2000;15:325–9

25. Salumets A, Hydèn-Granskog C, Suikkari AM, *et al.* The predictive value of pronuclear morphology of zygotes in the assessment of human embryo quality. *Hum Reprod* 2001;16:2177–81

26. Cummins JM, Breen TM, Harrison KL, *et al.* A formula for scoring human embryo growth rates in *in vitro* fertilization: its value in predicting pregnancy and in comparison with visual estimates of embryo quality. *J In Vitro Fertil Embryo Transf* 1986;3:284–95

27. Puissant F, Van Rysselberge M, Barlow P, *et al.* Embryo scoring as a prognostic tool in IVF treatment. *Hum Reprod* 1987;2:705–8

28. Steer CV, Mills CL, Tan SL, *et al.* The cumulative embryo score: a predictive embryo scoring technique to select the optimal number of embryos to transfer in an *in-vitro* fertilization and embryo transfer programme. *Hum Reprod* 1992;7:117–19

29. Visser DS, Fourie FR. The applicability of the cumulative embryo score system for embryo selection and quality control in an *in-vitro* fertilization/embryo transfer program. *Hum Reprod* 1993;8:1719–22

30. Hu Y, Maxson WS, Hoffman DI, *et al.* Maximizing pregnancy rates and limiting higher-order multiple conceptions by determining the optimal number of embryos to transfer based on quality. *Fertil Steril* 1998; 69:650–7

31. Ziebe S, Petersen K, Lindenberg S, *et al.* Embryo morphology or cleavage stage: how to select the best embryos for transfer after *in-vitro* fertilization. *Hum Reprod* 1997;12:1545–9

32. Giorgetti C, Terriou P, Auquier P, *et al.* Embryo score to predict implantation after *in-vitro* fertilization: based on 957 single embryo transfers. *Hum Reprod* 1995;10:2427–31

33. Pickering SJ, Taylor A, Johnson MH, *et al.* An analysis of multinucleated blastomere formation in human embryos. *Hum Reprod* 1995;10:1912–22

34. Laverge H, De Sutter P, Verschraegen-Spae MR, *et al.* Triple colour fluorescent *in-situ* hybridization for chromosomes X,Y and 1 on spare human embryos. *Hum Reprod* 1997;12: 809–14

35. Jackson KV, Ginsburg ES, Hornstein MD, *et al.* Multinucleation in normally fertilized embryos is associated with an accelerated ovulation induction response and lower implantation and pregnancy rates in *in vitro* fertilization–embryo transfer cycles. *Fertil Steril* 1998;70:60–6

36. Pelinck MJ, De Vos M, Dekens M, *et al.* Embryos cultured *in vitro* with multinucleated blastomeres have poor implantation potential in human *in-vitro* fertilization and intracytoplasmic sperm injection. *Hum Reprod* 1998;13:960–3

37. Van Royen E, Mangelschots K, De Neubourg D, *et al.* Characterization of a top quality embryo, a step towards single-embryo transfer. *Hum Reprod* 1999;14:2345–9

38. Van Royen E, Mangelschots K, Vercruyssen M, *et al.* Multinucleation in cleavage stage embryos. *Hum Reprod* 2003;18:1062–9

39. Hardarson T, Hanson C, Sjögren A, Lundin K. Human embryos with unevenly sized blastomeres have lower pregnancy and implantation rates: indications for aneuploidy and multinucleation. *Hum Reprod* 2001;16:313–18

40. Lundin K, Bergh C, Hardarson T. Early embryo cleavage is a strong indicator of embryo quality in human IVF. *Hum Reprod* 2001;16 2652–7

41. Salumets A, Hydèn-Granskog C, Makinen S, *et al.* Early cleavage predicts the viability of human embryos in elective single embryo transfer procedures. *Hum Reprod* 2003;18: 821–5

42. Desai NN , Goldstein J, Rowland DY, *et al.* Morphological evaluation of human embryos and derivation of an embryo quality scoring system specific for day 3 embryos: a preliminary study. *Hum Reprod* 2000;15:2190–6

43. Vilska S, Tiitinen A, Hydèn-Granskog C, *et al.* Elective transfer of one embryo results in an acceptable pregnancy rate and eliminates the risk of multiple birth. *Hum Reprod* 1999;14:2392–5

44. Martikainen H, Tiitinen A, Tomás C, *et al.* One versus two embryo transfer after IVF and ICSI: a randomized study. *Hum Reprod* 2001;16:1900–3

45. Gerris J, De Neubourg D, Mangelschots K, *et al.* Prevention of twin pregnancy after *in-vitro* fertilization or intracytoplasmic sperm injection based on strict embryo criteria: a prospective randomized clinical trial. *Hum Reprod* 1999;14:2581–7

46. De Neubourg D, Mangelschots K, Van Royen E, *et al.* Impact of patients' choice for single embryo transfer of a top quality embryo versus double embryo transfer in the first IVF/ICSI cycle. *Hum Reprod* 2002;17:2621–5

47. Huisman GJ, Alberda AT, Leerentveld RA, *et al.* A comparison of *in vitro* fertilization results after embryo transfer after 2, 3, and 4 days of embryo culture. *Fertil Steril* 1994;61:940–71

48. Shapiro BS, Harris DC, Richter KS. Predictive value of 72-hour blastomere cell number on blastocyst development and success of subsequent transfer based on the degree of blastocyst development. *Fertil Steril* 2000;73:582–6

49. Milki AA, Hinckley MD, Fisch JD, *et al*. Comparison of blastocyst transfer with day 3 embryo transfer in similar patient populations. *Fertil Steril* 2000;73:126–9

50. Gardner DK, Lane M, Stevens J, *et al*. Blastocyst score affects implantation and pregnancy outcome: towards a single blastocyst transfer. *Fertil Steril* 2000;73:1155–8

51. Behr B, Pool T, Milki A, Moore D, *et al*. Preliminary clinical experience with human blastocyst development *in vitro* without co-culture. *Hum Reprod* 1999;14:454–7

52. Coskun S, Hollanders J, Al-Hassan S, *et al*. Day 5 versus day 3 embryo transfer: a controlled randomized trial. *Hum Reprod* 2000;15:1947–52

53. Rienzi L, Ubaldi F, Iacobelli M, *et al*. Day 3 embryo transfer with combined evaluation at the pronuclear and cleavage stages compares favourably with day 5 blastocyst transfer. *Hum Reprod* 2002;17:1852–5

54. Utsunomiya T, Naitou T, Nagaki M. A prospective trial of blastocyst culture and transfer. *Hum Reprod* 2002;17:1846–51

55. Bungum M, Bungum L, Humaidan P, Yding Andersen C. Day 3 versus day 5 embryo transfer: a prospective randomized study. *Reprod BioMed Online* 2003;7:98–104

56. Peramo B, Ricciarelli E, Cuadros-Fernandez JM, *et al*. Blastocyst transfer and monozygotic twinning. *Fertil Steril* 1999;72:1116–7

57. Behr B, Fisch JD, Racowsky C, Miller K, *et al*. Blastocyst-ET and monozygotic twinning. *J Assist Reprod Genet* 2000;17:349–51

58. da Costa AL, Abdelmassih S, de Oliveira FG, *et al*. Monozygotic twins and transfer at the blastocyst stage after ICSI. *Hum Reprod* 2001;16:333–6

59. Blake D, Proctor M, Johnson N, *et al*. Cleavage stage versus blastocyst stage embryo transfer in assisted conception. *Cochrane Database Syst Rev* 2002;(2):CD0021188

60. Kolibianakis EM, Devroey P. Blastocyst culture: facts and fiction. *Reprod BioMed Online* 2002;5:285–93

61. Reynolds TM. Down's syndrome screening: a controversial test, with more controversy to come! *J Clin Pathol* 2000;53:893–8

62. Van Royen E, Mangelschots K, De Neubourg D, *et al*. Calculating the implantation potential of day 3 embryos in women younger than 38 years of age: a new model. *Hum Reprod* 2001;16:326–32

63. Huisman GJ, Fauser BC, Eijkemans MJ, Pieters MH. Implantation rates after *in vitro* fertilization and transfer of a maximum of two embryos that have undergone three to five days of culture. *Fertil Steril* 2000;73:117–22

64. Rijnders PM, Jansen CA. The predictive value of day 3 embryo morphology regarding blastocyst formation, pregnancy and implantation rate after day 5 transfer following *in-vitro* fertilization or intracytoplasmic sperm injection. *Hum Reprod* 1998;13:2869–73

7

Impact of elective single-embryo transfer on the total and multiple pregnancy rate

J. Gerris

THE PRACTICE OF IVF/ICSI

In the early days, *in vitro* fertilization (IVF) did not *have* a goal, it *was* a goal in itself. It was considered good medical practice to maximize the chances for 'success' (= a pregnancy) by transferring several embryos even at the price needed to 'treat' almost any complication in the mother and the newborn(s) by intensive care medicine. A twinning rate of 28%, a high-order pregnancy rate of 4% and a singleton pregnancy rate of 68% resulted in $56 + 12 + 68 = 136$ children born, of whom exactly half belonged to a set of multiples! Nevertheless, multiple pregnancy and its obstetric, neonatal, developmental and financial consequences represents the main iatrogenic complication of IVF/intracytoplasmic sperm injection (ICSI)[1–3].

As early as 1993, retrospective reports were published showing that the pregnancy rate did not change if two instead of three embryos were transferred[4]. Most convincingly, a large British study demonstrated that only the multiple birth rate and not the total birth rate increased when three instead of two embryos were transferred in cycles in which more than four eggs had been fertilized[5]. In some countries the incidence of triplets remains alarmingly high[6].

WHAT IS THE ESSENTIAL GOAL OF IVF/ICSI?

It should be realized that a normal, physiological pregnancy in the human female, as opposed to many other species, where multiple gestation is the rule, is a singleton pregnancy. The essential goal of IVF/ICSI, as a mature treatment for infertility, is to generate an optimal chance for a singleton live birth. An optimal chance is quite different from a maximal chance, which is in fact often suboptimal. Whereas maximization mainly looks at the chance for 'a pregnancy', 'accepting' (both by patients and by physicians and their team) almost any risk for its occurrence, optimization keeps a wise eye on the balance between the end result and the efforts, costs and complications of the treatment. The only way to strive towards that goal is to reduce the number of embryos transferred. A generalized introduction of single-embryo transfer is not feasible, because this would result in an unacceptable decrease in the overall efficacy of the treatment. The first published experience with the transfer of one embryo in patients who had only one embryo to transfer showed poor results[7]. The only way, therefore, to realize the essential goal of IVF/ICSI is to identify embryos with putative high competence and to define the twin-prone patient. Thus, the essence when applying elective single-embryo transfer is to be able actively to select (i.e. elect) the right embryo in the right patient, hence the term 'elective single-embryo transfer'. In doing so, there will always remain a substantial proportion of transfers of more than one embryo, hence there will always be a certain proportion of twin pregnancies. Therefore, the complete avoidance of twin pregnancies does not seem to be a realistic goal, as opposed to the prevention of triplets, which, apart from dizygotic triplets after two-embryo transfer, can be totally avoided. It is clear that other than purely scientific and rational clinical considerations are playing a role, e.g. the cost of the treatment, irrespective of who pays: the patient, the insurers or the government. In this contribution, we report the experience of one center with the progressive introduction of elective single-embryo transfer and its impact on overall and multiple pregnancy rates.

SELECTION OF PATIENTS SUITABLE FOR ELECTIVE SINGLE-EMBRYO TRANSFER

Several authors have contributed to our understanding of the clinical circumstances in which the number of embryos to be replaced should or could be limited. Until now, for most of these authors, 'to limit' still meant replacing two embryos instead of three. Several background characteristics of the patients as well as cycle characteristics of the particular cycle have been found to be correlated with the odds for a birth and/or with the odds for a multiple birth[5,8–12]. The conclusions of most of these reports are in agreement. Of all factors examined, the most important was the age of the female partner.

An important Swedish study found that the following factors correlated independently with birth and multiple birth, adjusted for the number of previous IVF cycles: female age, initial daily dose of follicle stimulating hormone (FSH), total dose of FSH, tubal versus other infertility, number of good-quality embryos available, number of good-quality embryos transferred and number of embryos available for freezing[11].

Tubal infertility, the original indication for IVF, is associated with a significantly lower pregnancy rate than the other indications. The risk for a multiple pregnancy and the chance to obtain a pregnancy are independently related to age. Older women have less chance to obtain a pregnancy but the proportion of them obtaining a multiple pregnancy is not lower than in young women (as in natural conception). The odds ratios of the factors examined are as a rule close to 1, suggesting a low impact of each individual variable. It is important to keep this in mind when looking at the importance of embryo characteristics. Whereas the UK report focused on the issue of two or three embryos, the Swedish study evaluated what would occur if, in certain cycles, only one embryo would have been transferred, assuming that at least one 'good-quality' embryo

was available[5,11]. They calculated that the chance of a multiple birth could be reduced from 26% to 13% of all births if elective single-embryo transfer were performed in selected cases. Data becoming available from an increasing number of centers show this calculation to be very close to observed multiple pregnancy rates.

INTRODUCTION OF SINGLE-EMBRYO TRANSFER

Recent experience in several countries such as Belgium and Finland has shown that the introduction of elective single-embryo transfer after IVF/ICSI has resulted in a dramatic reduction of the twinning rate and an almost complete disappearance of higher-order multiple pregnancies, without causing the much-dreaded decrease in the overall ongoing pregnancy rate of the program[13–19]. This is mainly the consequence of optimization of the various steps of the IVF/ICSI process: selection of the twin-prone patient, ovarian stimulation, oocyte recovery, embryo culture, embryo selection, embryo transfer and a coherent counseling of the patients. The two main determinants have been embryo selection and patient selection, in that order of impact.

In this contribution, we present the subsequent stages that led in our department to a reduction of the twinning rate after IVF/ICSI to < 50% of its initial incidence, while maintaining a stable overall ongoing pregnancy rate of > 30% per started cycle.

Step 1: Determination of the characteristics of a putative high-competence embryo prior to single-embryo transfer

In 1996, our standard embryo transfer policy consisted of the transfer of the two 'best-looking' day-3 embryos. Embryo selection criteria used at that time were the traditional morphological characteristics: number of blastomeres and percentage of fragmentation. A total of 337 IVF/ICSI cycles – for all accepted indications for treatment, including microsurgical epididymal sperm aspiration (MESA) and testicular sperm extraction (TESE) – resulted in 322 transfers of a mean number of 2.59 embryos, an ongoing pregnancy rate of 24% and an ongoing mean implantation rate of 13.5%; there were 57%

singletons, 40% twins and 3% high-order multiple pregnancies. When confronted with these figures, the clinicians, realizing that the obstetric and neonatal risk resulting from this high total proportion of multiple pregnancies was unacceptable, decided that something had to be done, even at the expense of a decrease in overall pregnancy rate. Logically, this 'something' could only be to introduce single-embryo transfer. At this stage, the embryologists had observed that twin pregnancies after two-embryo transfer coincided with the transfer of embryos with a particular combination of morphological characteristics. As a first step towards single-embryo transfer, they developed a rational system of embryo selection based on early cleaving embryo characteristics recorded systematically in a prospective embryo database.

A consecutive series of 23 ongoing twin pregnancies, originating in the year 1996, and resulting in the birth of 46 healthy babies, i.e. from 46 implanting embryos, were retrospectively analyzed. The details of this analysis have been published[20]. Crucial elements of this analysis were: strict time intervals for observation of each individual embryo, comprising the exact number of blastomeres, the percentage of fragmentation *and* the observation of multinucleation in any of the blastomeres at any stage of observation. On the basis of this analysis, strict criteria for a putative high-competence embryo were defined as follows: absence of multinucleated blastomeres, four or five blastomeres on day 2, a minimum of seven cells on day 3 and a maximum of 20% anucleated fragments.

Step 2: Validation of the characteristics of a putative high-competence embryo

In 1997, it was agreed that the standard procedure would still consist of the transfer of the two best looking embryos, defined according to traditional criteria, i.e. the two 'best looking' embryos using, this time, the 'strict' embryo characteristics as defined above. The whole IVF/ICSI population of that year was then analyzed retrospectively (400 cycles, of which 221 were with double-embryo transfer) in order to assess whether these 'strict putative high-competence embryo criteria' could be validated. Only women < 38 years of age had multiple pregnancies: after 221 transfers of two embryos, 45 out of 116 (39%) pregnancies were

multiple; and after 77 transfers of more than two embryos, 11 out of 31 (35%) pregnancies were multiple. We applied the above-mentioned putative high-competence embryo criteria to these 221 transfers of two embryos: 104 transfers with two putative high-competence embryos resulted in 65 (63%) ongoing pregnancies with 37 (57%) twins; 65 transfers with one top putative high-competence embryo and one non-high-competence embryo in 38 (58%) ongoing pregnancies with eight (21%) twins. In the two-embryo transfer group without putative high-competence embryos to transfer, there were 12 (23%) ongoing pregnancies in 52 transfers, but no twins. The ongoing implantation rates for these three groups were 49%, 35% and 12%, respectively. This analysis showed that these criteria could be used to consider single-embryo transfer with an acceptable pregnancy rate when such a top-quality embryo is available.

Step 3: Prospective randomized clinical trial comparing elective transfer of one putative high-competence embryo with elective transfer of two such embryos

After these two preparatory (retrospective) steps, a prospective randomized study was conducted comparing single- with double-embryo transfer[14]. We used the same characteristics of a putative high-competence embryo as delineated above. This first single-embryo transfer (SET-I) study was conducted in women < 34 years of age who were starting their first IVF/ICSI cycle, i.e. in a group with a very good prognosis. This was done because we found that > 80% of all twins occurred in this group of patients and our main goal was to eliminate a substantial proportion of twins. Study counseling included full explanation of the major risks of twin pregnancy and free choice to participate; the standard of treatment still consisted of the transfer of the best two embryos. Patients were clearly informed that they did not have the choice between one or two embryos but between participation in the study or not. It was also made clear that single-embryo transfer on request was possible, but in that case the patient was not included in the primary comparison of the study. Clearly, only patients actually producing at least two putative high-competence embryos could be included in the randomized comparison. Supernumerary embryos with > 7 blastomeres on day 3 were frozen. The study was limited to the first treatment cycle. The aim of this study was to obtain data on the ongoing implantation rate, the ongoing pregnancy rate and the ongoing multiple pregnancy rate in women receiving either one or two putative high-competence embryos. This study showed an ongoing pregnancy rate of 39% in the study arm receiving one embryo and of 67% in the study arm receiving two embryos. The group of patients who fell out of the primary analysis because they *requested* only one embryo and who did receive one also had an ongoing pregnancy rate of 39%. The outcome of the other groups in this study can be found in the published paper[14]. The main conclusion of this study was that elective (i.e. if at least one putative high-competence embryo is available) single-embryo transfer results in an acceptable ongoing pregnancy rate of about 40%. The study did not state that the result of *indiscriminate* single-embryo transfer versus double-embryo transfer gives similar results. It clearly showed that the number of embryos transferred was not the main determinant for 'success' (i.e. an ongoing pregnancy) but rather *which* embryo was transferred. It showed that elective single-embryo transfer is a feasible option to avoid a substantial proportion of twin pregnancies.

Step 4: Clinical impact study comparing elective single- with elective double-embryo transfer including a health-economic evaluation

Subsequently, another, non-randomized prospective impact study was conducted comparing the result of single-embryo transfer versus double-embryo transfer in women < 38 years of age in their first IVF/ICSI cycle both from a clinical and from a health-economic point of view (SET-II study; submitted for publication). This study is a two-center long-term health economic study with a follow-up of all children until 3 months after delivery. Its primary endpoint is a comparison between the maternal cost, the neonatal cost and the total of pregnancies obtained after elective single-embryo transfer versus pregnancies obtained after double-embryo transfer. The study was conducted simultaneously in the Middelheim Center for Reproductive Medicine in Antwerp and in the Ghent University Center for Reproductive Medicine. Prior to the

study, the embryologists of both centers agreed upon a similar interpretation of putative high-competence embryo characteristics. All patients were < 38 years of age and were undergoing their first ever IVF/ICSI treatment or their first IVF/ICSI treatment after a previous delivery. They were allowed to choose either a double transfer of the two best embryos (i.e. either two putative high-competence embryos, one high-competence plus one non-high-competence embryo, or two non-high-competence embryos) or a single embryo. If they chose single-embryo transfer, they received one embryo *only if* a putative high-competence embryo was available; if not, they received a double-embryo transfer of the two best (non-high-competence) embryos. A total of 367 embryo transfers were analyzed, leading to 181 (49.3%) cycles without conception and 186 (50.7%) with conception, of which 148 (40.3%) resulted in ongoing pregnancies (> 12 weeks) and 136 (37.1%) resulted in liveborn deliveries. Of 206 single-embryo transfers (56%) 83 resulted in an ongoing pregnancy (40.3%); of 161 double-embryo transfers (44%) 65 resulted in an ongoing pregnancy (40.4%). There were no twins in the SET group and 18 ongoing twins in the double-embryo transfer group (overall ongoing twinning rate 18/148; 12.1%), of which there were 15 live births. The health economic analysis showed a higher total cost (mother plus child) for pregnancies after double-embryo transfer, which was wholly attributable to a significant difference between the neonatal cost: $434 \pm 954€$ vs. $3414 \pm 8101€$ (Wilcoxon test; $p < 0.001$), explained by a significantly higher cost for the twin children.

In the course of these two studies, the original strict putative high-competence embryo criteria were further fine-tuned using a new model to calculate the implantation potential of day-3 embryos in women < 38 years of age, in which it was shown that embryos with multinucleated blastomeres have a very poor implantation potential. In this refinement, we analyzed the characteristics of embryos with documented implantation behavior, i.e. singletons after single-embryo transfer, twins after double-embryo transfer or cycles with negative serum human chorionic gonadotropin (hCG). This led to a ranking system of the implanted fraction[21]. This analysis showed that some categories of embryos with catch-up growth also have high implantation potential. It led to the insight that embryos cannot be categorically assigned to a group with high versus a group with low implantation potential, but rather that the implantation potential is a continuous variable that can to some extent be predicted for individual embryos, allowing one to pick *the one* embryo that will serve for a single-embryo transfer. The specific importance of multinucleation has been reported in detail in another publication[22]. These findings are in line with previous experience of other authors[23–25].

OVERALL EXPERIENCE WITH ELECTIVE SINGLE-EMBRYO TRANSFER

In summary, over a 5-year period (1998–2002), single-embryo transfer was applied in a gradual manner in three categories of patients: women participating in the SET-I study; women participating in the SET-II study; and women who did not fulfil the inclusion criteria of either study but nevertheless wanted only one embryo to be replaced, some of them > 38 years of age. It is essential to state that no patients were compelled to receive only one embryo. In all cases, they had the free choice between one or two embryos: either they could choose to participate in a randomized trial or not (SET-I) or they could directly choose one or two embryos (SET-II). Moreover, patients allotted by randomization (SET-I) or by their own choice (SET-II) to receive only one embryo received in principle only one embryo on the condition that it was a putative high-competence embryo, as strictly defined. If not, they received either one non-PHC embryo at their explicit request to receive only one embryo (usually women with children) or – in the large majority of cases – they received the two best non-high-competence embryos.

Of a total of 2007 ovum retrievals, 1882 (93.8%) transfers resulted, of which 578 were of a single embryo (30.1%); 461 (24.5%) were of a single putative high-competence embryo; and 117 (6.2%) were of a single non-high-competence embryo. We considered the complete population of patients receiving a single embryo and compared their outcome with all other patients receiving two or more embryos. The impact of the progressive

introduction of elective single-embryo transfer over these 5 years on the overall ongoing pregnancy rate and the multiple pregnancy rate (per year) was analyzed. Materials and methods are described elsewhere[15,26].

Table 1 illustrates the outcome of the transfer of a single top-quality embryo ($n = 461$), a single non-top quality embryo ($n = 117$), two embryos ($n = 1034$) or more than two embryos ($n = 270$) in our IVF/ICSI program (all ages) over the years 1998–2002.

Table 2 illustrates in more detail the clinical outcome variables in patients receiving one or two embryos, as a function of the number of putative high-competence embryos (all ages).

Figure 1 shows the progressive increase in the proportion of single-embryo transfers over these years.

Figure 2 shows the impact of elective single-embryo transfer on the ongoing implantation rate, the ongoing pregnancy rate and the multiple pregnancy rate over the years. Although the multiple pregnancy rate decreased from 33% (1998) to 11.7% in (2002), the ongoing implantation rate and the ongoing pregnancy rate remained stable at approximately 21% and 31%, respectively.

Figure 3 shows the evolution of the ongoing pregnancy rate, the multiple pregnancy rate and the mean number of embryos transferred over the period studied (from 2.54 in 1998 to 1.67 in 2002).

Table 3 shows the percentage of single-embryo transfers, the mean number of embryos transferred, the ongoing implantation rate, the ongoing pregnancy rate, the twinning rate and the total multiple pregnancy rate in an unselected IVF/ICSI population where elective single-embryo transfer was introduced over a 5-year period.

Figure 4 shows the evolution of the number of infants born as singletons or as part of a twin pair. In 1998, 80 singletons were born and $81 \times 2 = 162$ twin infants were born, for a total of 242 infants. In 2002 there were 120 singletons and $36 \times 2 = 72$ twin infants for a total of 192 children. Thus, there were 50 prevented twin children. In the same period, the ongoing pregnancy rate did not change significantly, implying that there were not fewer pregnancies, but only fewer twins.

Table 1 Outcome of the transfer of a single top-quality embryo ($n = 461$), a single non-top-quality embryo ($n = 117$), two embryos ($n = 1034$) or more than two embryos ($n = 270$) in an unselected population undergoing *in vitro* fertilization/intracytoplasmic sperm injection (all ages)

	SET top quality		SET non-top quality		All DET		> 2 ET		all non-SET		Total	
	n	%	n	%	n	%	n	%	n	%	n	%
Transfers	461	24.5	117	6.2	1034	54.9	270	14.4	1304	69.3	1882	
Conceptions	244	52.9	35	29.9	500	48.3	105	38.9	605	46.4	884	47.0
Ongoing pregnancies	174	37.7	24	20.5	363	35.1	64	23.7	427	32.7	625	33.2
Singletons*	172	98.9	23	95.8	253	69.7	44	68.8	297	69.6	492	78.7
Twins + triplets*	2	1.1	1	4.2	105 + 5	30.3	13 + 7	31.2	118 + 12	30.4	121 + 12	21.3

SET, single-embryo transfer; DET, double-embryo transfer; ET, embryo transfers
* The percentage of twins and triplets is expressed as a fraction of the total number of ongoing pregnancies

Table 2 Clinical outcome variables in patients receiving one (single-embryo transfer; SET) or two (double-embryo transfer; DET) embryos, as a function of the number of top-quality embryos in an unselected population undergoing in vitro fertilization/intracytoplasmic sperm injection (all ages)

	SET top-quality		SET non top-quality		DET 2 top-quality		DET 1 top-quality		DET 0 top-quality	
	n	%	n	%	n	%	n	%	n	%
Transfers	461		117		341		236		456	
Conceptions (A)	244	52.9	35	29.9	218	63.9	134	56.4	147	32.2
Ongoing pregnancy (B)	174	37.7	24	20.5	169	49.6	97	41.1	97	21.3
Biochemical pregnancies	40	16.4 (of A)	7	20	27	12.4 (of A)	24	17.9	29	19.7
Miscarriages	28	11.5	3	8.6	18	8.3	11	8.2	17	11.6
Ectopic pregnancies	4	1.6	0		4	1.8	2	1.5	4	2.7
Singletons	172	98.9 (of B)	23	95.8	97	57.4 (of B)	65	67.0	78	80.4
Twins	2	1.1	1	4.2	67	39.6	32	33.0	19	19.6
Dizygotic triplets	0		0		5	2.9	0		0	
Ongoing implantation rate	174/461 = 37.7%*		24/117 = 20.5%*		241/682 = 35.3%*		129/472 = 27.3%		116/912 = 12.7%	

* A monozygotic twinning is counted for one implantation; a dizygotic triplet is counted for two implantations

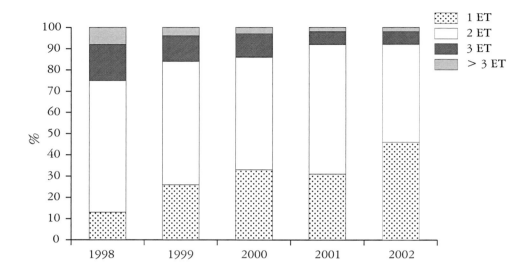

Figure 1   Evolution of the proportion of single-embryo transfers (ET) over a 5-year period (1998–2002) in an unselected population undergoing *in vitro* fertilization/intracytoplasmic sperm injection

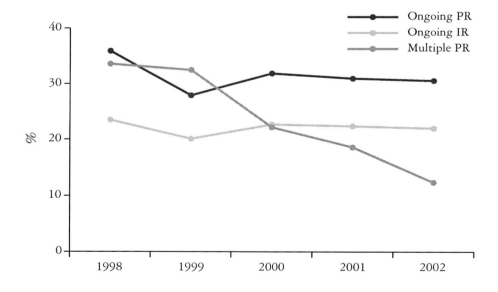

Figure 2   Evolution of the ongoing pregnancy rate (PR), the ongoing implantation rate (IR) and the multiple PR in an unselected population undergoing *in vitro* fertilization/intracytoplasmic sperm injection, where elective single-embryo transfer was gradually introduced over a 5-year period (1998–2002)

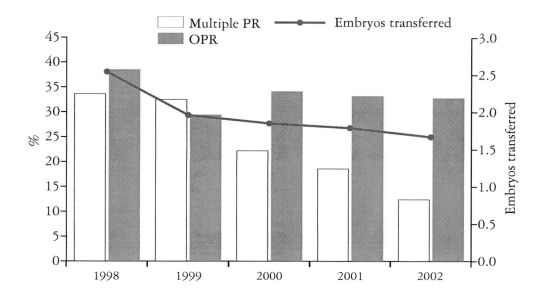

Figure 3 Evolution of the ongoing pregnancy rate (OPR), the multiple pregnancy rate (MPR) and the mean number of embryos transferred in an unselected population undergoing *in vitro* fertilization/intracytoplasmic sperm injection in which elective single-embryo transfer was gradually introduced over a 5-year period (1998–2002)

Table 3 Percentage of single-embryo transfers (SET), mean number of embryos transferred, ongoing implantation rate (OIR), ongoing pregnancy rate (OPR), twinning rate and total multiple pregnancy rate (MPR) in an unselected population undergoing *in vitro* fertilization/intracytoplasmic sperm injection where elective SET was introduced over a 5-year period (total 1882 cycles)

	1998	1999	2000	2001	2002	1998–2002
SET (%)	13	26	33	31	46	32
Embryos transferred	2.26	1.96	1.85	1.79	1.67	1.89
OIR (%)	23.5	20.1	22.7	22.4	22.0	22.1
OPR/OPU (%)	35.9	27.9	31.9	31.0	30.6	31.3
OPR/ET (%)	38.5	29.4	34.1	33.2	32.8	32.8
Twins (%)	29.5	30.7	20.6	16.3	12.4	21.5
Total MPR (%)	33.6	32.5	22.2	18.6	12.4	23.4

OPU, ovum pick-up

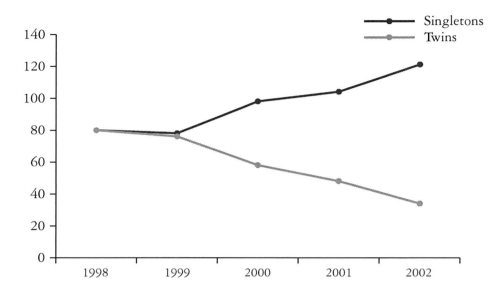

Figure 4 Evolution of the number of infants born as singletons or as twins from 1998 to 2002, illustrating the impact of elective single-embryo transfer

FURTHER REFLECTIONS

The group of patients suitable for elective single-embryo transfer may be smaller in other programs with older patients. It could also be larger if higher-rank treatment cycles with putative high-competence embryos are also included. The most suitable patients are young women in their first IVF/ICSI cycle. In 2002, 46% of all transfers in our program were single-embryo transfers. These results do not pertain to a small selected group of patients. The intention is to apply elective elective single-embryo transfer if a suitable embryo is present in the twin-prone patient. Combining validated, strict criteria of early cleaving embryos with a clinical profile of the twin-prone patient, as described by Strandell and colleagues, for example, results in a high and stable ongoing pregnancy rate of > 30% per started cycle[11]. This allows the transfer of a single top-quality embryo to be considered as the standard of care in these patients. The application of transfer of a single top-quality embryo could be extended to second and third treatment cycles, or perhaps to all cycles with at least one top-quality embryo. A patient who did not produce a putative high-competence embryo during her first cycle and who did not have an ongoing pregnancy after the transfer of two non-high-competence embryos, but who does produce a top-quality embryo in her second cycle, is probably also a good candidate for elective single-embryo transfer during that second cycle, as would be the patients who had a biochemical conception after the first transfer of one top-quality embryo. The feasibility of extending single-embryo transfer in a maximum number of cycles is also linked to the performance of the cryopreservation program. The role of cryopreservation is likely to become increasingly important as elective single-embryo transfer finds its way into the clinic, as has been demonstrated by others[11,18,19].

A debate is ongoing regarding the optimal stage at which embryo selection should take place, and this point is dealt with in more detail in other chapters. From the beginning, the quality of the oocyte is correlated with the implantation competence of the resulting embryo[27–29]. Pronuclear stage assessment has been advocated as well as the blastocyst stage[30–32]. Several prospective randomized trials have shown no superiority of day-5 over day-3 transfer[33–36]. These results are corroborated in a recent critical review, but the matter seems to remain unresolved until a prospective trial becomes available, comparing the transfer of one day-3 versus one day-5 embryo, with randomization prior to the initiation of ovarian stimulation[37].

Whatever the outcome of this debate, we must not err in choosing the wrong questions. The challenge is a primarily clinical one: how to reduce the excess number of multiple pregnancies after both IVF and non-IVF treatments. In IVF, embryologists should not lose themselves in largely academic discussions on how to select embryos. Clinicians should be aware that the ethical responsibility lies with them. New and expensive approaches such as systematic blastocyst culture, blastomere DNA fingerprinting, routine preimplantation aneuploidy screening, amino acid consumption patterns and other methods of 'improved' embryo selection, should be viewed with a cautious open mind as long as there are no prospective, randomized trials proving these methods to result in similar or rather better results than can be obtained by a committed and strict observance of some simple rules of good clinical and laboratory practice. This is not to oppose scientific research or advances in medical performance, but to listen at times and intervals to the more eternal voice of reason.

In order to see the twin incidence in national registries decrease, there is a need for national policies. At the interface of medicine and politics, however, not all is rational. In Belgium, until now, mainly two centers have been applying elective single-embryo transfer since 1997, to reach approximately 30–40% of all their transfers. These centers, taken together, represent no more than about 15–20% of all reported trials in Belgium. Therefore, the impact on national statistics until the year 2001 has not been noticeable, although it is likely to become evident in the years to come, because the reimbursement of IVF coupled with a strict transfer policy will induce all centers to apply elective single-embryo transfer. In this regulation, six cycles (in a lifetime) of IVF/ICSI will be refunded per patient, provided all participants comply with a restrictive embryo replacement policy. This policy requires the replacement of only one embryo in all first IVF/ICSI cycles in women < 36 years of age, and the replacement of one embryo in all second cycles if the embryo is of sufficient quality (if not, then two embryos can be replaced). Although this regulation will certainly result in a decrease in twins in the first cycle, it could also result in a decrease in the overall pregnancy rate, because no agreement has been reached with respect to the implantation potential of embryos. The regulation may displace the problem from twins in first cycles towards twins in second cycles, which is a pity, because it is easier to convince women to accept elective single-embryo transfer in a first cycle than it is in a second cycle. Moreover, reimbursement alone does not influence women's acceptance of a restrictive embryo transfer policy. Therefore, it can be predicted that the Belgian agreement on reimbursement will have to be reassessed. If not, the overall pregnancy rate of IVF/ICSI could decrease and multiples will simply be postponed to later cycles and not truly prevented. We recommend that, prior to later political discussions, data are collected and presented to those who take the decisions.

It is evident that our increased capacity in detecting, to a certain extent, embryos with a putative high implantation potential can be used in two ways.

If we adhere to our present attitude to transfer two embryos as a standard of care, we can certainly maximize pregnancy rates. In our program, if we had transferred two embryos in all of the 46% of cycles where we transferred only one embryo in the year 2002, the overall ongoing pregnancy rate would arguably have reached about 45%.

In contrast, and in our opinion more judiciously, we could also choose to optimize pregnancy rates, i.e. accept a wise trade-off between the efficacy and safety of IVF/ICSI.

Factors other than purely medical or scientific considerations come into play when making this decision. It can only be hoped that our daily practice will be dictated by high-quality data supported by common sense and the voice of reason emanating from our professional group and not by the threats of legal action, by political opportunism or by the superficial sensationalism of the mass media.

REFERENCES

1. Dhont M, De Sutter P, Ruyssinck G, *et al.* Perinatal outcome of pregnancies after assisted reproduction: a case–control study. *Am J Obstet Gynecol* 1999;181:688–95

2. Bergh T, Ericson A, Hillensjö T, *et al.* Deliveries and children born after *in-vitro* fertilization in Sweden 1982–95: a retrospective cohort study. *Lancet* 2000;354:1579–85

3. Schieve LA, Meikle SF, Ferre C, *et al.* Low and very low birth weight in infants conceived with the use of assisted reproductive technology. *N Engl J Med* 2002;346:731–7

4. Staessen C, Janssenswillen C, Van Den Abbeel E, *et al.* Avoidance of triplet pregnancies by elective transfer of two good quality embryos. *Hum Reprod* 1993;8:1650–3

5. Templeton A, Morris JK. Reducing the risk of multiple birth by transfer of two embryos after *in vitro* fertilization. *N Engl J Med* 1998;339:573–7

6. Martin JA, Park MM. Trends in twin and triplet births: 1980–97. *National Vital Statistics Report.* Hyattsville, MD: US Department of Health and Human Services, CDC, National Center for Statistics, 1999:24

7. Giorgetti C, Terriou P, Auquier P, *et al.* Embryo score to predict implantation after *in-vitro* fertilization: based on 957 single embryo transfers. *Hum Reprod* 1995;10:2427–31

8. Templeton A, Morris JK. Factors that affect outcome of *in-vitro* fertilization treatment. *Lancet* 1996;348:1402–6

9. Bassil S, Wyns C, Toussaint-Demylle D, *et al.* Predictive factors for multiple pregnancy in *in vitro* fertilization. *J Reprod Med* 1997;42:761–6

10. Minaretzis D, Harris D, Alper MM *et al.* Multivariate analysis of factors predictive of successful live births in *in vitro* fertilization (IVF) suggests strategies to improve IVF outcome. *J Assist Reprod Genet* 1998;15:365–71

11. Strandell A, Bergh C, Lundin K. Selection of patients suitable for one-embryo transfer may reduce the rate of multiple births by half without impairment of overall birth rates. *Hum Reprod* 2000;15:2520–5

12. Tur R, Barri P, Coroleu B, *et al.* Risk factors for high-order multiple implantation after ovarian stimulation with gonadotrophins: evidence from a large series of 1878 consecutive pregnancies in a single centre. *Hum Reprod* 2001;16:2124–9

13. Coetsier T, Dhont M. Avoiding multiple pregnancies in *in-vitro* fertilization: who's afraid of single embryo transfer? *Hum Reprod* 1998;13:2663–4

14. Gerris J, De Neubourg D, Mangelschots K, *et al.* Prevention of twin pregnancy after *in-vitro* fertilization or intracytoplasmic sperm injection based on strict embryo criteria: a prospective randomized clinical trial. *Hum Reprod* 1999;14:2581–7

15. Gerris J, De Neubourg D, Mangelschots K, *et al.* Elective single day 3 embryo transfer halves the multiple pregnancy rate without decrease in the total multiple pregnancy rates of an IVF/ICSI programme. *Hum Reprod* 2002;17:2626–31

16. De Sutter P, Van der Elst J, Coetsier T, *et al.* Single embryo transfer and multiple pregnancy rate reduction in IVF/ICSI: a 5 year appraisal. *Reprod Biomed Online* 2003;6:464–9

17. Vilska S, Tiitinen A, Hydèn-Granskog C, *et al.* Elective transfer of one embryo results in an acceptable pregnancy rate and eliminates the risk of multiple birth. *Hum Reprod* 1999;14:2392–5

18. Martikainen H, Tiitinen A, Tomàs C, *et al.* One versus two embryo transfers after IVF and ICSI: randomized study. *Hum Reprod* 2001;16:1900–3

19. Tiitinen A, Halttunen M, Härkki P, *et al.* Elective embryo transfer: the value of cryopreservation. *Hum Reprod* 2001;16:1140–4

20. Van Royen E, Mangelschots K, De Neubourg, et al. Characterization of a top quality embryo, a step towards single-embryo transfer. *Hum Reprod* 1999;14:2345–9

21. Van Royen E, Mangelschots K, De Neubourg D, et al. Calculating the implantation potential of day 3 in women younger than 38 years of age: a new model. *Hum Reprod* 2001;16:326–32

22. Van Royen E, Mangelschots K, Vercruyssen M, et al. Multinucleation in cleavage stage embryos. *Hum Reprod* 2003;18:1062–9

23. Pickering BJ, Taylor A, Johnson MH, et al. An analysis of multinucleated blastomere formation in human embryos. *Mol Hum Reprod* 1995;10:1912–22

24. Jackson KV, Ginsburg ES, Hornstein MD, et al. Multinucleation in normally fertilized embryos is associated with an accelerated ovulation induction response and lower implantation and pregnancy rates in *in vitro* fertilization–embryo transfer cycles. *Fertil Steril* 1998;70:60–6

25. Pelinck MJ, De Vos M, Dekens M, et al. Embryos cultured *in vitro* with multinucleated blastomeres have poor implantation potential in human *in-vitro* fertilization and intracytoplasmic sperm injection. *Hum Reprod* 1998;13:960–3

26. Gerris J, De Neubourg D, Van Royen E, et al. Impact of transfer of a single top quality embryo on overall and twin pregnancy rates of a IVF/ICSI program. *Reprod Biomed Online* 2001;3:172–7

27. Van Blerkom J, Davis PW, Lee J. ATP content of human oocytes and developmental potential and outcome after *in-vitro* fertilization and embryo transfer. *Hum Reprod* 1995;10:415–24

28. Van Blerkom J, Antczak J, Schrader R. The developmental potential of the human oocyte is related to the dissolved oxygen content of follicular fluid: association with vascular endothelial growth factor levels and perifollic-ular blood flow characteristics. *Hum Reprod* 1997;12:1047–55

29. Van Blerkom J. Epigenetic influences on oocyte developmental competence: perifollicular vascularity and intrafollicular oxygen. *J Assist Reprod Genet* 1998;15:226–34

30. Scott LA, Smith S. The successful use of pronuclear embryo transfers the day following oocyte retrieval. *Hum Reprod* 1998;13:1003–13

31. Tesarik J, Junca AM, Hazout A, et al. Embryos with high implantation potential after intracytoplasmic sperm injection can be recognized by a simple, non-invasive examination of pronuclear morphology. *Hum Reprod* 2000;15:1396–9

32. Gardner DK, Lane M, Stevens J, et al. Blastocyst score affects implantation and pregnancy outcome: towards a single blastocyst transfer. *Fertil Steril* 2000;73:1155–8

33. Coskun S, Hollanders J, Al-Hassan S, et al. Day 5 versus day 3 embryo transfer: a controlled randomized trial. *Hum Reprod* 2000;15:1947–52

34. Utsunomiya T, Naitou T, Nagaki M. A prospective trial of blastocyst culture and transfer. *Hum Reprod* 2002;17:1846–51

35. Rienzi L, Ubaldi F, Iacobelli M, et al. Day 3 embryo transfer with combined evaluation at the pronuclear and cleavage stages compares favourably with day 5 blastocyst transfer. *Hum Reprod* 2002;17:1852–5

36. Bungum M, Bungum L, Humaidan P, Uding Andersen C. Day 3 versus day 5 embryo transfer: a prospective randomized study. *Reprod Biomed Online* 2003;7:98–104

37. Kolibianakis EM, Devroey P. Blastocyst culture: facts and fiction. *Reprod Biomed Online* 2002;5:285–93

8

Elective single-embryo transfer in the first cycle of *in vitro* fertilization/intracytoplasmic sperm injection

D. De Neubourg

INTRODUCTION

Multiple pregnancies are now the most important complication of assisted reproductive technologies (ART). As has been described previously, multiple pregnancies have an important impact on obstetric outcome and can be responsible for neonatal complications[1]. The impact on the economic situation of the future parents, and the psychosocial impact of complicated multiple pregnancies and affected children are well known to treating physicians[2]. Efforts have been made to calculate the direct and indirect costs for the whole family and for society[3,4].

The relatively poor success rates after *in vitro* fertilization (IVF) in the early days have made multiple embryo transfer generally accepted to compensate for low implantation rates. The multiple pregnancies that originated from multiple embryo transfer have long been considered an unavoidable and acceptable price to be paid for a reasonable pregnancy rate. The quality of the IVF laboratory has gradually improved, increasing the success rates; however, the incidence of multiple pregnancies has also increased. The efforts initiated in the early 1990s by Staessen and colleagues have led to the complete disappearance of triplet pregnancies, while maintaining a steady pregnancy rate when, in a selected population, a reduction of three to two embryos for transfer was performed[5,6]. However, the twin pregnancy rate unfortunately remained unaffected.

By introducing single-embryo transfer, a significant reduction in the incidence of twin pregnancies can be achieved.

DEFINITIONS

Single-embryo transfer is the transfer of one embryo, without further qualifications. Elective single-embryo transfer is the transfer of an embryo of top quality, assumed to have a high implantation potential. In principle, this is chosen from among at least two, but usually several embryos; occasionally, a top-quality embryo may be the only embryo available for transfer. Double-embryo transfer, is the transfer of two embryos, without further qualifications. Elective double-embryo transfer is the transfer of the two embryos with the putative highest implantation potential, chosen from among several embryos. Conception is pregnancy defined by two subsequently increasing values of human chorionic gonadotropin (hCG) of > 5 IU/l each. Conception rate is the number of conceptions/number of embryo transfers. Ongoing pregnancy is a pregnancy that evolves beyond 25 weeks. Ongoing pregnancy rate is the number of ongoing pregnancies/number of embryo transfers.

APPLICATION OF SINGLE-EMBRYO TRANSFER

Key factors in the single-embryo transfer strategy are embryo selection and patient selection. One can argue about which is the most important, but in our experience, they both need to be taken into consideration. If only one embryo is transferred irrespective of its putative quality, as assessed by morphological criteria, pregnancy rates will drop and become unacceptably low to both patients and clinicians[7]. If single-embryo transfer is applied in the older age group (above 38 years of age), one is very likely to end with a similar important drop in pregnancy rate. Both patient selection and selection of the embryo with the highest implantation potential have been dealt with in previous chapters.

Patient selection

A review of the literature has shown that every major change in embryo transfer strategy has been successfully introduced because of the precise analysis of the patient population with regard to parameters such as age, indication and response profile to gonadotropin stimulation, and of the cohort of embryos present on the day of the transfer. In the early 1990s, the relationship between embryo quality and the occurrence of pregnancy and multiple pregnancies was clearly demonstrated[5]. These authors defined an IVF patient population at risk for multiple pregnancies as women < 37 years of age who had at least six good-quality embryos in the first three IVF cycles. Coetsier and Dhont considered patients at risk for multiple pregnancies as women younger than 36 years of age, in the first three IVF cycles with at least three embryos with a good embryo score[8]. In two studies a multivariate analysis of the risk for multiple pregnancies was performed. A Swedish study showed that the age of the patient and the number of embryos transferred were independent factors to predict multiple births[9]. A Dutch study showed that young age and high quality of the transferred embryos were the best predictors for increased risk of multiple pregnancies[10].

When analyzing our own patient population to define patients at risk for twin pregnancies, we found that 80% of the twin pregnancies occurred in first and second cycles of IVF/intracytoplasmic

sperm injection (ICSI). The overall implantation rate of all transferred embryos was stable (25% for patients younger than 35 and 23% for women between 35 and 38) but showed a steep fall from the age of 38 onwards, with an overall implantation rate of 11%. In combination with the data from the literature, it was clear that patients younger than 38 in their first IVF/ICSI cycle were the target group.

Embryo selection

The aim of embryo selection is to select the embryo with the highest implantation potential. From a study in our center it was concluded that embryos that had four or five cells on day 2 after fertilization and seven or more on day 3, that showed not more than 20% of fragmented cells and never showed the presence of multinucleated blastomeres could be considered as embryos with excellent implantation potential[11]. The ongoing implantation rate of these embryos was 49% and they were therefore named 'top-quality embryos'. Owing to subsequent continuous evaluation of embryos with documented implantation outcome (either no implantation or 100% implantation) the range of embryos with high implantation potential was broadened. Embryos with two blastomeres on day 2 and six or more cells on day 3; and embryos with six cells on day 2 and ten or more on day 3; always with absence of multinucleated blastomeres, also showed high implantation potential and were considered for single-embryo transfer.

Experience with elective single-embryo transfer in clinical practice

We first introduced single-embryo transfer into clinical practice in a prospective randomized trial[12]. Patients younger than 34 years, in their first IVF/ICSI cycle, who had at least two embryos of excellent quality, were randomized to have either one or two embryos transferred. A total of 53 patients were included in the final analysis – 26 in the single-embryo transfer study arm and 27 in the double-embryo transfer study arm (Table 1). After single-embryo transfer the ongoing pregnancy and implantation rate was 38.5%; there was one monozygotic twin pregnancy. For the double-embryo transfer group the ongoing pregnancy rate was 74.1% with an implantation rate of 48.1%. In this group there were six twin pregnancies for a multiple pregnancy rate of 30%. This study confirmed that the chance of conception and of multiple pregnancies was related to the number of excellent-quality embryos transferred, but the most important conclusion was that single-embryo transfer could lead to a conception and ongoing pregnancy rate comparable to those for the whole program. Therefore, single-embryo transfer could be introduced into IVF/ICSI without a decline in conception rate.

From January 2000 until December 2001 we introduced single-embryo transfer in the first IVF/ICSI cycle in all patients < 38 years of age. We evaluated the impact of the patients' choice for single-embryo transfer of a top-quality embryo versus double-embryo transfer in the first IVF/ICSI cycle[13]. This study analyzed the outcome of 243 transfers in 262 patients (Table 2). Of the patients, 64% chose transfer of a single top-quality embryo, if available, and two non-top-quality embryos if no top-quality embryo was available; 36% of the patients chose to have double-embryo transfer regardless of embryo quality. The first group of patients had an ongoing pregnancy rate of 40% with 2% twin pregnancies; the second group had an ongoing pregnancy rate of 44% with 26% twin pregnancies. This study showed single-embryo transfer of a top-quality embryo in the first IVF/ICSI cycle could systematically be introduced into the program, which has been carried out.

The following describes the impact of single-embryo transfer in the *first* IVF/ICSI cycle since its introduction in 1998 on the ongoing pregnancy rate and multiple pregnancy rates.

Table 1   Outcome of the prospective randomized single-embryo transfer (SET)/double-embryo transfer (DET) trial

	SET		DET	
	n	%	n	%
Patients	26		27	
Conceptions	17	65.4	22	81.5
Ongoing pregnancies	10	38.5	20	74.1
Twin pregnancies	1	10.0	6	30.0
Implantations	10	38.5	26	48.1

Table 2   Clinical outcome of patients after choice for single-embryo transfer (SET) of a top-quality embryo or double-embryo transfer (DET)

	SET		DET	
	n	%	n	%
Patients' choice	156	64	87	36
Ongoing pregnancies	63	40	38	44
Singleton pregnancies	62	98	28	74
Twin pregnancies	1	2	10	26

Characteristics of the first *in vitro* fertilization/intracytoplasmic sperm injection cycle

The introduction and the outcome of elective single-embryo transfer from January 1998 until December 2002 is evaluated. In this 5-year period, 1987 cycles were performed in our center of which 1882 underwent embryo transfer (95%). Of these embryo transfer cycles, 944 were first cycles (50%). Analysis of the age of the patients who received single-embryo transfer in the first cycle showed that 135/328 (41%) were < 30 years of age, 143/328 (44%) were between 30 and 35 years of age, 45/328 (14%) were between 35 and 38 years of age, and 5/328 (1%) were > 38 years of age. Obviously, women of > 38 years of age were not the target group for performing single-embryo transfer.

The indication for IVF/ICSI in the first cycle was female pathology in 78/328 (24%), male pathology in 172/328 (52%) cycles, mixed pathology in 38/328 (12%) and 40/328 (12%) were cases of unknown etiology. In 177/328 (54%) IVF was performed, and in 151/328 (46%) of first cycles ICSI was performed.

The type of embryo transfer in the first IVF/ICSI cycle is shown in Table 3. The number of first treatment cycles in which the patient chose to have single-embryo transfer of a top-quality embryo increased from 51% to 90% over this 5-year period. Consequently, the number of cycles in which a single-embryo of top quality was actually available and transferred increased from 15% to 51% over this 5-year period (Figure 1). There was a decrease in double-embryo transfers in favor of single-embryo transfers.

Table 3 Characteristics of first *in vitro* fertilization/intracytoplasmic sperm injection cycle

	1998	1999	2000	2001	2002
Total number of ovum pick-ups	335	406	395	410	441
Total number of transfers	317 (95%)	388 (96%)	370 (94%)	389 (95%)	418 (95%)
Total transfers in first cycles	171 (54%)	197 (51%)	177 (48%)	195 (50%)	204 (49%)
Number of patients with choice SET	87 (51%)	111 (56%)	93 (53%)	103 53%)	184 90%)
Number of cycles where a top-quality embryo was present	121 (71%)	134 (68%)	123 (69%)	112 (57%)	114 (56%)
Number of cycles with SET of a top-quality embryo	26 (15%)	56 (28%)	73 (41%)	68 (35%)	105 (51%)
Number of cycles with SET of a non-top-quality embryo	9 (5%)	17 (9%)	16 (9%)	14 (7%)	22 (11%)
Number of cycles with DET (two top-quality embryo)	43 (25%)	49 (25%)	27 (15%)	22 (11%)	2 (1%)
Number of cycles with DET (one top-quality embryo)	38 (22%)	20 (10%)	19 (11%)	18 (9%)	3 (1%)
Number of cycles with DET (no top-quality embryo)	35 (20%)	37 (19%)	36 (20%)	68 (35%)	66 (32%)
Number of cycles with transfer of > 2 embryos	20 (12%)	18 (9%)	6 (3%)	5 (3%)	6 (3%)

SET, single-embryo transfer; DET, double-embryo transfer

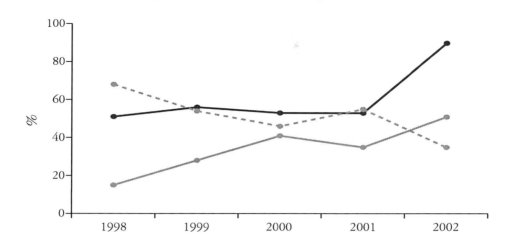

Figure 1   Type of transfer in the first *in vitro* fertilization/intracytoplasmic sperm injection cycle: choice of single-embryo transfer (SET) with a top-quality embryo (solid black); study SET with a top-quality embryo (gray); double-embryo transfer (dashed)

The percentage of first cycles in which a top-quality embryo was available and thus single-embryo transfer of a top-quality embryo could be considered varied between 71% in 1998 and 56% in 2002 (Table 3). Although the initial criteria for selection of an embryo with high implantation potential were broadened over this 5-year period in terms of cleavage speed and fragmentation rate, we noted a decrease in the number of cycles in which a top-quality embryo was available. This might be explained by the elaborate search for the presence of multinucleated blastomeres, the detection of which has increased from 17% to 40% since the importance for the prediction of implantation was recognized[14].

Outcome of single-embryo transfer of a top-quality embryo in the first cycle

When the outcome of the transfer of one top-quality embryo in the first cycle was analyzed in relation to age (Table 4) we observed a fairly stable conception rate, varying between 57% for patients of ≤ 30 years of age to 48.9% in the group between 35 and 38 years of age. There was an important decline in the patients of ≥ 38 of age, where a conception rate of only 20% was noted. As previously mentioned, this is not the target group for elective single-embryo transfer; however, some couples were so highly motivated to avoid the chance of a twin pregnancy that they requested elective single-embryo transfer even if a top-quality embryo was not available. The ongoing pregnancy rate was 38.1% for the whole group, but showed a decline with increasing age. There were two monozygotic twins in this elective single-embryo transfer group.

When the outcome of embryo transfers other than those of a single top-quality embryo in first treatment cycles was analyzed, we observed a fairly stable pregnancy rate of 50.5% for the women of ≤ 30 years of age and of 48.2% in those of 35–38 years of age. In the group of women of ≥ 38 years of age the conception rate was 37.9% (Table 5).

When the outcome of single top-quality embryo transfer was analyzed in the main twin-prevention target group of women of < 38 years of age, there were 181 conceptions in 323 first treatment cycles (56%); in the other than elective single-embryo transfer first treatment cycles there were 260 conceptions in 529 cycles (49%). The OR for a conception for elective single-embryo transfer cycles

Table 4   Outcome of transfer of a top-quality embryo in the first cycle

	Age (years)				
	≤ 30	30–35	35–38	≥ 38	Total
Total number of embryo transfers	135	143	45	5	328
Number of conceptions	77	82	22	1	182
Total conception rate (%)	57.0	57.3	48.9	20.0	55.5
Number of ongoing pregnancies	58	53	13	1	125
Ongoing singletons	56	53	13	1	123
Ongoing twins	2	0	0	0	2
Ongoing pregnancy rate (%)	43.0	37.1	28.9	20.0	38.1

Table 5   Outcome of other than top-quality embryo transfers in the first cycle

	Age (years)				
	≤ 30	30–35	35–38	≥ 38	Total
Total number of embryo transfers	196	248	85	87	616
Number of conceptions	99	120	41	33	293
Total conception rate (%)	50.5	48.4	48.2	37.9	47.6
Number of ongoing pregnancies	79	84	27	16	206
Ongoing singletons	52	59	16	11	138
Ongoing twins	26	25	10	4	65
Ongoing triplets	1	0	1	1	3
Multiple pregnancy rate (%)	34	30	41	31	33
Ongoing pregnancy rate (%)	40.3	33.9	31.8	18.4	33.4

versus other types of embryo transfer was 1.31 (95% CI 0.99–1.74). The multiple pregnancy rate in the first treatment cycle with other than elective single-embryo transfer was 33%. These data clearly show that after progressive implementation of single-embryo transfer in the target group for prevention of twin pregnancies, i.e. in the first IVF/ICSI cycle in patients < 38 years of age, the transfer of one embryo after careful selection of the embryo with the highest implantation potential did not decrease the chance for conception, whereas the double-embryo transfer group had a 33% risk of multiple pregnancy.

As expected, patients < 35 years of age had a high pregnancy rate as well as a high multiple pregnancy rate. However, women 35–38 years of age demonstrated a high conception rate in the elective single-embryo transfer group as well (48.9%), comparable to that after other than elective single-embryo transfers (48.2%). It is therefore not surprising that they also showed a high multiple pregnancy rate (41%). These data clearly demonstrate that this group of patients should also be offered single-embryo transfer if a top-quality embryo is available. The recommendation to transfer a top-quality embryo, if available, to women in this age group, should not be lightly dismissed.

When single-embryo transfer of a top-quality embryo is compared to other transfers in the first cycle, the data show that the chance of conception as well as the chance for multiple pregnancies are related to the number of top-quality embryos (Table 6).

Elective single-embryo transfer in subsequent cycles

These excellent conception rates after elective single-embryo transfer encouraged us further to implement elective single-embryo transfer in the second and higher-rank cycles. From our own data and from the analysis of the characteristics of patients at risk for twin and multiple pregnancies, it was clear that second and third cycles were also at risk. The question was raised whether the criteria for selection of the embryo with the highest implantation potential would yield similar high conception rates in second and higher-rank cycles. Therefore, we compared single-embryo transfer of a top-quality embryo in the first cycle with single-embryo transfer of a top-quality embryo in the second or higher-rank cycle (Table 7). Although the number

of cycles analyzed was limited, elective single-embryo transfer cycles in second or higher-rank cycles also yielded a high pregnancy rate of 47.4% (76.3% of these cycles were second IVF/ICSI cycles). This is not significantly different from the conception rate of 55.5% in the first cycle (OR 1.38; 95% CI 0.92–2.06). These are important data to be taken into account when further implementation of single-embryo transfer in the general program is considered. Second cycles particularly should be the target for further implementation of single-embryo transfer of a top-quality embryo, since we and others found that the first and second cycles carried a high risk for multiple pregnancies. The impact of further implementation of single-embryo transfer of a top-quality embryo in other than first cycles on the multiple pregnancy rate of the whole program is discussed elsewhere.

Counseling towards elective single-embryo transfer

These data have been collected over a 5-year period, during which elective single-embryo transfer has been gradually implemented. The selection of the embryo with the highest implantation potential was the milestone to start the successful introduction of

Table 6 Outcome of transfer of a top-quality embryo in first cycle compared to other embryo transfers

	SET top-quality	SET non-top-quality	DET 2 top-quality	DET 1 top-quality	DET 0 top-quality
Total number of embryo transfers	328	78	143	98	242
Number of conceptions	182	25	103	56	86
Total conception rate (%)	55.5	32	72	57	36
Number of ongoing pregnancies	125	18	82	44	55
Ongoing singletons	123	17	51	21	45
Ongoing twins	2	1	29	22	10
Ongoing triplets	0	0	2	1	0
Multiple pregnancy rate (%)	0.01	4	30	41	11
Ongoing pregnancy rate (%)	38.1	23	57	45	23

SET, single-embryo transfer; DET, double-embryo transfer

Table 7   Outcome of transfer of a top-quality embryo in second or higher-rank cycles

	Age (years)				
	≤ 30	*30–35*	*35–38*	*≥ 38*	*Total*
Total number of embryo transfers	40	64	25	6	135
Number of conceptions	16	29	17	2	64
Total conception rate (%)	40	45.3	68	33.3	47.4
Number of ongoing conceptions	13	14	10	2	39
Ongoing singletons	13	14	10	2	39
Ongoing twins	0	0	0	0	0
Ongoing pregnancy rate (%)	32.5	21.9	40.0	33.3	28.9

elective single-embryo transfer. A prospective randomized study in a selected young motivated population confirmed the possibilities of elective single-embryo transfer[12]. These data provided strong arguments which we could use for the counseling of young patients in their first IVF/ICSI cycle. Although many patients had become aware of the possible risks and complications of twin pregnancies, many couples still felt that they had to take all their chances by choosing double-embryo transfer. Because it was not our aim to impose the elective single-embryo transfer strategy, we started a study in which we evaluated the patients' choice of single-embryo transfer of a top-quality embryo versus double-embryo transfer in their first IVF/ICSI cycle[13]. The patients whose choice was single-embryo transfer, on the condition that one top-quality embryo was available, received one top-quality embryo or two embryos if there was no top-quality embryo available; this group had an ongoing pregnancy rate of 40% with 2% twin pregnancies. The patient group who chose two embryos regardless of the embryo quality had an ongoing pregnancy rate of 44% with 26% twin pregnancies (Table 2). Since this large study with 262 patients in their first cycle showed that elective single-embryo transfer did not decrease the patients' chance of success and protected them from a 26% chance of twin pregnancies, we feel it is our medical duty to convince the patients to have only one embryo transferred if an embryo with high implantation

potential is available. After this study was completed, 90% of the patients in their first IVF/ICSI cycle chose elective single-embryo transfer.

Augmenting the impact of a cryopreservation program

First IVF/ICSI cycles in which elective single-embryo transfer was applied yielded on average 1.5 embryos for cryopreservation versus 0.5 embryos in the group of patients choosing double-embryo transfer[13]. To fully appreciate the chances of pregnancy after elective single-embryo transfer, pregnancies occurring after frozen–thawed cycles should be added to pregnancies from fresh transfer. This was shown in a Finnish study[15]. These authors analyzed 127 fresh single-embryo transfer cycles (clinical pregnancy rate of 38.6%) and 129 frozen–thawed cycles in 83 patients. In 46 frozen–thawed cycles one embryo was transferred (clinical pregnancy rate of 17%) and in 83 frozen–thawed cycles two embryos were transferred (clinical pregnancy rate of 37.3%). The cumulative delivery rate per oocyte retrieval was 52.8% with a twin pregnancy rate of 7.6%. These authors clearly showed the importance of a good cryopreservation program by its ability to augment the success obtained with fresh single-embryo transfer. Full implementation of elective single-embryo transfer will become easier if a well-performing cryopreservation program can be combined with it.

REFERENCES

1. Bergh T, Ericsson A, Hillensjö T, *et al.* Deliveries and children born after *in-vitro* fertilisation in Sweden 1982–95: a retrospective cohort study. *Lancet* 1999;453:1579–85

2. Scholz T, Bartholomaus S, Grimmer I, *et al.* Problems of multiple birth after ART: medical, psychological, social and financial aspects. *Hum Reprod* 1999;14:2932–7

3. Collins J. An international survey of health economics of IVF and ICSI. *Hum Reprod Update* 2002;8:265–77

4. De Sutter P, Gerris J, Dhont M. A health-economic decision-analytic model comparing double with single embryo transfer in IVF/ICSI. *Hum Reprod* 2002;17:2891–6

5. Staessen C, Camus M, Bollen N, *et al.* The relationship between embryo quality and the occurrence of multiple pregnancies. *Fertil Steril* 1992;57:626–30

6. Staessen C, Janssenswillen C, Van Den Abbeel E, *et al.* Avoidance of triplet pregnancies by elective transfer of two good quality embryos. *Hum Reprod* 1993;8:1650–3

7. Giorgetti C, Terriou P, Auquie RP, *et al.* Embryo score to predict implantation after *in-vitro* fertilization based on 957 single embryo transfers. *Hum Reprod* 1995;10:2427–31

8. Coetsier T, Dhont M. Avoiding multiple pregnancies in *in-vitro* fertilization: who's afraid of single embryo transfer? *Hum Reprod* 1998;13:2663–70

9. Strandell A, Bergh C, Lundin K. Selection of patients suitable for one-embryo transfer may reduce the rate of multiple births by half without impairment of overall birth rates. *Hum Reprod* 2000;15:2520–5

10. Hunault CC, Eijkemans MJC, Pieters MHEC, *et al.* A prediction model for selecting patients undergoing *in vitro* fertilization for elective single embryo transfer. *Fertil Steril* 2002;77:725–32

11. Van Royen E, Mangelschots K, De Neubourg D, *et al.* Characterization of a top quality embryo, a step towards single-embryo transfer. *Hum Reprod* 1999;14:2345–9

12. Gerris J, De Neubourg D, Mangelschots K, *et al.* Prevention of twin pregnancy after *in-vitro* fertilization or intracytoplasmic sperm injection based on strict embryo criteria: a prospective randomized clinical trial. *Hum Reprod* 1999;14:2581–7

13. De Neubourg D, Mangelschots K, Van Royen E, *et al.* Impact of patients' choice for single embryo transfer of a top quality embryo versus double embryo transfer in the first IVF/ICSI cycle. *Hum Reprod* 2002;17:2621–5

14. Van Royen E, Mangelschots K, Vercruyssen M, *et al.* Multinucleation in cleavage stage embryos. *Hum Reprod* 2003;18:1062–9

15. Tiitinen A, Halttunen M, Härkki P, *et al.* Elective single embryo transfer: the value of cryopreservation. *Hum Reprod* 2001;16:1140–4

9

National experience with elective single-embryo transfer

Introduction

J. Gerris

In this chapter, the experience to date with elective single-embryo transfer is described in four European countries, in two of which (Finland and Belgium) the idea was pioneered, and in two of which (Sweden and The Netherlands) the *in vitro* fertilization (IVF) community was quick to follow. It is clear that others also have taken the way of elective single-embryo transfer. A Slovenian group has published a retrospective randomized trial comparing the transfer of one or two day-2 versus one or two day-5 embryos obtained after IVF/intracytoplasmic sperm injection (ICSI)[1]. They did not find a difference between day-2 versus day-5 transfers but failed to mention the results in the subsets of patients receiving only one embryo ($n = 62$ for day-2 and $n = 46$ for day-5 single-embryo transfers). A Spanish group reported their experience with the transfer of one versus two embryos, showing a pregnancy rate of 42.2% with elective single-embryo transfer versus 68.6% for elective double-embryo transfer with 54.2% twins[2]. An Australian group compared elective single-embryo transfer on day 5 with two-embryo transfer on day 5 and did not find a diminished live birth rate[3]. The live birth rate per embryo was 36% in both groups; however, the twinning rate was 50% in the double-embryo transfer group. Using frozen–thawed embryos the cumulative pregnancy rate was 60% for both groups. Other centers have initial experience with elective single-embryo transfer confirming ongoing pregnancy rates of around 35%.

This is the place to express the hope that, from now onwards, national, supranational and world registries of IVF/ICSI will include in their figures the percentage of elective single-embryo transfers performed and the results obtained in that group of patients. This will allow for the much-needed long-term follow-up of declining twin (and high-order) pregnancy rates worldwide, while keeping an eye on the overall pregnancy rates. These figures will yield the ultimate criterion for an improvement of the clinical safety of these treatments. In parallel, ART results should no longer be expressed as crude frequency rates, but as the percentage of started cycles ending in the birth of one healthy child.

REFERENCES

1. Kovacic B, Vlaisavljevic V, Reljic M, *et al.* Clinical outcome of day 2 versus day 5 transfer in cycles with one or two developed embryos. *Fertil Steril* 2002;77:529–33

2. Tur R, Coroleu B, Veiga A, *et al.* Elective single embryo transfer: one versus two embryos. *Abstracts Book for the 19th ESHRE Annual Meeting*, Madrid, O-391. *Hum Reprod* 2003;18:133

3. Catt J, Henman M, Wood T, Jansen R. Elective single embryo transfer on day 5 does not diminish live birth rates. *Abstracts Book for the 19th ESHRE Annual Meeting*, Madrid, O-015. *Hum Reprod* 2003;18:5

a. Finland

S. Vilska and A. Tiitinen

INTRODUCTION

In comparison with the incidence of twins after spontaneous conception (about 1%), the incidence of multiple pregnancies is more than 20 times higher after the use of assisted reproductive technologies (ART). In Europe, the overall multiple pregnancy rate in 1999 was 26.3%. Of all multiple pregnancies, 24% were twins, 2.2% triplets and 0.1% quadruplets[1]. Thus, nearly half of the children conceived with ART have originated from multiple pregnancies.

In the early 1990s many European countries accepted the strategy of transferring only two embryos at a time, in order to avoid multiple pregnancies. In Finland the transition to the two-embryo-transfer policy took place in 1993–94; since then triplet pregnancies following ART have occurred only occasionally. However, in spite of this change in embryo transfer (ET) policy, the proportion of twin births has still remained high, accounting for 20–25% of all births after ART.

Multiple gestation should be considered as the main complication of ART. Compared to singletons, not only triplets but also twin pregnancies carry more maternal, fetal and neonatal risks. Prematurity is the most frequent and the most serious risk for the newborn. Almost half of the twin pregnancies after ART have resulted in birth before the 37th gestational week, and about 40% of twin newborns are of low birth weight (< 2500 g). The perinatal mortality rate in twins is nearly five times as high as that in singletons. Perinatal complications may lead to long-term consequences resulting in a variety of disabilities. Multiple birth, even twins, is the main factor affecting the health of the children conceived with ART[2,3].

In addition, prematurity and perinatal problems of the children as well as the twin birth itself may cause impaired psychosocial well-being of the family. Moreover, the health-economic concerns are important. The World Health Organization (WHO) recommends that, during ART, attention be paid to the impact of multiple gestation[4]. With respect to the medical and psychosocial risks, the high total number of twin pregnancies following ART is no longer acceptable, and reduction of the number of twins has become one of the main challenges in ART.

FACTORS INFLUENCING THE RISK FOR A TWIN PREGNANCY AFTER ART

The age of the mother, the number of good-quality embryos, the rank of the ART cycle and the number of embryos transferred as well as previous birth all predict good prognosis in ART[5,6]. If more than one embryo is transferred, the age of the mother, the number of good-quality embryos and the number of previous ART cycles are the most significant factors affecting the risk of a multiple gestation[6,7]. In a Finnish retrospective analysis of 2223 fresh *in vitro* fertilization (IVF)/intracytoplasmic sperm injection (ICSI) cycles, the correlation between the twinning rate and the age of the woman was found to be very clear. After two-embryo transfer the twinning rate was 39% in women aged < 30 years, 27% in women aged 30–35 years and 15% in women aged > 35 years[8]. The multiple pregnancy rate clearly correlates with the number of embryos transferred[5]. If three to six embryos were transferred, the pregnancy rate per ET was 37.5–50%, but the multiple pregnancy rate was 34–50%. In earlier studies the pregnancy rate after one-embryo transfer in cycles where only one embryo was available was as low as < 10%, which has further encouraged clinicians to transfer more embryos at a time if available[9].

TOWARDS ELECTIVE SINGLE-EMBRYO TRANSFER

In Finland the application of elective single-embryo transfer started in 1997. In the beginning, this was recommended to women in whom a twin pregnancy could be predicted to carry special obstetric and/or neonatal risk. This is the case for women with a chronic illness such as diabetes mellitus, or women with a history of hysterotomy who are exposed to an increased risk of obstetric complications. Apart from offering elective single-embryo transfer to these women with a specific medical contraindication for a twin pregnancy, this was also proposed to couples with an indication for prenatal diagnosis and to couples who expressed a clear wish of their own to avoid a twin pregnancy. The results of elective single-embryo transfer in these special groups of patients were encouraging[10]. The results of these initial data revealed a different prognosis between cases of elective single-embryo transfer and cases of single-embryo transfer when only one embryo was available (Table 1).

In a prospective randomized study carried out in three large clinics in Finland, 144 couples were randomized to elective single-embryo or double-embryo transfer[11]. Inclusion criteria were: at least four good-quality embryos and no more than one previous failed IVF or ICSI cycle. The pregnancy rate per ET after elective single-embryo transfer was 32%, and 47% after double-embryo transfer. This difference was not statistically significant. The twin pregnancy rate in the double-embryo group was 39% whereas in the elective single-embryo group there was only one pair of monozygotic twins. The cumulative pregnancy rate per patient after the transfer of fresh and frozen embryos was 47.3% in the single-embryo group and 58.5% in the double-embryo group.

In a retrospective follow-up study all the embryo transfers carried out at the Infertility Clinic of

Helsinki University Central Hospital during 1998–99 were analyzed[12]. The pregnancy rate per ET in 127 women receiving an elective single-embryo transfer was 38.6%; after the transfer of two embryos it was 40.0%. The twin birth rate after double-embryo transfer was 26.2%. There was again one pair of monozygotic twins after single-embryo transfer in this group. The cumulative pregnancy rate per oocyte retrieval after both fresh and frozen transfers was 58.5% in the single-embryo group and 62.2% in the double-embryo group (NS).

ELECTIVE SINGLE-EMBRYO TRANSFER IN CLINICAL PRACTICE

After this preliminary experience with elective single-embryo transfer in 1997, it has been accepted as a part of embryo transfer policy at the Infertility Clinic of the Helsinki University Central Hospital and at the Infertility Clinic of the Family Federation of Finland. Since 1998 the proportion of elective single-embryo transfers has increased progressively. Now, approximately half of day-2 or day-3 fresh embryo transfers are elective single-embryo transfers. The increased application of elective single-embryo transfer has resulted in a substantial reduction in the twin delivery rate after ART without affecting the pregnancy and delivery rates. In 2001 a total of 623 fresh IVF/ICSI cycles with ET on day 2 or 3 were performed. Of these, 307 (49.3%) were elective single-embryo transfers. The twin delivery rate was only 7.8%, whereas the overall pregnancy rate and delivery rates remained unchanged (Table 2).

Table 1   Pregnancy rate (PR) per embryo transfer (ET) and multiple delivery rate following the transfer of two embryos, elective single-embryo transfer and transfer of one embryo, when only one embryo was available

	Number of ETs	Clinical PR/ET		Twin PR	
		n	%	n	%
Double-embryo transfer	742	218	29.4	52	23.9
Elective single-embryo transfer	74	22	29.7	0	
Only one embryo	94	19	20.2	0	

Table 2   The number of elective single-embryo transfers (eSET), two-embryo transfers (two ET) and only one ET in the case when only one embryo is available, clinical pregnancies and the twin birth rate in *in vitro* fertilization and intracytoplasmic sperm injection cycles performed during 1998–2001 at the infertility clinic of Helsinki University Central Hospital and at the Family Federation of Finland

	1998	1999	2000	2001
All fresh ETs (*n*)	869	857	773	623
Pregnancies (*n*)	286	307	267	196
%	32.9	35.8	34.5	31.5
eSET (*n*)	136	196	303	307
% of all ETs	15.7	22.9	39.2	49.3
Pregnancies (*n*)	48	68	118	105
%	35.3	34.7	38.9	34.2
Only one ET (*n*)	113	98	88	69
% of all ETs	13.0	11.4	11.4	11.1
Pregnancies (*n*)	16	18	13	12
%	14.2	18.4	14.8	17.4
Two ETs (*n*)	620	563	382	247
% of all ETs	71.3	65.7	49.4	39.6
Pregnancies (*n*)	222	221	136	79
%	35.8	39.3	35.6	32.0
Twins/births	49/215	62/240	27/214	12/154
% of all births	22.8	25.8	12.6	7.8

ELECTIVE SINGLE-EMBRYO TRANSFER IN A COUNTRY-WIDE PERSPECTIVE

There are 17 IVF clinics in Finland. Thirteen of these perform more than 100 IVF/ICSI cycles per year. In Finland 4280 IVF/ICSI cycles were carried out in 2001. The number of frozen ETs was 2436.

Three large clinics in Finland have accepted the elective single-embryo transfer policy to some extent; about half of their fresh ETs are elective single-embryo transfers. Using this policy clinical pregnancy and delivery rates have remained unchanged, and the twin birth rate has been lower than 10%[13]. According to the Finnish IVF registry the proportion of single-embryo transfers has increased since 1997 (Figure 1). Because the proportion of IVF cycles where there is only one embryo available is fairly stable, it is expected that other Finnish IVF clinics will follow the tendency to increase the number of elective single-embryo transfers. The effect of the increased application of elec-

tive single-embryo transfer is already reflected in the significant decrease in the proportion of twin deliveries after ART in the IVF statistics of the whole of Finland (Figure 2) as well as in the proportion of multiple deliveries in the country (Figure 3).

ELECTIVE SINGLE-EMBRYO TRANSFER IN AN OVUM-DONATION PROGRAM

High pregnancy and delivery rates are reported in most ovum-donation programs. Oocyte recipients are at high risk of obstetric complications, which is an important indication to avoid twins in this special group of patients[14].

In the ovum-donation program at the Infertility Clinic of the Family Federation of Finland, the application of elective single-embryo transfer has increased progressively. During 1998–99 the proportion of elective single-embryo transfers in oocyte recipients was 17% (13/76) of fresh embryo

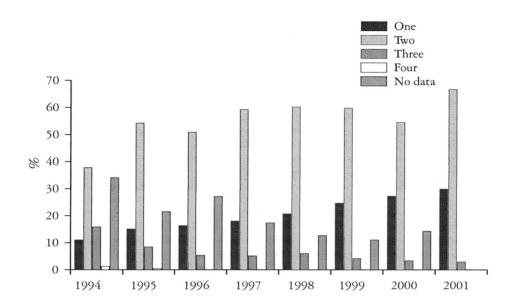

Figure 1 The number of embryos used per transfer in Finland, 1994–2000. From National Research and Development Center for Welfare and Health/IVF statistics 2003

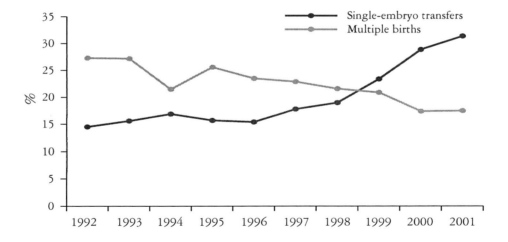

Figure 2 The percentage of single-embryo transfers of all embryo transfers and the percentage of multiple births of all births after assisted reproductive technologies in Finland 1992–2001. From National Research and Development Centre for Welfare and Health/IVF Statistics 2003

transfers. The clinical pregnancy rate per ET was 36.8% and the delivery rate per ET was 31.6%. The twin birth rate was 29.2%. During the subsequent period, between 2000 and 2001, the proportion of elective single-embryo transfers increased to 61% (36/59) of fresh embryo transfers. The clinical preg-nancy rate per ET was 45.8% and the delivery rate per ET was 33.9%. Only 10% of the deliveries were twins. A three-fold increase in the proportion of elective single-embryo transfers in our ovum-dona-tion program resulted in a substantial decrease in the twin birth rate without affecting the overall

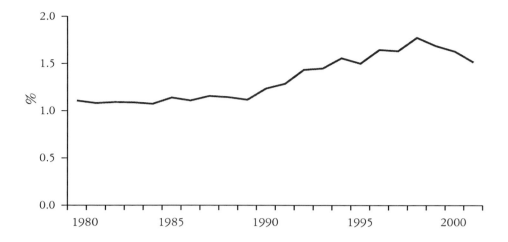

Figure 3 The percentage of multiple deliveries out of all deliveries, Finland, 1980–2001. From Medical Birth Register

clinical pregnancy and delivery rates. Now we recommend elective single-embryo transfer as the first choice to couples treated with ovum donation[15].

THE EMBRYOLOGICAL BASIS FOR ELECTIVE SINGLE-EMBRYO TRANSFER

Embryo quality is obviously the most significant single factor predicting a successful outcome of ART. Our initial data on elective single-embryo transfer showed that the implantation rate for day-2 embryos with four cells was significantly higher than that for two- or three-cell embryos. The degree of fragmentation of the blastomeres was also shown to correlate with the implantation rate of the embryos[10]. The top-quality embryo with < 20% fragmentation and no multinucleated blastomeres had an implantation rate of 39.8%[12]. In an analysis of 178 elective single-embryo transfer cycles, a correlation between an early first cleavage of the embryo and the pregnancy rate as well as the morphology of the embryo was found[16]. In this study the clinical pregnancy rate was significantly higher after the transfer of an embryo with early first cleavage than of an embryo with late first cleavage (50.0 vs. 26.4%). The proportion of embryos with fragmentation of < 20% as well as the propor-

tion of embryos with mononucleated blastomeres were significantly higher among embryos with early first cleavage. In addition, early-cleaved embryos possessed significantly more blastomeres on day 2 after fertilization[16]. In contrast, pronuclear morphology of zygotes did not have any predictive value with regard to embryo morphology or implantation or pregnancy rates in 144 cycles with single-embryo transfer[17].

Based on our experience we have defined a good-quality embryo as follows: an embryo with early first cleavage (approximately 25 h after fertilization) resulting in the four-cell stage on day 2 or at least in the six-cell stage on day 3 after ovum pick-up, with mononucleated blastomeres and with a degree of fragmentation of < 20%.

THE VALUE OF CRYOPRESERVATION IN ELECTIVE SINGLE-EMBRYO TRANSFER PROGRAMS

A successful cryopreservation program to preserve supernumerary embryos is necessary and of great importance when elective single-embryo transfer is used. As presented before, the cumulative pregnancy rate per oocyte harvest after the combination of a fresh elective single embryo and subsequent frozen embryo transfers is acceptable. In comparison with other European countries the number of frozen embryo transfers in Finland is high[1]. According to the Finnish IVF registry, 39% (2436/6254) of all embryo transfers in 2001 were frozen embryo transfers and 31.1% (362/1165) of all IVF/ICSI deliveries were the result of frozen embryo transfers. In the randomized study by the Finnish ET Study Group the proportion of pregnancies following frozen embryo transfer was 33% after elective single-embryo transfer and 19% after double-embryo transfer[11]. Based on these Finnish data, frozen embryo transfer is an effective treatment, especially in patients with a good prognosis and suitable for elective single-embryo transfer. The significance of cryopreservation should be considered when the total effectiveness of elective single-embryo transfer is evaluated.

IN WHOM SHOULD WE PERFORM ELECTIVE SINGLE-EMBRYO TRANSFER?

Optimally, elective single-embryo transfer should be offered to women who are at risk of a twin pregnancy. Both clinical and embryological factors should be considered in decision-making. The age of the woman younger than 36 years and the number of good-quality embryos available are factors predicting a twin pregnancy after two-embryo transfer[6,7]. However, regarding the prognosis of elective single-embryo transfer, the most important factor is obviously the quality of the embryo.

Initially we recommended elective single-embryo transfer in women younger than 36 years of age, during the first or second IVF or ICSI cycle and if there was at least one good-quality embryo available. However, with increasing experience the recommendations for elective single-embryo transfer have widened. When there is a medical indication to avoid a multiple gestation or if the couple has expressed a clear wish to avoid a multiple pregnancy, elective single-embryo transfer is performed even more liberally.

COUNSELING OF THE COUPLE

Many couples do not consider a twin or even a high-order pregnancy as a failure of ART[18]. However, after careful counseling giving the results after elec-tive single-embryo transfer followed by frozen embryo transfer as well as information regarding the risks of multiple pregnancy, the majority of couples in our experience want to minimize the risk of a twin pregnancy. Since we began to perform elective single-embryo transfers, the attitude of the patients has changed. Many of them ask for the transfer of one embryo. However, most of the couples will leave the final decision to be made by the team of clinicians and embryologists, when the result of the ovarian stimulation and especially the quality of the embryos is known. According to our experience, it is important that the principles of the number of the embryos to be transferred are discussed with the couple when the treatment is planned, well before the embryo transfer.

SUMMARY

The Finnish experience confirms the significance of elective single-embryo transfer as a method for reducing the proportion of twin pregnancies resulting from ART. In clinics where elective single-embryo transfer is performed in approximately half of the IVF/ICSI cycles, the twin birth rate has decreased below 10%, whereas the pregnancy and delivery rates have remained unchanged at a very acceptable overall level of approximately 30% ongoing pregnancies per egg retrieval. The effect of the increased use of elective single-embryo transfer has already been observed as a reduction in the proportion of twin deliveries following ART in Finland, as well as in a reduction of the proportion of multiple births in the Finnish Medical Birth Register.

ACKNOWLEDGEMENTS

We would like to acknowledge Professsor Outi Hovatta, Hannu Martikainen, Viveca Söderström-Anttila, Sirpa Mäkinen, Christel Hydén-Granskog, Mika Gissler and all the other staff of the IVF teams at the Family Federation of Finland, at the Helsinki University Hospital and Oulu University Hospital for their collaboration.

REFERENCES

1. ESHRE. The European IVF-monitoring programme (EIM) for the European Society of Human Reproduction and Embryology (ESHRE). Assisted reproductive technology in Europe, 1999. Results generated from registers by ESHRE. *Hum Reprod* 2002;17:3260–74

2. Klemetti R, Gissler M. Comparison of perinatal health of children born from IVF in Finland in the early and late 1990s. *Hum Reprod* 2002;17:2192–8

3. Koivurova S, Hartikainen A-L, Gissler M, *et al*. Neonatal outcome and congenital malformations in children born after *in-vitro* fertilization. *Hum Reprod* 2002;17:1391–8

4. WHO. Current practices and controversies in assisted reproduction. In Vayena E, Rowe PJ, Griffin PD, eds. *Report of a Meeting on Medical, Ethical and Social Aspects of Assisted Reproduction*. Geneva, Switzerland: WHO, 2001

5. Elsner CW, Tucker MJ, Sweitzer CL, *et al*. Multiple pregnancy rate and embryo number transferred during *in vitro* fertilization. *Am J Obstet Gynecol* 1997;177:350–7

6. Templeton A, Morris JK. Reducing the risk of multiple births by transfer of two embryos after *in vitro* fertilization. *N Engl J Med* 1998;339:573–7

7. Strandell A, Bergh C, Lundin K. Selection of patients suitable for one-embryo transfer may reduce the rate of multiple births by half without impairment of overall birth rates. *Hum Reprod* 2000;15:2520–5

8. Martikainen H. Single-embryo transfer after *in vitro* fertilization and intracytoplasmic sperm injection. In *Reproductive Medicine in the Twenty-first Century. Proceedings of the 17th World Congress on Fertility and Sterility*, Melbourne, Australia. London: Parthenon Publishing, 2002:194–200

9. Giorgetti C, Terriou P, Auquier P, *et al*. Embryo score to predict implantation after *in-vitro* fertilization: based on 957 single embryo transfers. *Hum Reprod* 1995;10:2427–31

10. Vilska S, Tiitinen A, Hydén-Granskog C, *et al*. Elective transfer of one embryo results in an acceptable pregnancy rate and eliminates the risk of multiple birth. *Hum Reprod* 1999;14:2392–5

11. Martikainen H, Tiitinen A, Tomás C, *et al*. One versus two embryo transfer after IVF and ICSI: a randomized study. *Hum Reprod* 2001;16:1900–3

12. Tiitinen A, Halttunen M, Härkki P, *et al*. Elective single embryo transfer: the value of cryopreservation. *Hum Reprod* 2001;16:1140–4

13. Tiitinen A, Unkila-Kallio L, Halttunen M, Hydén-Granskog C. Significant impact of elective single embryo transfer on the twin pregnancy rate. *Hum Reprod* 2003;18:1449–53

14. Söderström-Anttila V, Vilska S, Mäkinen S, *et al*. Elective single embryo transfer yields good delivery rates in oocyte donation. *Hum Reprod* 2003;18:1858–63

15. Söderström-Anttila V, Tiitinen A, Foudila T, *et al*. Obstetric and perinatal outcome after oocyte donation – comparison with *in vitro* fertilization pregnancies. *Hum Reprod* 1998;13:483–90

16. Salumets A, Hydén-Granskog C, Mäkinen S, *et al*. Early cleavage predicts the viability of human embryos in elective single embryo transfer procedures. *Hum Reprod* 2003;18:821–5

17. Salumets A, Hydén-Granskog C, Suikkari A-M, *et al*. The predictive value of pronuclear morphology of zygotes in the assessment of human embryo quality. *Hum Reprod* 2001;16:2177–81

18. Pinborg A, Loft A, Schmidt L, *et al*. Attitudes of IVF/ICSI-twin mothers towards twins and single embryo transfer. *Hum Reprod* 2003;18:621–7

b. Belgium

P. De Sutter and M. Dhont

INTRODUCTION

Together with the Scandinavian countries, a few centers in Belgium were amongst the first to launch the principle of single-embryo transfer and to implement it into clinical practice. In 1998, Coetsier and Dhont published a theoretical calculation suggesting that single-embryo transfer could easily lead to a substantial drop in multiple pregnancy rates in assisted reproductive technologies (ART), without a significant decrease in the overall pregnancy results[1]. In the Ghent University Center for Reproductive Medicine, SET has been gradually introduced from 1997 onwards and is currently being performed in about 20% of all cycles. Simultaneously, single-embryo transfer has been introduced and studied in the Antwerp Middelheim Hospital where single-embryo transfer accounted for > 40% of all transfers in 2002[2]. Both centers have actively promoted single-embryo transfer on a national level, directly leading to a reimbursement regulation. Together, we have developed a health-economic model comparing single-embryo transfer with double-embryo transfer and performed a real-life health-economic impact study[3] (and manuscript submitted for publication). The impact of the application of single-embryo transfer on the pregnancy and multiple pregnancy rates in both centers has been reported previously and will be discussed in depth in other chapters of this book. It has clearly been shown that implementation of single-embryo transfer in a group of patients with a good prognosis leads to a 50% reduction in multiple pregnancy rates, while preserving the overall pregnancy results[4,5]. The specific aim of this chapter was to analyze the introduction of the single-embryo transfer practice in Belgium as a whole and how this has influenced the national results.

THE BELGIAN REGISTER FOR ASSISTED PROCREATION (BELRAP)

At the end of the 1980s, most Belgian fertility centers voluntarily began to register their results on a yearly basis. This lasted until 1993, when the Belgian Register for Assisted Procreation (BELRAP) was officially created. Originally, BELRAP was a voluntary association and aimed to analyze the national ART results in Belgium and publish them. All infertility centers could submit their results on a cycle-by-cycle basis, and gradually more than 90% of all in vitro fertilization (IVF)/intracytoplasmic sperm injection (ICSI) cycles performed in Belgium were thus registered and stored in a single database. Since 1999 registration of ART activities in Belgium is no longer voluntary, but regulated by law. A special 'College of Physicians in Reproductive Medicine' (CPRM) was installed with members appointed by the Ministry of Social Affairs. The CPRM has been given the responsibility, though not yet all the necessary means, for quality control (including registration) of ART in Belgium. The expertise and much of the voluntary effort contained within BELRAP has been preserved by integrating it as a functional part of the CPRM. BELRAP is controlled by the College and now functions as a special sub-commission for the ART registration created within the College. A further improvement of the quality of the Belgian register was obtained by the introduction in 2001 of an on-line registration system, so that each individual ART cycle initiated is recorded in a prospective manner. This allows for a more complete and a more reliable registration of all cycles initiated, and also of cancelled cycles. All cycle data are to be submitted to the register per trimester. The Belgian register therefore accounts for 100% of all ART activities covered by the public health insurance system in Belgium. Cycles performed in foreign patients are not included in the analysis of this register, although they are registered.

SINGLE-EMBRYO TRANSFER IN THE BELRAP REGISTER

Figure 1 shows the evolution of the number of embryos transferred between 1990 and 2002 in Belgium. It can clearly be seen that single-embryo transfer constituted no more than about 10% of all transfers until around 1998. Indeed, until that year almost all single-embryo transfers were compulsory (non-elective) single-embryo transfers and consequently were usually followed by poor results, as previously published. This was before single-embryo transfer was performed as a desired option[6].

Table 1 shows the national results of 2001 in terms of the number of transferred embryos. It is clear that elective single-embryo transfer yielded a higher pregnancy rate than non-elective SET (ongoing pregnancy rates per transfer, 19% vs. 8%). Similarly and expectedly, elective double-embryo transfer led to a higher pregnancy rate (26%) than non-elective double-embryo transfer (13%). The fact that three or more than three embryos are

mostly transferred in patients with a poor prognosis was reflected in relatively low pregnancy rates (23% and 16%, respectively).

Since 1998, however, a steady rise in the incidence of SET has been witnessed, as illustrated in Figure 1. In 2002 single-embryo transfer was already performed in 17% of all cycles nationwide. Because of a new law regulating quality control of ART in Belgium from 1 July 2003 onwards, it can be expected that the proportion of single-embryo transfer cycles will rapidly increase in the coming years. This law forbids the transfer of more than one embryo in the first treatment cycle in all women under 36 years of age, and in the second cycle if a top-quality embryo is available. It will be extremely interesting to observe the impact of this nationally regulated policy on the ART results in our country. The weak point of the regulation resides in the fact that no strict definition is given of a 'top-quality' embryo. Obviously, what is meant is an embryo with a high putative implantation potential. It was considered that it would be better not to define a putative high-competence embryo too strictly, thereby allowing all centers to improve their own efficacy to select the 'best' embryo. However, this point will need long-term follow-up to avoid a mere shift of twinning from first or second cycles to second or subsequent cycles.

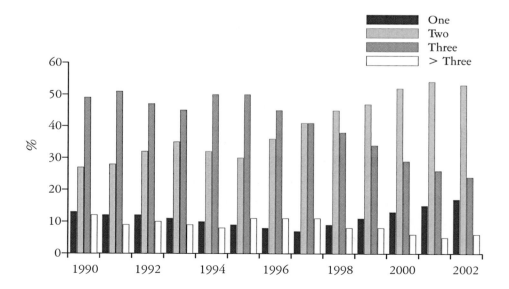

Figure 1   Number of embryos transferred in Belgium from 1990 to 2002. Data from BELRAP

Another interesting observation that can be derived from Figure 1 is the continuous decline in triple-embryo transfer rates since 1995 (from 50% of all transfers to 24% in 2002). Parallel with this evolution in the single- and triple-embryo transfer rates, one can observe a rise in the incidence of double-embryo transfers until 2001, whereas since 2002 this incidence is also beginning to decline in favor of single-embryo transfer. Figure 1 therefore illustrates the shift in one decade from triple to double to single embryo transfer in Belgium. The main question, of course, is whether this change in transfer policy is being reflected in a change in pregnancy results over the same decade.

Figure 2 shows the evolution of the live birth rate per started cycle between 1990 and 2001. It

Table 1   Belgian Register for Assisted Procreation (BELRAP) data for 2001: ongoing pregnancy rates following different number of embryos transferred (elective versus non-elective). Data on 8002 transfers

Number of embryos transferred	n	Frequency (%)	Ongoing pregnancies	Ongoing pregnancies/ numbers transferred (%)
One	1123	14	160	14
elective*	643		123	19
non-elective	480		37	8
Two	4269	53	1052	25
elective*	3647		968	26
non-elective	622		84	13
Three	2176	27	499	23
More than three	434	5	68	16
Total	8002	100	1779	22

* When more embryos were available than were actually transferred

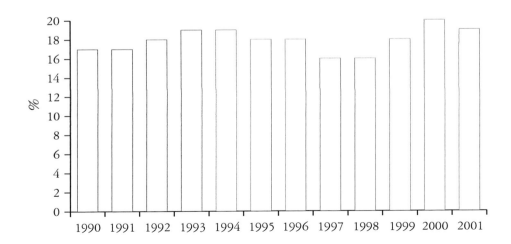

Figure 2   Evolution of the live birth rate per started cycle in Belgium from 1990 to 2001

does not seem from this figure that the change in transfer strategy has affected the live birth rate, which stays between 16 and 20% per started cycle. Although these data are purely observational and subject to many possible biases, they are an epidemiological piece of evidence that the implementation of single-embryo transfer has not led to a dramatic decrease in pregnancy rates nationwide. Of course, the most dramatic impact of the increased single-embryo transfer practice in Belgium should be a decrease in multiple pregnancy rates after ART. The incidences of singleton, twin and triplet births in Belgium between 1990 and 2000 are depicted in Figure 3. It is clear that the incidence of triplets has drastically decreased since 1998 and has become marginal. This is the result of the decrease in the rates of triple-embryo transfers, which are currently only performed in patients with a poor prognosis.

Figure 4 shows the evolution of *elective* single-embryo transfer in Belgium from 1996 until 2001 per center. On average, elective single-embryo transfer has almost reached the level of 10% of all transfers in 2001, coming from about 2% in previous years. From this figure it can be seen that the national increase in single-embryo transfer frequency results from the efforts of only a few

centers, which now have reached a 20–40% single-embryo transfer rate. These centers have actively promoted and implemented the single-embryo transfer strategy in Belgium since 1998, while the majority of clinics have been slow in changing their transfer policy towards elective single-embryo transfer. Of course, such a policy change takes time, and it can be expected that most centers will finally follow, in view of the new law regulating embryo transfer in Belgium. However, this explains why the substantial drop in twinning rate after IVF, as is observed in Finland, has not yet been observed in Belgium, but this is likely to become visible in the data from 2002 to 2003 onwards.

However, since 1998 the twin birth rates after ART have shown some decrease, and the singleton births have conversely been slowly increasing, showing that the practice of single-embryo transfer slowly but gradually bears its fruits. It is known that around 40% of all multiple births in Belgium result from infertility therapy, of which two-thirds result from IVF/ICSI treatment (and one-third from non-IVF treatments). We therefore analyzed the Flemish perinatal register (SPE), which registers all births in Flanders (about 60 000 per year) independently from BELRAP, to look for an effect of the

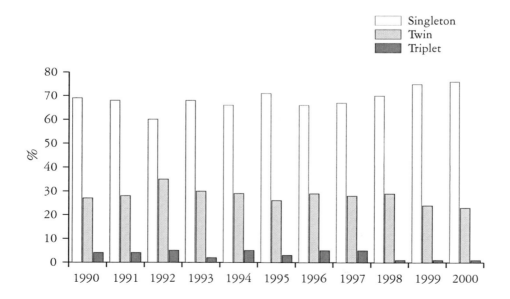

Figure 3   Evolution of singleton, twin and triplet births after assisted reproductive technologies in Belgium from 1990 to 2000

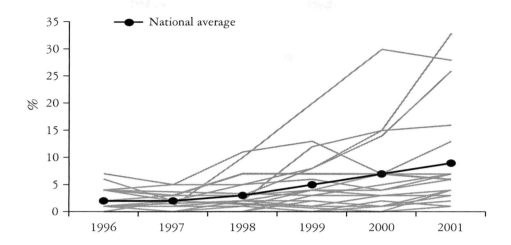

Figure 4　Evolution of the percentage of elective single-embryo transfers of the total number of embryo transfers in all registering Belgian centers from 1996 to 2001

emerging single-embryo transfer practice in our country. The SPE covers only deliveries in Flanders (the Flemish speaking part of the country) which account for about 60% of all births in Belgium. Since no similar registration exists for Wallony and the French-speaking part of Brussels, there is unfortunately no national perinatal register in Belgium. Indeed, for the first time for decades, from 1998 onwards the percentage of overall twin births in Flanders has shown a tendency towards a decrease, strongly suggesting an incipient impact of the change in ART practice. In 1998, 1.88% of all births were twin births; this figure dropped to 1.82% in 1999, 1.80% in 2000 and 1.74% in 2001[7]. This may also reflect changes in policies of non-IVF treatment (careful stimulation and monitoring, cancellations or escape from IVF if there are more than three follicles, etc.), but the influence of single-embryo transfer practice is allegedly more important. It will indeed be exciting to observe the evolution in multiple pregnancy rates in the coming years. We may have found one of the solutions to the multiple pregnancy epidemic that has occurred because of ART over the past 20 years.

CONCLUSION

Data from the national Belgian register show that the introduction of elective single-embryo transfer

in Belgium has not caused a decline in the overall birth rates after ART, whereas multiple birth rates have started a discrete but steady decline. The impact of this (r)evolution will be tremendous from a medical, psychological, social and financial point of view. The new law regulating ART practice in our country from 1 July 2003 onwards is expected to reinforce this development.

REFERENCES

1.　Coetsier T, Dhont M. Avoiding multiple pregnancies in *in-vitro* fertilization: who's afraid of single embryo transfer? *Hum Reprod* 1998;13:2663–4

2.　Gerris J, De Neubourg D, Mangelschots K, *et al*. Elective single day 3 embryo transfer halves the twinning rate without decrease in the ongoing pregnancy rate of an IVF/ICSI programme. *Hum Reprod* 2002;17:2626–31

3.　De Sutter P, Gerris J, Dhont M. A health-economic decision-analytic model comparing double with single embryo transfer in IVF/ICSI. *Hum Reprod* 2002;17:2891–6

4. Gerris J, De Neubourg D, Mangelschots K, *et al.* Prevention of twin pregnancy after *in-vitro* fertilization or intracytoplasmatic sperm injection based on strict criteria: a prospective randomized clinical trial. *Hum Reprod* 1999;14:2581–7

5. De Sutter P, Van der Elst J, Coetsier T, Dhont M. Single embryo transfer and multiple pregnancy rate reduction in IVF/ICSI: a 5 year appraisal. *Reprod Biomed Online* 2003;6:464–9

6. Giorgetti C, Terriou P, Auquier P, *et al.* Embryo score to predict implantation after *in-vitro* fertilization: based on 957 single embryo transfers. *Hum Reprod* 1995;10:2427–31

7. Cammu H, Martens G, Bekaert A, *et al. Perinatal Activities in Flanders 2001*. Brussels: SPE (Studiecentrum voor Perinatale Epidemiologie), 2001

c. Sweden

C. Bergh

BACKGROUND

Despite the great success in *in vitro* fertilization (IVF), considerable concerns have been raised worldwide about the greatly increased multiple pregnancy rate after IVF and side-effects associated with multiple birth[1,2]. Sweden has long had several well-functioning population registries, e.g. the Swedish Medical Birth Registry, the Swedish Registry of Congenital Malformations and the Swedish Cancer Registry. These registries are among the most complete registries in the world, thereby making Sweden a suitable country for high-quality epidemiological studies. With permission from the Swedish Data Inspection Board an IVF Registry has been created covering all children born after assisted reproduction technologies (ART) since the first baby was born in 1982. Based on this IVF registry and other population registries, several large epidemiological studies have been performed and published concerning ART children and compared to children born after spontaneous conception[3–6]. These studies have shown that IVF children have a higher rate of prematurity (< 37 weeks) and low birth weight (< 2500 g) compared to controls. A higher mortality rate, malformation rate and rate of neurological sequelae have also been observed in some studies. A considerable part of this increased risk of adverse outcome can be explained by the higher rate of multiple births after IVF.

GENERALIZED SINGLE-EMBRYO TRANSFER

The results of the above-mentioned epidemiological studies have been intensively discussed in the Swedish Society for Obstetrics and Gynecology. An overall change to a one-embryo transfer policy would certainly result in mainly singletons. In fact, a generalized single-embryo transfer policy has been stated in Swedish law to be the normal routine since the beginning of 2003. The Swedish National Board of Health and Welfare has advocated single-embryo transfers and stated in particular that singletons should be the overall goal in IVF. However, without an increase in the number of subsidized IVF cycles per couple, an overall change to single-embryo transfers would probably result in a substantial decrease in pregnancy and birth rates and would hardly be acceptable for both patients and physicians.

INDIVIDUALIZED SINGLE-EMBRYO TRANSFER

In the meanwhile, several studies have been published showing that single-embryo transfers give satisfactory clinical pregnancy rates in selected groups of patients. In the first published study from Finland the pregnancy rate after elective embryo transfer in 74 cycles was 29.7%[7]. The cumulative pregnancy rate, when including additional freeze cycles from the same oocyte retrieval, was 47.3%. In contrast, when only one embryo was available, the pregnancy rate was 20.2%. From this study it was concluded that single-embryo transfers could be recommended for women younger than 35 years of age and who have grade-1 or grade-2 embryos available for transfer. Two randomized, controlled studies have been published comparing the pregnancy rate between one versus two embryo transfers. In a study from Belgium, 26 single-embryo transfers resulted in 17 conceptions, and 27 double-embryo transfers resulted in 20 conceptions, giving an ongoing clinical pregnancy rate of 38.5% and 74%, respectively[8]. In the other randomized study, which originated from Finland, women younger than 36 years and undergoing their first IVF cycle were included if four good-quality embryos were available[9]. A total of 74 women were randomized to one-embryo transfer and 70 women to two-embryo transfers. The clinical pregnancy rates in the two groups were 32.4% and 47.1%, respectively, which did not differ significantly, but of course the confidence intervals for the difference was wide. The authors supported one-embryo transfers in selected women. Despite being of limited size, these two studies showed that satisfactory pregnancy rates could be achieved with single-embryo transfers in selected women while limiting the twin pregnancy rate in these women to its natural incidence of about 1%. Another Finnish follow-up study of 127 single-embryo transfers reported a pregnancy rate of 38.6%[10]. The cumulative delivery rate for this cohort of women, when including freeze cycles, was 52.8% per retrieval and the twin rate was 7.6%.

SCANDINAVIAN PROSPECTIVE MULTICENTER RANDOMIZED STUDY COMPARING ONE- VERSUS TWO-EMBRYO TRANSFERS

Owing to the limited availability of studies, a large prospective, randomized study comparing one- versus two-embryo transfers was initiated in Sweden 2000. The aim of the study was to show that one fresh single-embryo transfer and (if pregnancy was not achieved) one additional single-embryo frozen–thawed transfer would give a similar birth rate to that of a fresh two-embryo transfer. The simple hypothesis is thereby that $1 + 1 = 2$. A retrospective study from Gothenburg University had identified female age and number of good-quality embryos transferred as independent predictors of multiple birth[11]. Based on the results of that study and aiming to reduce the overall multiple birth rate by half (26% to 13%) it was calculated that 330 patients would be needed in each arm of the study, assuming a birth rate of 30% per fresh treatment cycle started and an upper limit of the confidence interval for the difference in birth rates between groups of 10%. Both IVF and intracytoplasmic sperm injection (ICSI) patients are included in the study, undergoing their first and second IVF cycles, with female age below 36 years and at least two good-quality embryos available. The study has been running in 11 Scandinavian clinics and recruitment of patients is soon to be completed. Recruitment has been time-consuming, in the beginning owing to patients' unwillingness to be randomized and fear of a lower birth rate when having only one embryo transferred. In the past year recruitment has been troublesome for opposite

reasons: patients have themselves wished for single-embryo transfers, owing to fear/risk of a twin pregnancy. The study will be completed in the course of 2003 and results will soon be available.

NUMBER OF EMBRYOS TRANSFERRED AT PRESENT

Since 1993 the routine in Sweden has been to transfer two embryos (Figure 1). While almost eliminating triplets, the twinning rate after IVF has remained constant, at around 25%. A change in the number of embryos transferred has taken place in 2002–03, reflecting the change in the law and the general debate. For the year 2001 the rate of single-embryo transfers was still low, around 15% for the whole country, whereas it has increased in 2002 and particularly in 2003 (Figure 2 and unpublished results). However, at the moment there are huge differences between different clinics with respect to the application of elective single-embryo transfer, reflecting different attitudes among clinicians towards its risks and benefits. There is a strong need for more scientific evidence. The ongoing randomized study will give us much knowledge on how to advise our patients and will help us to establish more general rules for IVF clinics and society. Preliminary results for clinics practicing elective single-embryo transfer in a considerable number of cycles show that it seems possible to achieve satisfactory birth rates with elective single-embryo transfer, without lowering the overall birth rate and at the same time reducing the multiple birth rate considerably.

SUMMARY

The challenge for IVF clinics is to introduce single-embryo transfer into clinical practice without a significant drop in delivery rates. Studies to date have shown that this strategy is possible for a large group of women. Larger randomized studies are underway that will help us better to select this group of women. Among patients themselves, there is a growing awareness of the risks involved in a twin pregnancy. Many patients no longer consider the high incidence of iatrogenic multiples as an acceptable 'price to be paid' in order to achieve high

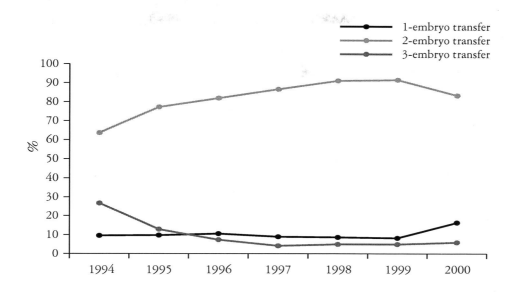

Figure 1 Number of embryos per transfer, Sweden, 1994–2000. Reproduced with permission from P. O. Karlström

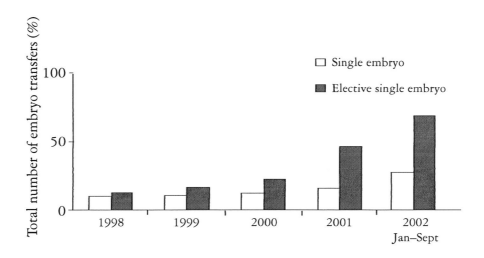

Figure 2 Proportion of single-embryo transfers in Sweden, 1998–2002. Reproduced with permission from J. Olofsson

pregnancy rates. In fact, it is not the patients who need to be convinced about the need to decrease the number of embryos per transfer but the clinicians working in IVF units. Most IVF clinicians are involved only in IVF and have no or very limited contact with obstetricians, neonatologists or women pregnant with twins. They might therefore not have

the possibility of fully realizing all the consequences of a multiple pregnancy. The habit of presenting the success of IVF as pregnancy per cycle or pregnancy per transfer has surely also contributed to the current situation. A debate, initiated by Scandinavian IVF doctors on how to present success, was recently published in *Human*

Reproduction[12]. Until results are available from controlled studies, a strategy for single-embryo transfer has recently been adopted by Swedish IVF doctors. Single-embryo transfer is currently recommended in the first or second IVF/ICSI cycle in women ≤ 36 years of age if at least two good-quality embryos are available. Similar strategies have recently been discussed in Europe and reported as a European Society of Human Reproduction and Embryology (ESHRE) consensus statement. According to this recommendation, single-embryo transfer should be proposed in the first or second IVF/ICSI cycle in women ≤ 36 years of age if at least one good-quality embryo is available[13].

REFERENCES

1. Nygren KG, Andersen AN. Assisted reproductive technology in Europe, 1998. Results generated from European registers by ESHRE. *Hum Reprod* 2001;16:2459–71

2. ASRM/SART Registry 1999. *Fertil Steril* 2002;78:918–27

3. Bergh T, Ericsson A, Hillensjö T, *et al.* Deliveries and children born after *in-vitro* fertilization in Sweden 1982–95: a retrospective cohort study. *Lancet* 1999;354:1579–85

4. Wennerholm UB, Bergh C, Hamberger L, *et al.* Incidence of congenital malformations in children born after ICSI. *Hum Reprod* 2000;15:944–8

5. Ericsson A, Källen B. Congenital malformations in infants born after IVF: a population-based study. *Hum Reprod* 2001;16:504-9

6. Strömberg B, Dahlquist G, Ericson A, *et al.* Neurological sequelae in children born after *in-vitro* fertilization: a population-based study. *Lancet* 2002;359:461–5

7. Vilska S, Tiitinen A, Hyden-Granskog C, Hovatta O. Elective transfer of one embryo results in acceptable pregnancy rate and eliminates the risk of multiple birth. *Hum Reprod* 1999;14:2392–5

8. Gerris J, De Neubourg D, Mangelschots K, *et al.* Prevention of twin pregnancy after *in-vitro* fertilization or intracytoplasmic sperm injection based on strict embryo criteria: a prospective randomized clinical trial. *Hum Reprod* 1999;14:2581–7

9. Martikainen H, Tiitinen A, Tomas C, *et al.* One versus two embryo transfer after IVF and ICSI: a randomized study. *Hum Reprod* 2001; 16:1900–3

10. Tiitinen A, Haltunen M, Härkki P, *et al.* Elective single embryo transfer: the value of cryopreservation. *Hum Reprod* 2001;16: 1140–4

11. Strandell A, Bergh C, Lundin K. Selection of patients suitable for one-embryo transfer may reduce the rate of multiple births by half without impairment of overall birth rates. *Hum Reprod* 2000;15:2520–5

12. Hazekamp J, Bergh C, Wennerholm UB, *et al.* Avoiding multiple pregnancies in ART: consideration of new strategies. *Hum Reprod* 2000;15:1217–19

13. Land JA, Evers JLH. Risks and complications in assisted reproduction techniques: report of an ESHRE consensus meeting. *Hum Reprod* 2003;18:455–7

d. The Netherlands

D. Braat and J. Kremer

INTRODUCTION

Dutch women are leading worldwide in delaying childbirth. From 1972 onwards in The Netherlands the mean age of a mother having her first child increased from 24.5 years up to 29.2 in 2001[1]. In recent years there seems to have been a stabilization (29.1 in 1998, 1999 and 2000, and 29.2 in 2001), but unfortunately no decrease has yet been observed. This is one of the major reasons for the increase in couples seeking help for infertility. Although there is an increasing knowledge of the relationship between infertility and higher age, social factors such as the difficulties women experience in combining making a career for themselves with starting a family still have an impact on the age at which women begin trying for a pregnancy. The first successful *in vitro* fertilization (IVF) treatment in The Netherlands took place in 1983. Since then the number of IVF and intracytoplasmic sperm injection (ICSI) cycles has increased enormously. From 1996 onwards the Dutch Society of Obstetrics and Gynecology has registered the number of IVF and ICSI cycles in all 13 IVF centers in The Netherlands and their outcome per center[2]. This information is open to the general public (www.nvog.nl). In 2001 13 975 cycles were performed, divisible into 9379 IVF and 4596 ICSI cycles; this is approximately 875 cycles per 1 000 000 inhabitants. Unfortunately, there is still no central registration of the number of multiples, but using the reported percentages of multiples per center allows one to calculate the mean percentage of multiples (almost all twins) for 2001 (between 20 and 25%). The number of initiated cycles in relation to the population is relatively high in The Netherlands, although Denmark, Finland, Iceland and Sweden report higher numbers[3]. This may be related to the fact that Dutch health insurance companies reimburse no more than up to three cycles of IVF. In case a child is born, another three cycles are paid for. On the other hand, even if not reimbursed, IVF treatment in The Netherlands is relatively cheap, costing approximately 1200 euro excluding medication.

COST ANALYSIS OF SINGLETON PREGNANCIES COMPARED WITH TWINS

Multiple pregnancies are associated with more obstetric and perinatal complications than singleton pregnancies. Therefore, medical costs are expected to be higher for multiple pregnancies compared with singleton pregnancies. To investigate whether single-embryo transfer might be cost effective, a retrospective cost analysis in the IVF Department at the University Medical Center Nijmegen was performed. In this study only cost drivers from pregnancy until 6 weeks after delivery were determined in a representative sample of singleton and twin pregnancies occurring after IVF treatment between 1995 and 2001. Maternal and neonatal hospital admissions were the major cost drivers. The cost per twin pregnancy was found to be more than five times higher than per singleton pregnancy (13.469 euro versus 2.550 euro, respectively) (H.G. Lukassen and colleagues, unpublished data). In this study the long-term costs due to extra costs for disabilities or handicaps were not taken into account. Prospective cost-analysis studies comparing single-embryo transfer with double-embryo transfer should be performed. Meanwhile, the 10 000 euro difference in our study indicates that there is enough money to be saved by the reduction of twin pregnancies by single-embryo transfer to compensate for the additional IVF cycles necessitated by single-embryo transfer.

DATA ON SINGLE-EMBRYO TRANSFER

As a rule in Dutch IVF centers, a maximum of two embryos are transferred; single-embryo transfer studies are ongoing in different centers in The Netherlands.

Natural-cycle *in vitro* fertilization/intracytoplasmic sperm injection

Although less successful than conventional – stimulated – IVF, this might be an option for reducing the number of multiples as well as for preventing complications such as ovarian hyperstimulation syndrome (OHSS) and other adverse effects of ovarian hyperstimulation[4].

Two Dutch pilot studies were performed. The first took place in the Vrije Universiteit Medical Center of Amsterdam; in this prospective study in 50 patients with tubal infertility, 75 cycles were needed to obtain one oocyte from each patient. In 33 patients the oocyte was obtained in the first cycle, 11 patients needed two, four patients three and two patients needed four consecutive cycles before an egg was obtained. This resulted in a cumulative ongoing pregnancy rate of 9.8% per cycle, 11.9% per egg retrieval and 19.5% per embryo transfer[4].

The second study was performed in the University Medical Center Nijmegen[5]. Couples with severe male infertility with an indication for ICSI and no female fertility problems were included. Female age was < 37 years. In 25 couples 29 cycles were started. In 16 cases one oocyte was obtained; in one case two oocytes were obtained; resulting in an oocyte recovery rate of 58.6% per cycle. In three cases, ICSI could not be performed (once because of ejaculatory failure, twice because of morphological abnormalities of the oocyte). ICSI was performed in 14 cases, all leading to fertilization. In two cases no embryo transfer was performed because of abnormal fertilization, resulting in transfer in 12 patients, i.e. 41.4% per cycle. Three patients conceived and had a child (25% per embryo transfer). The live birth rate per started cycle was 10.3%.

These two Dutch studies illustrate that natural-cycle IVF or ICSI might be an alternative to IVF or ICSI in stimulated cycles. It has the advantage of a low patient burden, low costs and low risks. During the same period in the University Medical Center Nijmegen an ongoing pregnancy rate of 32% per started ICSI cycle in women aged < 37 years was observed (unpublished data). Extrapolation of the observed 10.3% ongoing pregnancy rate after one natural cycle yields a calculated cumulative live birth rate after three natural cycles of 28%.

Therefore, natural-cycle IVF might be a suitable alternative, since a stimulation cycle with a long gonadotropin releasing hormone (GnRH) agonist protocol takes 3 months. To investigate whether this is a realistic alternative, a study was performed to determine the preferences of patients and physicians for IVF in three natural cycles compared to one stimulated cycle. A questionnaire was sent to patients as well as to physicians. In both groups a majority preferred IVF in a natural cycle, given an equivalent success rate of 17%. A substantial number of patients as well as physicians were willing to trade off 6% success in live birth for their treatment of choice, i.e. IVF in a natural cycle. Anxiety about hormone injections was a predictor of patient preferences.

A third study in a large number of patients is ongoing at the Fertility Department of the University of Groningen. In this study 'minimal-stimulation IVF' is performed: late follicular phase GnRH antagonist plus 150 IU recombinant follicle stimulating hormone (FSH), human chorionic gonadotropin (hCG) to trigger ovulation and hCG for luteal support. In a pilot study, 78 cycles were started in 33 women, resulting in 14 ongoing pregnancies, i.e. 17.9% per started cycle[6]. Results of the large study have not yet been published; however, the Groningen group has already published a review of natural-cycle IVF/ICSI reports worldwide[7].

Elective single-embryo transfer in stimulated cycles

In the University Medical Center Nijmegen a prospective randomized study was performed comparing the pregnancy rate after a maximum of two consecutive IVF or ICSI cycles with elective single-embryo transfer (2 × 1) with the pregnancy rate after one IVF or ICSI cycle with elective double-embryo transfer (1 × 2). Only women < 35 years of age, with basal serum FSH level < 10 IU/l and starting their first IVF/ICSI treatment were randomized. They had to have at least one good-quality embryo on day 3 after fertilization. If the patient did not become pregnant in the first cycle of the 2 × 1 group, a further single embryo was transferred in the following cycle. Preliminary results showed no statistical differences between groups[8]. The clinical pregnancy rate in the 2 × 1 group was 27.3% after one cycle and 36.4% after two cycles

($n = 22$), compared with 28.2% after one cycle in the 1×2 group ($n = 21$). In the 1×2 group two twin pregnancies were established. The study was closed after inclusion of 104 (2×52) women. No significantly different pregnancy rates were observed between the groups (manuscript in preparation).

Another Dutch group evaluated the results of elective single-embryo transfer in the first three treatment cycles[9]. A total of 326 patients were treated for 574 treatment cycles. The policy was to perform elective single-embryo transfer whenever at least two embryos were available, of which at least one was a top-quality embryo. In the other cycles, two embryos were transferred. In 61 cycles, elective single-embryo transfer could not be applied, because there was either no fertilization, or only one available embryo. In the remaining 513 cycles, elective single-embryo transfer policy led, in 108 cycles (21%), to the elective transfer of only one embryo. No significant differences were observed between ongoing pregnancy rates of embryo transfer groups in each treatment cycle rank. The ongoing pregnancy rates after elective single-embryo transfer were 33%, 36% and 18% for first, second and third rank cycles, respectively. After double-embryo transfer the pregnancy rates were 32%, 22% and 24%, respectively. These rates were further augmented by the transfer of frozen–thawed embryos to a cumulative pregnancy rate of 47%, 39% and 29% for the elective single-embryo transfer groups in the first, second and third trial, respectively; and 34%, 24% and 24% for the double-embryo transfer groups, respectively. The authors concluded that elective single-embryo transfer could be the policy of choice in at least the first three treatment cycles without compromising pregnancy results in this selected group of patients.

CONCLUSION

Although in The Netherlands the standard IVF protocol still consists of ovarian hyperstimulation and double-embryo transfer, many clinics are studying single-embryo transfer or natural-cycle IVF. Pressure is increasing on health insurance companies to reimburse the costs of six attempts instead of three, with one embryo to be transferred whenever appropriate.

REFERENCES

1. Centraal Bureau voor de Statistiek (CBS) [Central Statistical Office]

2. Kremer JA, Beekhuizen W, Bots RSGM, *et al.* The results of *in vitro* fertilisation in the Netherlands, 1996–2000. *Ned Tijdschr Geneeskd* 2002;146:2358–63

3. Nygren KG, Nyboe Andersen A. Assisted reproductive technology in Europe, 1998. Results generated from European registers by ESHRE. *Hum Reprod* 2001;16:2459–71

4. Janssens RM, Lambalk CB, Vermeiden JPW, *et al. In-vitro* fertilization in a spontaneous cycle: easy, cheap and realistic. *Hum Reprod* 2000;15:314–18

5. Lukassen HG, Kremer JAM, Lindeman EJM, *et al.* A pilot study of the efficacy of intracytoplasmic sperm injection in a natural cycle. *Fertil Steril* 2003;79:231–2

6. Pelinck MJ, Arts EGJM, Hoek A, *et al.* Natural cycle IVF with late follicular phase GnRH antagonist administration: a pilot study. *Abstract Book of the 18th Annual Meeting of the ESHRE*, O-050. *Hum Reprod* 2002;17:18

7. Pelinck MJ, Hoek A, Simons AHM, Heineman MJ. Efficacy of natural cycle IVF: a review of the literature. *Hum Reprod Update* 2002;8:129–39

8. Lukassen HG, *et al.* 2×1 versus 1×2, a randomized study. *Abstract Book of the 18th Annual Meeting of the ESHRE*, O-005. *Hum Reprod* 2002;17:2

9. Dumoulin JCM, Van Montfoort APA, Land JA, *et al.* Results of elective single embryo transfer (eSET) in the first three treatment cycles. *Abstracts of the 19th Annual Meeting of the ESHRE*, P-392. *Hum Reprod* 2003;18 (Suppl 1):133

10

Laboratory-related risks in assisted reproductive technologies

J. P. W. Vermeiden

INTRODUCTION

When analyzing the risks that can be incurred during the laboratory procedures in *in vitro* fertilization (IVF)/intracytoplasmic sperm injection (ICSI) treatments, three different levels can be distinguished, leading to first-, second- and third-order risks. First-order risks are related to the quality system of an assisted reproductive technology (ART) laboratory; second-order risks are related to the state of the art of ART and third-order risks are related to ART laboratory procedures affecting gametes, embryos and as a consequence the quality of life of the children.

First-order risks deal with deviations from well-defined procedures, i.e. deviations in matters we can and have to control. Examples of these types of risk are insemination with the wrong semen sample or the use of embryotoxic transfer catheters.

Second-order risks deal with the state of the art of laboratory procedures. Here we are dealing with risks related to lack of evidence-based scientific knowledge. As an example: the exact composition of the optimal culture medium is not known. Nevertheless, we have to make the decision to use a particular medium in order to grow embryos. This kind of decision is often based on local historical factors, sometimes on consensus, but rarely on solid evidence-based scientific knowledge. This can be explained by the 'never change a winning horse' approach: the ART center is thought to perform well, meaning that the pregnancy rate is considered satisfactory, and that the children are apparently healthy. When we analyze the ART procedures it will become clear that many aspects are not under-

stood. It is a black box, but it works. It will also be clear that often we do not know precisely how well we perform, because good models for comparison of the results (pregnancy rates, patient satisfaction) with those of other ART centers are lacking.

Third-order risks are defined as unwanted side-effects of the ART laboratory procedures on the gametes or the embryos, resulting in the birth of disabled children. When, in experimental animals, embryonic development, DNA structure and chromosomal constitution of embryos developed *in vivo* are compared with those of embryos developed *in vitro*, it is clear that ART procedures affect the embryos. Because of ethical reasons this type of research is not possible with human embryos; hence, our knowledge of the impact of ART laboratory procedures on human embryos is sparse, but it is possible that these laboratory procedures could affect human embryos in a comparable way. ART procedures can have a large impact on the health of the offspring of mice, sheep and cows. In this respect humans appear to be different. Besides marginal effects on birth weight, a small increase in the incidence of chromosomal abnormalities after ICSI and an increase in the incidence of rare diseases, ART laboratory procedures do not appear to have a clear intrinsic negative effect on the health of the children at the time of birth, during the first years of life and up to the period of adolescence. However, the number of children studied in the age group between 2 years of age and adolescence is very small in comparison with the number of people born after ART. In addition, we know nothing yet about the aging of adults born after ART, which is easy to understand because the first *in vitro* fertilization (IVF) child was born in 1978. Therefore, final conclusions with respect to the health effects of ART treatments on the children thus conceived cannot be made.

In this chapter the risks of ART laboratory procedures are identified and categorized. The question is asked whether they can be quantified, minimized or prevented. After analyzing the risks factors a final problem is left: what are our responsibilities and what are our duties? It will be obvious that we have to inform our patients about the risks and the uncertainties of ART.

FIRST-ORDER RISKS

Most couples feel confident with most aspects of the ART treatment. The women can follow the response of the ovaries to the hormonal treatment by watching the screen of the ultrasound machine; her partner deposits his semen sample in a properly labeled jar. However, at a certain moment, they

have to hand over their gametes to the laboratory personnel: into the unknown. After a few days, (or after a few years when cryopreserved embryos are involved) they have to trust that their own embryos are transferred and that we have offered them optimal care. When interviewed, couples often appear to display a certain fear that there is a risk that they could be the victims of something that may have happened in that unknown. This fear is fed by reports in the news, such as the birth of a Black baby out of a White woman, because of a mistake in the IVF procedure (Figure 1). Other examples are reports on lost embryos or on documented criminal acts perpetrated by embryologists.

Not only do patients fear being a victim of a mistake; technicians involved in ART, and working in a center that performs many ART treatments, can also have feelings of doubt (whether they have inseminated with the proper semen sample, whether they have chosen the best embryos, whether truly no mistake has been made).

These obvious risks are examples of potential human failure. When analyzing ART procedures it

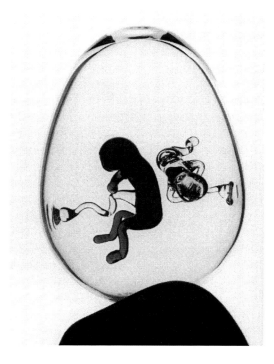

Figure 1   Artist's impression of a twin pregnancy of a White and Black fetus. The intention of the artist was to express the brotherhood of man. For embryologists it is a symbol that they can make mistakes (courtesy of Nel Bottema, 1992)

is clear that different equipment and instruments are used, and that each step of the procedure has to be validated and has to be performed properly. The only way to be in control of these aspects of ART is a quality system that describes all laboratory procedures in detail and that dictates that all crucial manipulations are performed under the witness of a qualified colleague. A quality system also involves careful follow-up of all incidents and deviations. A good-quality system will provide the best guarantee that the ART procedures are performed according to defined standards and that the risks for deviations will be small. It will protect the patients, the personnel and the center. A good-quality system is a self-teaching system: one learns from incidents and deviations and the procedures will be adapted to prevent them occurring again. It will quantify and reduce the risks. Essential for a quality system is an external, independent control (audit) by a quality agency.

Although essential for well-controlled functioning of the ART laboratory, relatively little attention has been paid to this in the literature. Wikland and Sjöblom were the first to advocate the introduction of the ISO 9000 and the EN 4500 quality systems for ART laboratories[1]. Local organizations have published handbooks for ART laboratory quality, but there are only very few ART laboratories that have implemented a quality system that matches the quality system of ISO 9001. It is essential that each ART laboratory implement a quality system that ensures all aspects of quality, and the application of ISO 15189 for all ART laboratories is advocated[2].

SECOND-ORDER RISKS

First-orders risks are related to the question of how the ART procedure has to be performed. Second-order risks are related to the question of why the procedures are performed as they are performed. Are they performed according to the state of the art, according to the newest results of science?

A problem with these questions is that there are many differences between ART laboratories and that the answer to some questions is seemingly irrelevant, because the results (pregnancy rates) are comparable. Some conclude that the human gametes and embryos are versatile and that many of the differences in ART procedures are of no great importance.

However, there are three reasons why we should be concerned. First, there actually is a difference in pregnancy rates. Pregnancy rate depends on many variables, such as patient particulars (age of the women, causes of infertility, smoking behavior, etc.), method of embryo transfer, number of embryos transferred and the quality of the ART laboratory. Second, there is the question of whether the ART procedures influence the quality of the gametes and the embryos, affecting the pregnancy rate and the health of the offspring (see following paragraph). Third, it is our moral obligation to offer the best possible treatment to our patients.

There truly is a difference in pregnancy rates between ART centers. This is demonstrated in the yearbook of the Human Fertilisation and Embryology Authority. The center performing the worst had a pregnancy rate of < 4% per treatment cycle, and the center performing the best had a rate

Table 1 Frequency distribution of live birth rate per *in vitro* fertilization/intracytoplasmic sperm injection treatment cycle (based on data from the Human Fertilisation and Embryo Authority, *Eleventh Annual Report and Account*)

	Pregnancy rate (%)						
	< 5	6–10	10–15	16–20	21–25	26–30	> 31
Frequency	1	0	15	11	17	13	4

This table shows the large differences in pregnancy rates per assisted reproduction technology (ART) center. These differences can be explained, in part, by differences in patient selection, but also by differences in the quality of the ART laboratories

of > 40% (Table 1). Obviously, ART centers can learn from each other, but the value of a figure that expresses a crude pregnancy rate is dubious. We have to express our results in such a way that they are comparable. This requires that corrections be made for the patient factors that affect the pregnancy rate, for the number of embryos transferred and for unwanted side-effects. As an example, we can grade ART centers using a figure that expresses singleton birth rate per started cycle per single-embryo transfer including cryopreserved embryos of non-smoking women at the age of 35 with a body mass index of < 25 kg/m² with or without male factor. It would be optimal if this figure were furthermore corrected for the cost of the ART treatment, for the cost of the failures and for the cost related to the complications of multiple births and lifetime health care related to congenital malformations and premature birth because of ART. If these figures are known, then a meaningful and useful comparison between ART centers will be possible. The deviation of the figures of a particular ART center from the figure of the best performing ART center can be defined as the risk of not obtaining the optimal treatment. It can be anticipated that not many ART centers will participate voluntarily in such a system of quality assessment.

A serious problem is the complexity of the ART laboratory procedures and the lack of scientific knowledge regarding many aspects of the laboratory phase. At this moment ART is more art than science. The general public thinks that ART is the result of the advancement of science. We know better; it is a technique that luckily works, with many open questions regarding why it works or why it does not work. As an example, let us consider the composition of the culture medium and just one component of it – glucose[3]. There is no consensus in the scientific community about the optimal concentration of glucose in the culture medium on the various culture days. Culture medium often has 20 or more components; many of these components will interact. When, of ten components, three different concentrations are studied, we have a factorial number of possibilities $(30!/(30 − 1))$. Mimicking tubal fluid is no option, because we do not know the effect of the various growth factors secreted by the oviduct and the cross talk between

tubal and endometrial cells and the embryo. It will be clear from these examples that we are far from an optimal culture system for human embryos. The composition of culture media is mainly based on intuition, but as soon as we have composed a new culture medium we can compare it with the old one, according to the rules of a good prospective randomized control study. Often we have to accept that there is no improvement, and we have to conclude that intuition failed[4]. Hopefully, a systematic approach will be fruitful, and step-by-step improvement of our system will be realized[5]. We have to accept that many aspects of the ART procedures are art and not science and that we can improve our art only by learning from other better performing ART centers. What we do not have to accept is that some commercial media are sold without the manufacturer clearly documenting their precise composition. What should also make us suspicious are claims of allegedly superior culture media or culture systems, e.g. sequential media, made on the basis of erroneous methodological assumptions.

This does not mean that ART procedures cannot be performed according to scientific principles. Various parts of the ART procedure can be distinguished and each part can be the subject of scientific research. For example, it is clear that the meticulous evaluation and prospective validation of embryo implantation potential adds to the quality of the ART laboratory procedures[6]. This allows elective single-embryo transfer without reduction of the pregnancy rate and preventing multiple pregnancies.

There is sufficient scientific evidence that ART laboratory procedures affect the quality of the embryos. Viuff and co-workers compared the incidence of chromosomal abnormalities between cattle embryos at 2–5 days after insemination (in vitro-produced) with in vivo-developed embryos at days 2–5 after ovulation[7,8]. These authors used fluorescence in situ hybridization (FISH) with chromosome 6- and chromosome 7-specific probes and counted the cell number on the various days. They concluded that the in vivo-developed embryos were significantly more advanced than the in vitro-produced embryos. They also observed a significantly lower frequency of chromosomal abnormalities in the in vivo-produced embryos. They concluded that these chromosomal abnormalities may be inherent to the process of *in vitro* production in cattle.

There is no reason to presume that human embryos behave differently in culture, but we do not know this. A problem in human ART is that it is not possible to compare *in vivo*- and *in vitro*-produced embryos. We have to address the problem of effects of the culture system in a different way. Bielanska and associates analyzed the chromosomal constitution of human embryos produced *in vitro* on the various days of culture up to the blastocyst stage[9]. These authors analyzed the presence of nine different chromosomes with FISH. With each culture day the number of genetically normal cells decreased dramatically. Of the 216 analyzed embryos 64 (29.6%) were completely normal for the nine chromosomes. Of the analyzed blastocysts only 3/33 (9.1%) were fully normal. These findings demonstrate that there are two types of chromosomal abnormality: those caused by faulty meiotic chromosomal separation and those caused by postzygotic mitotic errors. The meiotic errors are probably intrinsic to the gametes and are not affected by the culture system. It is presumed that mitotic errors are affected by the ART procedure and can be reduced by improved culture systems. This will be a matter for future research.

Problems related to embryonic development may not be caused only by imperfect culture systems. Some authors compared DNA methylation patterns of two-cell murine embryos from superovulated and non-superovulated females and related their rate of development up to the blastocyst stage with aberrant DNA methylation patterns[10]. It appeared that superovulation caused aberrant DNA methylation patterns, which affected the developmental potential of embryos negatively. Other authors found an increased incidence of multinucleation in embryos generated in cycles in which higher doses of gonadotropins were needed[11].

Since, in our opinion, there is no reason to presume that bovine and murine embryos are essentially different from human embryos, it can be hypothesized that both ovarian hyperstimulation and the culture procedure can affect the quality of embryos and the chances to conceive.

THIRD-ORDER RISKS

These risks are defined as unwanted side-effects of the ART procedures to gametes and embryos resulting in the birth of disabled children, or children with health hazards in later life, including poor school results, reproductive impairment and increased health problems when aging.

Effect of ART on the children

It is clear that the population of children born after ART differs from the population of spontaneously conceived children. To date, a 20–30% twin pregnancy rate is common after IVF or ICSI. Therefore, 30–40% of all children born after IVF/ICSI belong to a set of multiples. As a consequence, many health complications of ART children are related to multiple pregnancies and premature birth.

Another aspect of ART is that the population which needs ART differs from the population which can conceive naturally. We have a complex situation where differences in the population of ART children can be caused by the ART procedures, by multiple pregnancies and by the background of the parents.

Another serious problem to be taken into account when making a final judgement of the effect of ART on the children is the lack of sufficient good-quality data and the lack of the proper controls. Each year more than 100 000 children are born worldwide because of ART treatments, but the number of children in which systematic health data are collected is a relatively small part of this number. Also, there is no systematic information on school results and there is only fragmentary information on adolescence. There is only minimal interest in investing public or corporate money into answering these questions. One can only guess at the reason why that is; one explanation is that, up to now, most ART children are healthy.

The largest study of the incidence of chromosomal abnormalities after ICSI was performed by Bonduelle and colleagues, who reported 1586 karyotypes of ICSI fetuses[12]. They concluded that there is an increased chance of about 1% of *de novo* chromosomal abnormalities, mainly related to sex chromosomes (0.6%). The cause of this increase might be the genetic background of the parents but it cannot be excluded that the ICSI laboratory procedures are related to this increase.

ART has a small but significant effect on birth weight. A large Dutch study analyzed the birth weight of singletons born after IVF, comparing 1465 IVF children with 2061 controls[13]. The uncorrected difference in birth weight was 186 g; after correction for lifestyle factors, infant sex and gestational age, the birth weight of IVF children was 90 g less ($p < 0.02$) than that of spontaneously conceived children. It can be concluded that, after correction for confounding factors, IVF children still have a lower average birth weight, indicating that the ART procedures can affect fetal growth.

IVF has no significant effect on congenital malformations. Another Dutch study analyzed a cohort of 4224 children born after IVF (including 380 children born after ICSI) and compared the incidence of congenital malformations with that among 314 605 naturally conceived children[14]. Before correction for confounding factors there was a significantly higher incidence of the risk of any malformation (OR 1.20; 95% CI 1.01–1.43). After correction for differences in maternal age, parity and ethnicity, the OR was 1.03 (95% CI 0.86–1.23). The authors concluded that the small increase in overall congenital malformations observed in IVF children appears to be attributable to differences in maternal characteristics and not to the IVF procedure itself.

There is one report on a slightly negative effect of ICSI on motor development at 1 year of age[15]. The study was repeated when these children were 5 years old. At that age no differences from the controls was found[16]. Another study compared the development at 2 years of age of children born after ICSI or born after IVF, and no differences could be detected[17]. Reports on school results and adolescent behavior also showed no negative effects of ART[18,19]. However, these studies were performed with relatively small groups, and it is too early for final conclusions to be drawn.

From the collected evidence one could conclude that ART has no or only minor health effects on the children. However, before this conclusion can be finally adopted, two additional issues should be addressed: the potential effects of ART on imprinted genes and on the process of aging.

Diseases caused by errors in genomic imprinting

It is known from studies in cattle that the more invasive the ART procedure, the more frequent and the more severe the health effects[20]. In cattle and sheep this health effect is known as the large offspring syndrome. Large offspring syndrome, also called fetal overgrowth syndrome, is characterized by an average increase in birth weight of 10–100%, by prolonged gestational age, increased amniotic fluid production, claw problems, sudden postnatal death, and heart and liver enlargement. It appeared that the severity of the large offspring syndrome could be tempered by omitting fetal calf serum from the culture medium. Large offspring syndrome can in part be explained by errors in genomic imprinting.

What is genomic imprinting? Mammals are diploid (their cells contain two sets of chromosomes); each parent has supplied one set. Most autosomal genes show the same transcription status. The loss of one copy can be easily tolerated for the majority of genes. Some genes, however, are different. The transcription of these genes is determined by their parental origin. The two parental alleles can be either maternally expressed and paternally silent or vice versa. This is called genomic imprinting. Genomic imprinting takes place during gamete formation and early embryonic development. It is estimated that there are 60–80 imprinted genes[21]. It is presumed that imprinted genes are of importance in the regulation of fetal growth and in the development of the placenta. Genomic imprinting assures that the gametes of both the female and the male are involved in the genesis of the offspring. DNA methylation is the mechanism of genomic imprinting. Some examples of imprinted genes are *H19*, *IGF2* and *IFG2R*. It has been shown that large offspring syndrome is associated with reduced methylation and expression of the imprinted gene *IFG2R* and with different expression of other genes[22].

It is generally accepted that ART procedures can affect the expression of imprinted genes in animal experiments[23]. It would be highly exceptional if the human embryo behaved differently, hence genetic diseases related to imprinting defects could be expected, but not easily observed[24]. This has by chance happened recently. Four papers have been published on the occurrence of syndromes caused by imprinting errors in ART children. Two papers report on the sporadic form of Angelman syndrome and two on the Beckwith–Wiedemann syndrome.

The Angelman syndrome is a neurogenic disorder characterized by severe mental retardation, delayed motor development, poor balance, absence of speech and a happy disposition. It is caused by loss of function of the maternal allele of the *UBE3A* gene on chromosome 15. This loss is due to a point mutation, uniparental disomy (UPD) or an imprinting defect. This means that there is a paternal imprint on the maternal chromosome or an inherited imprinting-center deletion. Two girls with Angelman syndrome have been described, both caused by an imprinting defect[25]. In both girls the imprinting center was normal. This rare form of Angelman syndrome occurs in 1 : 300 000 newborns. The authors concluded that, in these two girls, the Angelman syndrome was caused by a postzygotic epigenetic defect, associated with the ICSI procedure. Another author published a comparable case of a girl with Angelman syndrome with the sporadic imprinting error[26]. All three were girls and were about 3 years old when the Angelman syndrome was diagnosed.

Children with Beckwith–Wiedemann syndrome have macroglossia, pre- and/or postnatal overgrowth and anterior wall defects. Beckwith–Wiedemann syndrome is a model imprinting disorder located at chromosome 11p15.5. Of the sufferers, 5–15% have epigenetic alterations at the *H19/IGF2* loci (the maternal *H19* and *IGF2* alleles display paternal allele methylation and expression patterns with biallelic *IFG2* expression and silencing of *H19* expression), 40–50% have loss of imprinting of the maternal allele *LIT1*, an untranslated RNA within the *KVLQT1* gene and 20% is caused by UPD. The children grow up normally but are at an increased risk of embryonic tumors. Six children with Beckwith–Wiedemann syndrome were identified in a cohort of 43 074 IVF/ICSI children, whereas 1.7 would have been expected normally, therefore showing an increase of almost four times[27]. The authors concluded that there was a significant over-representation of Beckwith–Wiedemann syndrome in children after IVF or ICSI. In four of the six children, UPD was excluded; two children had hypomethylation within the *KVLQT1*

gene, but no information on the other two was available.

Other authors recently reported seven children with Beckwith–Wiedemann syndrome[28]; four were born after ICSI and three after IVF. Six out of seven had a DNA analysis of the DNA regions involved. Five had aberrant methylation of the *LIT1* gene; the methylation of *H19* was affected in another child. These observations showed that imprinting errors did cause the syndrome. The authors presumed that the population of IVF/ICSI children had a six-fold increase in the incidence in Beckwith–Wiedemann syndrome. The incidence in the normal population is 1 : 15 000. If the authors mentioned above, reporting in the UK and the USA, respectively[27,28], are correct then we can expect a child with Beckwith–Wiedemann syndrome in every 2500 to 5000 births. In The Netherlands, > 4000 IVF/ICSI children are born each year; however, in the national Beckwith–Wiedemann syndrome registry, no children born after assisted reproduction have been found to date. However, this is a voluntary registry and only recently were the parents asked to notify the method of conception. A problem with these registries in both the UK and the USA is that they are voluntary, and we do not know whether there are any unregistered cases. The suggested increase in the Beckwith–Wiedemann syndrome incidence four- to six-fold in IVF/ICSI children is uncertain, but we can conclude that IVF/ICSI possibly increases the incidence of the syndrome significantly. The cause is unknown, but we know from work in mice, cattle and sheep that the ART laboratory procedures can affect imprinted genes. We have to conclude that the four mentioned papers give good evidence that ART laboratory procedures can possibly affect these genes in humans as well. To date, 16 children have been reported with diseases related to genomic imprinting. We have no information about the size of the population of ART children they represent, but this will be at least 90 000. In such a population, six cases would reflect the natural incidence. If these estimations are correct, ART will cause an increase from 1 : 15 000 to 1 : 5500 in the incidence of rare diseases. It must be possible to check this figure in the registries of Beckwith–Wiedemann syndrome, Angelman syndrome and other rare diseases. Even if ART results in a four- to six-fold increase in the incidence of rare diseases, the absolute number will still be small in comparison with the baseline risk of giving birth to an affected child. Large offspring syndrome occurs in 7–30% in *in vitro*-produced lambs and calves. The question is how it is possible that ART causes such a high incidence of affected imprinted genes in these animals, whereas the incidences in the human seem to be low.

Retinoblastoma

Retinoblastoma is a malignant tumor of the retina occurring in childhood. The incidence of the disease is around 1 : 17 000 live births. In The Netherlands in the period November 2000 to February 2002 five children born after IVF or ICSI treatment had retinoblastoma[29]. It is concluded that IVF/ICSI results in an increased risk ratio of at least 4.9 (95% CI 1.6–11.3) for retinoblastoma (the incidence is increased from 1 : 17 000 to 1 : 3500). It is possible that this is just a coincidence, but there has been a previous paper in which it was concluded that children born after IVF or ICSI had an increased risk of ocular anomalies[30]. These two reports suggest that IVF or ICSI can affect the eyes of the children. Retinoblastomas are not caused by imprinting errors. The mechanism of how IVF or ICSI may cause retinoblastoma is not known.

Effect of ART on the process of aging of the offspring

There are no data about the process of aging of children born after ART. The oldest child, Louise Brown, was born in 1978 and has just turned 25. To imagine what ART means for the process of aging we have to use experiments of human history and the results achieved in experimental animals.

Barker formulated his hypothesis of the fetal origin of diseases in later life[31]. This hypothesis is based on many observations, of which one will be mentioned. During World War II in the West of Holland there was a period of famine, with a well-defined beginning and a well-defined end. In the Academic Hospital of Amsterdam, records were kept of pregnant women and of all children born in the period of the famine. Records are also available of the period before and after the famine, to be used as controls. All these records were available for research. It appeared that malnutrition during the

period of conception and during the first trimester of pregnancy, followed by normal energy intake during the rest of the pregnancy, resulted in babies with a normal birth weight (average 3470 g, not different from controls). More than 50 years later, these individuals were traced and participated in a health survey. It appeared that the group of people of whom the mother had suffered malnutrition during conception and early pregnancy had significantly poorer general health, a higher incidence of coronary heart diseases, a lower concentration of high-density lipoprotein (HDL) cholesterol and an increased ratio of low-density lipoprotein (LDL)/HDL cholesterol than the control group[32]. Similar results were achieved with the offspring of experimental animals who were kept on a low-calorie diet at the period of conception and during preimplantation embryonic development.

ART laboratory procedures affect the aging of the offspring in a comparable way, as is demonstrated in the three following examples. Eppig and O'Brien described the history of Eggbirth. A male mouse, born from an *in vitro*-matured primordial follicle, Eggbirth was normally fertile and died prematurely because of severe neurological problems: diabetes type II and too much body fat[33]. Dulioust and co-workers flushed two-cell embryos from tubes of superovulated mice, and divided them into control and experimental groups[34]. The embryos of the control group were kept in culture for several hours and the embryos of the experimental group were cryopreserved and thawed. The embryos were then transferred to foster mothers. The growth, development and learning behavior of both groups was investigated. It appeared that cryopreservation and thawing resulted in an increased body weight at adult age. It also affected learning behavior negatively.

Oganuki and colleagues performed an experiment with three groups of mice[35]: one group was naturally mated, one group was conceived by ICSI with spermatids and one group was cloned and had its origin in Sertoli cells. These authors observed the groups for more than 800 days (Figure 2). The first cloned animal died at the age of 300 days. The first ICSI animal died at the age of 500 days and the first animal of the natural conception group died at the age of 650 days. At the age of 800 days, ten out of 12 cloned animals had died and two of the ICSI

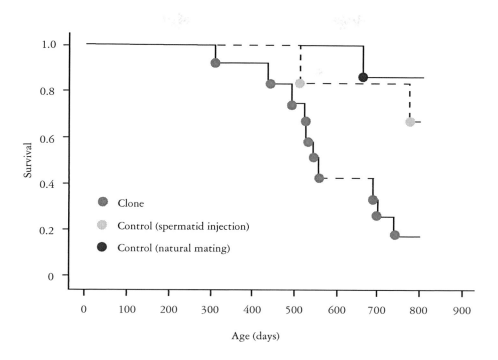

Figure 2 The survival of three groups of mice, after natural mating, intracytoplasmic sperm injection (ICSI) with spermatids and cloning with nuclei from Sertoli cells. Cloning caused premature death, ICSI did not. From reference 33 with permission

group. Only one animal in the natural conception group had died at that age. Although the groups were small, it was concluded that ICSI with spermatids did not result in premature death, as did cloning.

ART affects aging in experimental animals in comparable ways, causing an increased incidence of high blood pressure, too much body fat, an increased incidence of type II diabetes mellitus, comparable with the diseases predicted by the Barker hypothesis. It is advocated that we carry out research in glucose and cholesterol metabolism in children born because of ART treatments. This will indicate whether these children will have increased risks related to impaired glucose metabolism and an increased ratio of LDL/HDL cholesterol.

CLOSING REMARKS

A new pharmaceutical is introduced according to very well-defined protocols and pharmaceutical companies are responsible for the unforeseen side-effects. ART procedures have not been and are not being introduced according to well-defined protocols and are introduced without knowledge of the risks. We, the professionals performing ART, are responsible, but what are the risks?

Begetting children involves taking a risk. About 2.7% of children born after natural conception have congenital malformations. ICSI children have an increased risk for chromosomal abnormalities (+0.6%) and there is a small increase in the incidence of rare diseases such as Angelman syndrome, Beckwith–Wiedemann syndrome and retinoblastomas. The total increase of the incidence of rare disease is less than a fraction of a per cent. IVF/ICSI children have a slightly smaller average birth weight (−90 g) after correction for confounding factors, demonstrating that ART procedures can potentially affect the children, but there are no indications that this small decrease in birth weight affects the health of the children. Besides the three mentioned effects (+0.6% chromosomal abnormalities after ICSI, increased incidence of rare diseases by ±0.02%, decrease of birth weight by 90 g), there do not seem to be intrinsic risks in ART procedures. However, the effects on the process of aging are not known. If there are obvious iatrogenic risks to ART, they are mainly related to multiple birth, to the human factor in performing the ART laboratory procedures and to a pregnancy rate that is too low, because the ART procedures are not performed according to the state of the art. The risks of the human factor can be reduced by the introduction of a good-quality system. The risks of a pregnancy rate that is too low can be reduced by meticulously comparing the ART procedures with the way they are performed in ART centers with optimal results. As a scientific community we can reduce these risks by transforming the art of ART into the science of ART. This will be a long path because of the many variables involved.

To know the risks of ART for the offspring we have to start to register all health problems of ART children. We need all ART children to be registered in order to detect the potential effects of ART on the incidence of rare diseases, and we need proper registries of naturally conceived children as well, to know whether the effect is indeed caused by ART. We are responsible for the quality of ART treatments. We have to know the risks and we have to counsel our patients honestly about the risks and the uncertainties.

To date, all new ART laboratory procedures have been introduced according to the same pattern. The first IVF babies born from 1978 were apparently healthy and IVF spread rapidly throughout the world. ICSI followed the same pattern (first baby born in 1992), as did microsurgical epididymal sperm aspiration, testicular sperm extraction and preimplantation genetic diagnosis. The introduction of new culture media and the decision to transfer blastocysts instead of day-2 or day-3 embryos – all new procedures – were introduced without questioning the impact on the newborns. Semicloning (haploidization) and cloning are now being advocated, once again without knowing the health effects on the children and the effects on their health in later life. Not many ART centers are concerned about the health of the children, nor are the health authorities. This is remarkable, if one realizes that in the Western world between 0.5 and 4% (in The Netherlands, 2%) of the newborn babies are the result of ART treatments.

It is time that we accept our responsibilities[36]. We have to know the health effects of ART in later life. ART will remain a 'black box' for a long time, but we can make the black box smaller. To date, we have been lucky; let us not challenge our luck any longer.

REFERENCES

1. Wikland M, Sjöblom C. The application of quality systems in ART programs. *Mol Cell Endocrinol* 2000;166:3–7

2. Kastrop PM, Weima SM. International standard for IVF centres. *Hum Reprod* 2003;18:460–1

3. Coates A, Rutherford AJ, Hunter H, Leese HJ. Glucose-free medium in human *in vitro* fertilization and embryo transfer: a large-scale, prospective, randomized clinical trial. *Fertil Steril* 1999;72:229–32

4. Macklon NS, Pieters MH, Hassan MA, *et al.* A prospective randomized comparison of sequential versus monoculture systems for *in-vitro* human blastocyst development. *Hum Reprod* 2002;17:2700–5

5. Leese HJ. Quiet please, do not disturb: a hypothesis of embryo metabolism and viability. *Bioessays* 2002;24:845–9

6. Gerris J, De Neubourg D, Mangelschots K, *et al.* Elective single day 3 embryo transfer halves the twinning rate without decrease in the ongoing pregnancy rate of an IVF/ICSI programme. *Hum Reprod* 2002;17:2626–31

7. Viuff D, Greve T, Avery B, *et al.* Chromosome aberrations in *in vitro*-produced bovine embryos at days 2–5 post-insemination. *Biol Reprod* 2000;63:1143–8

8. Viuff D, Hendriksen PJ, Vos PL, *et al.* Chromosomal abnormalities and developmental kinetics in *in vivo*-developed cattle embryos

at days 2 to 5 after ovulation. *Biol Reprod* 2001;65:204–8

9. Bielanska M, Tan SL, Ao A. High rate of mixoploidy among human blastocysts cultured *in vitro*. *Fertil Steril* 2002;78:1248–53

10. Shi W, Haaf T. Aberrant methylation patterns at the two-cell stage as an indicator of early developmental failure. *Mol Reprod Dev* 2002; 63:329–34

11. Van Royen E, Mangelschots K, Vercruyssen M, *et al.* Multinucleation in cleavage stage embryos. *Hum Reprod* 2003;18:1062–9

12. Bonduelle M, Van Assche E, Joris H, *et al.* Prenatal testing in ICSI pregnancies: incidence of chromosomal anomalies in 1586 karyotypes and relation to sperm parameters. *Hum Reprod* 2002;17:2600–14

13. Buitendijk SE. IVF pregnancies: outcome and follow-up. PhD Thesis, Leiden, 2000

14. Anthony S, Buitendijk SE, Dorrepaal CA, *et al.* Congenital malformations in 4224 children conceived after IVF. *Hum Reprod* 2002;17: 2089–95

15. Bowen JR, Gibson FL, Leslie GI, Saunders DM. Medical and developmental outcome at 1 year for children conceived by intracytoplasmic sperm injection. *Lancet* 1998;351: 1529–34

16. Leslie GI, Cohen J, Gibson FL, *et al.* ICSI children have normal development at school age. *Hum Reprod* 2002;17: *Abstract Book* 1, O–009

17. Bonduelle M, Ponjaert I, Steirteghem AV, *et al.* Developmental outcome at 2 years of age for children born after ICSI compared with children born after IVF. *Hum Reprod* 2003;18: 342–50

18. Cederblad M, Friberg B, Ploman F, *et al.* Intelligence and behaviour in children born

after *in-vitro* fertilization treatment. *Hum Reprod* 1996;11:2052–7

19. Golombok S, Brewaeys A, Giavazzi MT, *et al.* The European study of assisted reproduction families: the transition to adolescence. *Hum Reprod* 2002;17:830–40

20. van Wagtendonk-de Leeuw AM, Mullaart E, de Roos AP, *et al.* Effects of different reproduction techniques: AI MOET or IVP, on health and welfare of bovine offspring. *Theriogenology* 2000;53:575–97

21. Sleutels F, Barlow DP. The origins of genomic imprinting in mammals. *Adv Genet* 2002;46:119–63

22. Young LE, Fernandes K, McEvoy TG, *et al.* Epigenetic change in IGF2R is associated with fetal overgrowth after sheep embryo culture. *Nature Genet* 2001;27:153–4

23. Khosla S, Dean W, Reik W, Feil R. Culture of preimplantation embryos and its long-term effects on gene expression and phenotype. *Hum Reprod Update* 2001;7:419–27

24. Leese HJ, Donnay I, Thompson JG. Human assisted conception: a cautionary tale. Lessons from domestic animals. *Hum Reprod* 1998;13:184–202

25. Cox GF, Burger J, Lip V, *et al.* Intracytoplasmic sperm injection may increase the risk of imprinting defects. *Am J Hum Genet* 2002;71:162–4

26. Orstavik KH, Eiklid K, van der Hagen CB, *et al.* Another case of imprinting defect in a girl with Angelman syndrome who was conceived by intracytoplasmic semen injection. *Am J Hum Genet* 2003;72:218–19

27. Maher ER, Brueton LA, Bowdin SC, *et al.* Beckwith–Wiedemann syndrome and assisted reproduction technology (ART). *J Med Genet* 2003;40:62–4

28. DeBaun MR, Niemitz EL, Feinberg AP. Association of *in vitro* fertilization with Beckwith–Wiedemann syndrome and epigenetic alterations of LIT1 and H19. *Am J Hum Genet* 2003;72:156–60

29. Moll AC, Imhof SM, Schouten-van Meeteren AY, van Leeuwen FE. *In vitro* fertilization and retinoblastoma. *Lancet* 2003;361:1392

30. Anteby I, Cohen E, Anteby E, BenEzra D. Ocular manifestations in children born after *in vitro* fertilization. *Arch Ophthalmol* 2001;119: 1525–9

31. Barker DJ, Clark PM. Fetal undernutrition and disease in later life. *Rev Reprod* 1997;2: 105–12

32. Roseboom TJ. The fetal origins hypothesis. *Twin Res* 2001;4:iii

33. Eppig JJ, O'Brien MJ. Comparison of preimplantation developmental competence after mouse oocyte growth and development *in vitro* and *in vivo*. *Theriogenology* 1998;49:415–22

34. Dulioust E, Toyama K, Busnel MC, *et al.* Long-term effects of embryo freezing in mice. *Proc Natl Acad Sci USA* 1995;92:589–93

35. Ogonuki N, Inoue K, Yamamoto Y, *et al.* Early death of mice cloned from somatic cells. *Nature Genet* 2002;30:253–4

36. Lambert RD. Safety issues in assisted reproduction technology: the children of assisted reproduction confront the responsible conduct of assisted reproductive technologies. *Hum Reprod* 2002;17:3011–15

11

Timing of embryo transfer as relevant to twin prevention

P. De Sutter and J. Gerris

INTRODUCTION

Since the beginning of *in vitro* fertilization (IVF), it has been unclear on what day after fertilization embryo transfer should best take place. In 1984, Edwards and colleagues performed a controlled trial comparing day-2 with day-3 transfers, and concluded that day-3 transfer led to an increased (although not statistically significant) pregnancy rate, when compared to day-2 transfer[1]. On the other hand, they observed significantly higher abortion rates after day-3 than after day-2 transfers, and this may have been the reason why, over the years, most people continued to transfer embryos on the second day after fertilization. In the 1990s, however, many laboratories shifted to day-3 transfers, although there was no conclusive evidence supporting this decision. Surprisingly, only a very low number of studies have been performed to compare day-2 with day-3 transfer in IVF, in contrast to the substantial number of trials comparing day-2 and day-3 (or early cleaving stage) embryo transfers with blastocyst transfers. Owing to the very high ongoing pregnancy rates obtained by some authors in the 1990s after the transfer of more than one (two and often more than two) day-5 embryos, usually in selected groups of patients, blastocyst culture and transfer in many centers has become the unquestioned default procedure.

There are some theoretical considerations that support the idea that delaying embryo transfer could increase pregnancy and implantation rates in human assisted reproductive technologies (ART). First, delaying the time of transfer could optimize the synchronization of the uterine environment with the developmental stage of the embryos. Indeed, it does not appear to be physiological to replace early cleavage embryos in the uterus 2 or 3 days after ovulation; this is the stage of development in which, under normal physiological circumstances of a spontaneous conception, these embryos are supposedly to be found no further down the feminine tract than the Fallopian tubes. Second, delaying the moment of transfer theoretically allows the possibility of selecting the embryo(s) with the highest implantation potential, the underlying assumption being that time itself acts as a selection mechanism, avoiding the necessity of any form of selection at an earlier stage. Different embryo evaluation systems have been designed[2-7]. Some of them are intrinsically scoring systems, i.e. they do not address the predictability of ongoing implantation of specific individual embryos, but they try to correlate the odds for a pregnancy with a 'total embryo score', whereas others have from the beginning addressed a potential correlation between the implantation of individual embryos and their morphological characteristics. All of them, to some extent have been shown to predict IVF outcome. It has been hypothesized that evaluation at a later stage could increase the efficiency of the selection procedure: embryos could show arrest in their development; embryo characteristics could deteriorate; cellular fragmentation could increase; and multinucleation could become more prominently visible[7]. The embryonic genome has been shown to be activated between the four-cell (day 2) and the eight-cell stage (day 3)[8]. However, the precise biological meaning of all these morphological phenomena has not been unequivocally clear, whereas the latter argument has always sounded rather spurious in favor of blastocyst transfer, because, if anything, it implies that day-3 embryos, in which embryonic genes have been switched on, are at the stage of choice for transfer.

A third theoretical argument in favor of delaying the transfer has been suggested, introducing the rather contentious notion that blastocyst culture and transfer allow the reduction of the number of embryos to be transferred, ultimately leading to a much desired decrease in the multiple birth rate following ART[9], as if selection at an earlier stage could not be combined with single-embryo transfer. This chapter will deal with the following question: does the delay of embryo transfer increase embryo implantation rates and is blastocyst transfer therefore a prerequisite for elective single-embryo transfer?

DAY-2 VERSUS DAY-3 TRANSFER

Only eight studies have been published on this subject to date. Two are fully randomized prospective trials[10,11], two are prospective pseudo-randomized studies and four are retrospective studies[1,12–16]. Seven out of the eight trials showed no significant difference between day-2 and day-3 transfer in terms of clinical and ongoing pregnancy rates and embryo implantation rates. Odds ratios (OR) for ongoing pregnancy rates per transfer were 1.29 (95% CI 0.75–2.22) for the trial of Ertzeid and colleagues[10] and 0.93 (95% CI 0.69–1.25) for the trial of Laverge and colleagues[11]. Only one trial demonstrated a higher implantation and pregnancy rate in the day-3 versus the day-2 group[16]. However, this study was not randomized and the patients who underwent transfer on day 3 were younger, had more oocytes and more often underwent intracytoplasmic sperm injection (ICSI) than the patients in the day-2 group. In conclusion, although there is not much evidence in the literature, there certainly is no reason to conclude from the available evidence that day-3 transfer increases pregnancy and implantation rates compared to day-2 transfer. One might therefore wonder why intuitively most clinicians and laboratories prefer day-3 to day-2 transfers. It should be emphasized that, in all of these studies, selection of day-2 and day-3 embryos was performed on the basis of 'traditional'

morphological characteristics of the embryos, i.e. the number of blastomeres and the percentage of fragmentation. More subtle characteristics (e.g. early onset of the first mitotic cleavage, blastomere symmetry, the percentage of observed multinucleation) were not taken into consideration. If they had been, the result of a prospective comparison might have been different, but such a study has apparently lost its scientific attraction.

DAY 2/3 VERSUS DAY 5/6 TRANSFER

In the 1990s, culture media improved. Especially the advent of sequential media on the IVF market claimed to be able to result in successful prolonged culture of embryos until the blastocyst stage. Under the influence of other than merely scientific interests, trials have been designed to demonstrate the superiority of blastocyst culture in human ART and the scientific literature has known an outburst of blastocyst trials. However, recently some authors have shown the alleged superiority of so-called sequential culture media to be questionable[17]. Severe criticism has been voiced regarding commercialized culture media of which the precise composition has been kept 'secret', which is a doubtful if not unethical practice. Some clinical reviews have provided excellent summaries of all published trials to date[18,19], and we here provide only a synopsis of the available evidence.

The Cochrane Review, which has performed a meta-analysis of published randomized trials[19], shows no significant differences between day 2/3 and day 5/6 in live birth rate (OR 1.59; 95% CI 0.80–3.15), nor could these authors conclude that there is a difference in pregnancy rate (both overall and in different subgroups) between the transfer groups (OR 0.86; 95% CI 0.57–1.29). Implantation rates per embryos transferred were equally not significantly different (day 2/3, 17.1% versus day 5/6, 18.9%). In a subgroup of trials using the newer sequential media, implantation rates for blastocyst transfers were higher, but not significantly so (day 2/3, 22.6% versus day 5/6, 32%), which was also found in a recent Dutch study[17]. Furthermore, there were no differences between groups regarding miscarriage rates. The results of embryo freezing were better in the day 2/3 group (but at the limit of statistical significance) and there were also fewer cancellations in this group. Curiously, and of special interest to our subject, there was no significant difference in the rate of multiple pregnancies nor in the rate of high-order pregnancies. The reviewers therefore concluded that the routine practice of blastocyst culture should be offered to patients with caution, and they suggested that more data be collected using sequential media.

Kolibianakis and Devroey have also looked at all the evidence from the literature, and they concluded that higher implantation rates of blastocysts as compared to early cleavage embryos are in fact only reported in retrospective comparative studies[18]. Most of these studies were not controlled and looked at effects in small groups of selected patients; often a different number of embryos was transferred in both groups[20–26]. The same reviewers also pointed out that the argument of better synchronization of the embryo with the endometrium on day 5/6 does not hold in stimulated cycles[27]. From eight randomized controlled trials comparing day 3 with day 5, there were only five in which the number of embryos transferred was the same in both groups (Table 1)[28–32]. In three other trials a different number of embryos was transferred[33–35]. Among these eight trials, none demonstrated higher pregnancy rates in the blastocyst transfer group. Only two studies reported higher implantation rates in the blastocyst group, but it was in these trials that a different number of embryos was transferred[33,34]. Kolibianakis and Devroey concluded that there is currently no evidence supporting the switch from day 2 or 3 to blastocyst transfer, because of a similar outcome between both procedures, and an increased cost of culturing embryos until day 5[18].

More recent to this review, two more randomized trials were published comparing day-3 with day-5 transfer. One found a significant advantage in the blastocyst group[36], but unfortunately the number of transferred embryos was once again different between the day-3 and day-5 groups. The other trial found no difference in implantation or pregnancy rates between day-3 and day-5 transfers[37], both groups receiving two embryos at transfer, thereby confirming similar results found in an earlier study by Coskun and associates[30].

OPTIMAL TIME FOR EMBRYO SELECTION FOR TRANSFER

One of the intuitive but totally unproven arguments in favor of delaying the time of transfer is that embryos undergo a process of natural elimination in culture. Evaluation at a later stage could therefore render the process of embryo selection more efficient, since fewer embryos remain available in culture, which are assumed to be the 'best', and this could be the basis for higher implantation rates. However, studies that have described embryo scoring as early as the zygote stage[38,39], and certainly at the four- and eight-cell stages[7], have convincingly demonstrated that selection of the 'best' embryo for transfer does not have to be performed at the blastocyst stage to yield excellent implantation rates. Indeed, the later study[40] obtained implantation rates of 48.1% on day 3. This is a similar percentage to the 50.5%[42], the 47%[22] and the 42%[26] obtained on day 5, and these are the highest implantation rates for blastocysts published to date (with the exclusion of oocyte donation cycles). Of course, these figures (also in the study by Gerris and colleagues[40]) apply only to a highly selected group of patients with a good prognosis. In retrospect, not much remains of the theoretical assumption of blastocysts being 'by definition' the best embryos. In fact, *all* embryos that will ultimately lead to the birth of a healthy child must necessarily pass through all the early cleavage stages. The challenge is not to wait for time to passively select the 'best' embryos by assuming that blastocysts are, by definition, 'the best' embryos, but by actively recognizing those embryos that have the highest implantation potential, keeping in mind that the optimal selection technique must be not only efficacious, but also easy to learn, easy and swift to perform, preferably non-invasive, as cheap as possible, easy to repeat, easy to compare between different centers and applicable in all IVF centers of the world. Moreover, one should remember that, when a day 2 plus day 3 procedure is able to detect those embryos that possess the potential to result in an ongoing implantation of about 40%, one probably has reached the upper limit of detection of the subpopulation of euploid embryos that are generated, even in the most fertile woman. This does not exclude new developments that may be still more efficacious, perhaps in specific subgroups of patients (e.g. the older patient, the patient with

Table 1 Randomized trials comparing day (2 or) 3 versus day 5 (or 6) transfer

Authors and number of patients enroled	Inclusion criteria	Culture media	Number of embryos transferred		Pregnancy rate (%)		Implantation rate (%)		Multiple pregnancy rate (%)	
			Day 2/3	Day 5/6	Day 2/3	Day 5/6	Day 2/3	Day 5/6	Day 2/3	Day 5/6
Scholtes and Zeilmaker (1996)[28] Day 3: 233 Day 5: 410	all IVF patients	single	2.4	2.1	26	25	13	21	15	20
Gardner et al. (1998)[33] Day 3: 47 Day 5: 45	patients with > 10 follicles	sequential	3.7	2.2	66	71	30.1*	50.5	–	–
Motta et al. (1998)[45] Day 2: 58 Day 5: 58	all ICSI patients	sequential	4.6	2.3	36.8	40.4	19.4*	30.1	57	14
Huisman et al. (2000)[29] Day 3: 590 Day 5: 709	all IVF patients	single	1.9	1.9	21.7	22.1	14.4	15.5	26	32
Plachot et al. (2000)[46] Day 2: 60 Day 5: 50	excess embryos on day 2	sequential	3.03	2.24	41.7	42	18.9	24.1	25.8	31.6
Coskun et al. (2000)[30] Day 3: 101 Day 5: 100	≥ 4 zygotes	sequential	2.3	2.2	39	39	21.3	23.8	33	38

continued

Table 1   continued

Authors and number of patients enroled	Inclusion criteria	Culture media	Number of embryos transferred		Pregnancy rate (%)		Implantation rate (%)		Multiple pregnancy rate (%)	
			Day 2/3	Day 5/6	Day 2/3	Day 5/6	Day 2/3	Day 5/6	Day 2/3	Day 5/6
Karaki et al. (2002)[34] Day 3: 82 Day 5: 80	> 4 zygotes	sequential	3.5	2.0	26	29	12.7*	26.1	48	39
Levron et al. (2002)[35] Day 3: 44 Day 5: 46	> 5 zygotes	sequential	3.1	2.3	45.5*	18.6	38.7*	20.2	40	50
Utsunomiya et al. (2002)[31] Day 3: 184 Day 5: 180	all patients	sequential	2.9	3.0	26.3	24.8	11.7	9.2	–	–
Rienzi et al. (2002)[32] Day 3: 48 Day 5: 50	< 38 years, > 7 zygotes	sequential	2.0	2.0	56	58	35	38	–	–
Bungum et al. (2003)[37] Day 3: 57 Day 5: 61	< 40 years at least three 8-cell embryos	sequential	2.00	1.96	63.2	52.5	43.9	36.7	41.6	40.6
Frattarelli et al. (2003)[36] Day 3: 23 Day 5: 26	< 35 years at least six good embryos on day 3	sequential	2.96	2.04	57.1	43.5	26.1*	43.4	70*	27.7

IVF, in vitro fertilization; ICSI, intracytoplasmic sperm injection
*Significantly different from corresponding day 5 rate ($p < 0.05$)

repeated miscarriage, etc.) but when speaking about a reduction in twin pregnancies, we should first look where these occur most readily, i.e. in young women during their first treatment cycles.

SINGLE-EMBRYO TRANSFER OR SINGLE-BLASTOCYST TRANSFER?

To date, no results have been published of a prospective randomized trial comparing the transfer of a single day-3 embryo with a single day-5 embryo, which could settle the issue. However, some recommendations are to be made. Such a trial should address an unselected population of patients, below a preset age (e.g. 38 years of age) and all in their first trial of IVF/ICSI treatment. Randomization must be performed prior to the initiation of ovarian stimulation, if the aim is to demonstrate or refute equipoise for the general IVF/ICSI patient population. If this is not done, one is again looking at selected patients. Furthermore, the details of the selection procedure both for day-3 and for day-5 embryos must be described in detail and must be performed optimally. There is no point in comparing blastocyst transfer with poorly selected day-3 embryo transfer. This is probably why blastocyst transfer has appealed to many centers: if early-cleavage embryo selection is poorly performed, there is a good chance that switching to blastocyst transfer will improve the results of a particular center. However, such personal experiences should not be taken for results of prospectively randomized trials.

From the available evidence in the literature and after refuting all hypothetical arguments in favor of delayed transfer, it seems clear that the secret of twin prevention lies in the transfer of one embryo, and that the timing of transfer in this respect does not seem the most important factor. The only prerequisite is that a top-quality embryo is available and how this is achieved is a matter of patient selection, laboratory skill in embryo culture and selection and, perhaps to some extent, to subjective appreciation.

Given the fact that literature data do not sustain the superiority of blastocyst transfer in terms of pregnancy rates, there are some indications that blastocyst culture may even be less effective than early-cleavage transfer. In one randomized trial, implantation rates on day 5 were lower than on day

3[35], but again, this was a study with different numbers of embryos transferred in both groups. The Rienzi trial[32] also concluded that day-3 transfers were superior to day-5 transfers if one freeze–thaw cycle was added to the fresh results, because cryopreservation of day-3 embryos in their hands had appeared more successful. Moreover, in terms of cost-effectiveness it may well be expected that blastocyst culture and transfer will be inferior to day-3 transfer, because of the elevated cost of sequential media and because of the extension of the culture period and the need for more laboratory infrastructure (the need for more incubator space) and man-hours.

With respect to the issue of twin prevention, it has been suggested that monozygotic twinning rates may be increased after blastocyst transfers in comparison with day-3 transfers[41–43]. This would imply that the transfer of a single blastocyst could lead to a higher (monozygotic) twinning rate than the transfer of a single early-cleavage embryo.

Finally, a very important aspect that has not been taken into consideration in most trials to date is the aspect of cryopreservation. If fewer embryos remain available for transfer on day 5/6, it can be expected that fewer blastocysts will be frozen than if freezing had been performed on day 3. On the other hand, freezing techniques are different for blastocysts and cleavage-stage embryos, and both survival and implantation rates may be different. Langley and co-workers have shown higher implantation rates for frozen–thawed blastocysts (21.9%) than for day-3 embryos (10.1%)[44], but this was in a retrospective comparison. The cryo-augmentation potential of day-3 and blastocyst transfer cycles will therefore depend on both the number of embryos available for freezing and post-thaw survival and implantation rates. Only prospective randomized studies including this outcome parameter will be able to answer the question of whether single-embryo transfer or single-blastocyst transfer is the answer to twin prevention in human ART.

In the meanwhile, nothing forbids individual centers from following their own course to provide the service they deem to be the best for their patients. It is most likely that each stage of embryo development can give some information that is useful for optimizing selection with a view to transferring, as frequently as possible, only one embryo. We should probably use all possible selection criteria in a complementary, not a competitive, fashion. The point made in this contribution is that it is not a prerequisite to culture all embryos in all patients to the blastocyst stage in order to introduce single-embryo transfer.

REFERENCES

1. Edwards RG, Fishel SB, Cohen J, *et al*. Factors influencing the success of *in-vitro* fertilization for alleviating human infertility. *J In Vitro Fert Embryo Transf* 1984;1:3–23

2. Puissant F, Van Rysselberge M, Barlow P, Deweze J, Leroy F. Embryo scoring as a prognostic tool in IVF treatment. *Hum Reprod* 1987;2:705–8

3. Steer CV, Mills CL, Tan SL, Campbell S, Edwards RG. The cumulative embryo score: a predictive embryo scoring technique to select the optimal number of embryos to transfer in an *in-vitro* fertilization and embryo transfer programme. *Hum Reprod* 1992;7:117–19

4. Roseboom TJ, Vermeiden JP, Schoute E, Lens JW, Schats R. The probability of pregnancy after embryo transfer is affected by the age of the patient, cause of infertility, number of embryos transferred and the average morphology score, as revealed by multiple logistic regression analysis. *Hum Reprod* 1995;10:3035–41

5. Palmstierna M, Murkes D, Csemizdy G, Andersson O, Wramsby H. Zona pellucida thickness variation and occurrence of visible mononucleated blastomeres in preembryos are associated with a high pregnancy rate in IVF treatments. *J Assist Reprod Genet* 1998;15:70–5

6. Rijnders PM, Jansen CAM. The predictive value of day 3 embryo morphology regarding blastocyst formation, pregnancy and implantation rate after day 5 transfer following *in-vitro* fertilizaton or intracytoplasmic sperm injection. *Hum Reprod* 1998;13:2869–73

7. Van Royen E, Mangelschots K, De Neubourg D, *et al*. Characterization of a top quality embryo, a step towards single-embryo transfer. *Hum Reprod* 1999;14:2345–9

8. Braude P, Bolton V, Moore S. Human gene expression first occurs between the four and eight-cell stages of preimplantation development. *Nature (London)* 1988;332:459–61

9. ESHRE Capri Workshop Group. Multiple gestation pregnancy. *Hum Reprod* 2000;15:1856–64

10. Ertzeid G, Dale PO, Tanbo T, Storeng R, Kjekshus E, Abyholm T. Clinical outcome of day 2 versus day 3 embryo transfer using serum-free culture media: a prospective randomized study. *J Assist Reprod Genet* 1999;16:529–34

11. Laverge H, De Sutter P, Van der Elst J, Dhont M. A prospective, randomized study comparing day 2 and day 3 embryo transfer in human IVF. *Hum Reprod* 2001;16:476–80

12. Van Os HC, Alberda AT, Janssen-Caspers HAB, Leerentveld RA, Scholtes MCW, Zeilmaker GH. The influence of the interval between *in vitro* fertilization and embryo transfer and some other variables on treatment outcome. *Fertil Steril* 1989;51:360–2

13. Huisman GJ, Alberda AT, Leerentveld RA, Verhoeff A, Zeilmaker GH. A comparison of *in vitro* fertilization results after embryo transfer after 2, 3, and 4 days of embryo culture. *Fertil Steril* 1994;61:970–1

14. Goto Y, Kanzaki H, Nakayama T, *et al*. Relationship between the day of embryo transfer and the outcome in human *in vitro* fertilization and embryo transfer. *J Assist Reprod Genet* 1994;11:401–4

15. Dawson KJ, Conaghan J, Ostera GR, Winston RML, Hardy K. Delaying transfer to the third day post-insemination, to select non-arrested

embryos, increases development to the fetal heart stage. *Hum Reprod* 1995;10:177–82

16. Carillo AJ, Lane B, Pridham DD, *et al*. Improved clinical outcomes for *in vitro* fertilization with delay of embryo transfer from 48 to 72 hours after oocyte retrieval: use of glucose- and phosphate-free media. *Fertil Steril* 1998;69:329–34

17. Macklon NS, Pieters MHEC, Hassan MA, *et al*. A prospective randomized comparison of sequential versus monoculture systems for *in-vitro* human blastocyst development. *Hum Reprod* 2002;17:2700–5

18. Kolibianakis EM, Devroey P. Blastocyst culture: facts and fiction. *Reprod Biomed Online* 2002;5:285–93

19. Blake D, Proctor M, Johnson N, Olive D. Cleavage stage versus blastocyst stage embryo transfer in assisted conception (Cochrane Review). In *The Cochrane Library*, Issue 1. Oxford: Update Software, 2003

20. Cruz JR, Dubey AK, Patel J, *et al*. Is blastocyst transfer useful as an alternative treatment for patients with multiple *in vitro* fertilization failures? *Fertil Steril* 1999;72:218–20

21. Marek D, Langley M, Gardner DK, *et al*. Introduction of blastocyst culture and transfer for all patients in an *in vitro* fertilization program. *Fertil Steril* 1999;72:1035–40

22. Milki AA, Hinckley MD, Fisch JD, *et al*. Comparison of blastocyst transfer with day 3 embryo transfer in similar patient populations. *Fertil Steril* 2000;73:126–9

23. Racowsky C, Jackson KV, Cekleniak NA, *et al*. The number of eight-cell embryos is a key determinant for selecting day 3 or day 5 transfer. *Fertil Steril* 2000;73:558–64

24. Balaban B, Urman B, Alatas C, *et al*. Blastocyst-stage transfer of poor-quality cleav-

age-stage embryos results in higher implantation rates. *Fertil Steril* 2001;75:514–18

25. Abdelmassih V, Balmaceda J, Nagy Z, *et al*. ICSI and day 5 embryo transfers: higher implantation rates and lower rate of multiple pregnancy with prolonged culture. *Reprod BioMed Online* 2001;3:216–20

26. Wilson M, Hartke K, Kiehl M, *et al*. Integration of blastocyst transfer for all patients. *Fertil Steril* 2002;77:693–6

27. Nikas G, Develioglu OH, Toner JP, *et al*. Endometrial pinopodes indicate a shift in the window of receptivity in IVF cycles. *Hum Reprod* 1999;14:787–92

28. Scholtes MC, Zeilmaker GH. A prospective, randomized study of embryo transfer results after 3 or 5 days of embryo culture in *in vitro* fertilization. *Fertil Steril* 1996;65:1245–8

29. Huisman GJ, Fauser BC, Eijkemans MJ, *et al*. Implantation rates after *in vitro* fertilization and transfer of a maximum of two embryos that have undergone three to five days of culture. *Fertil Steril* 2000;73:117–22

30. Coskun S, Hollanders J, Al-Hassan S, *et al*. Day 5 versus day 3 embryo transfer: a controlled randomized trial. *Hum Reprod* 2000;15:1947–52

31. Utsunomiya T, Naitou T, Nagaki M. A prospective trial of blastocyst culture and transfer. *Hum Reprod* 2002;17:1846–51

32. Rienzi L, Ubaldi F, Iacobeli M, *et al*. Day 3 embryo transfer with combined evaluation at the pronuclear and cleavage stages compares favourably with day 5 blastocyst transfer. *Hum Reprod* 2002;17:1852–5

33. Gardner DK, Schoolcraft WB, Wagley L, *et al*. A prospective randomized trial of blastocyst culture and transfer in *in-vitro* fertilization. *Hum Reprod* 1998;13:3434–40

34. Karaki RZ, Samarraie SS, Younis NA, *et al*. Blastocyst culture and transfer: a step toward improved *in vitro* fertilization outcome. *Fertil Steril* 2002;77:114–18

35. Levron J, Shulman A, Bider D, *et al*. A prospective randomized study comparing day 3 with blastocyst-stage embryo transfer. *Fertil Steril* 2002;77:1300–1

36. Frattarelli JL, Leondires MP, McKeeby JL, Miller BT, Segars JH. Blastocyst transfer decreases multiple pregnancy rates in *in vitro* fertilization cycles: a randomized controlled trial. *Fertil Steril* 2003;79:228–30

37. Bungum M, Bungum L, Humaidan P, *et al*. Day 3 versus day 5 embryo transfer: a prospective randomized study. *RBM Online* 2003;7:98–104

38. Scott LA, Smith S. The successful use of pronuclear embryo transfers the day following oocyte retrieval. *Hum Reprod* 1998;13: 1003–13

39. Scott L, Alvero R, Leondires M, Miller B. The morphology of human pronuclear embryos is positively related to blastocyst development and implantation. *Hum Reprod* 2000;15: 2394–403

40. Gerris J, De Neubourg D, Mangelschots K, *et al*. Prevention of twin pregnancy after *in-vitro* fertilization or intracytoplasmic sperm injection based on strict embryo criteria: a prospective randomized clinical trial. *Hum Reprod* 1999;14:2581–7

41. Peramo B, Ricciarelli E, Cuadros-Fernandez JM, *et al*. Blastocyst transfer and monozygotic twinning. *Fertil Steril* 1999;72:1116–17

42. Behr B, Fisch JD, Racowsky C, *et al*. Blastocyst-ET and monozygotic twinning. *J Assist Reprod Genet* 2000;17:349–51

43. da Costa al AL, Abdelmassih S, de Oliveira FG, *et al*. Monozygotic twins and transfer at the blastocyst stage after ICSI. *Hum Reprod* 2001;16:333–6

44. Langley MT, Marek DM, Gardner DK, *et al*. Extended embryo culture in human assisted reproduction treatments. *Hum Reprod* 2001;16:902–8

45. Motta LA, Alegretti JR, Pico M, Sousa JW, Baracat EC, Serafini P. Blastocyst vs. cleaving embryo transfer: a prospective randomized trial. *Fertil Steril* 1998;70(3Suppl 1):S17

46. Plachot M, Belaisch-Allart J, Mayenga JM, Chouraqui A, Serkine AM, Tesquier L. Blastocyst stage transfer: the real benefits compared with early embryo transfer. *Hum Reprod* 2000;15(Suppl 6):24–30

12

Epidemiology and pathophysiology of ovarian hyperstimulation syndrome

A. Delvigne

EPIDEMIOLOGY

Incidence

Global incidence

The reported incidence of ovarian hyperstimulation syndrome (OHSS) is extremely variable, according to different studies, because various classifications have been used. Furthermore, these studies relate to very different clinical situations such as controlled ovarian stimulation or ovarian stimulation during *in vitro* fertilization (IVF), which are not comparable in terms of therapeutic goals and strategies. When considering IVF treatment, the reported incidence lies between 3 and 6% for the moderate and between 0.1 and 2% for the severe form of OHSS[1]. The mild forms of OHSS, which have little clinical relevance, constitute about 20–33% of IVF cycles[2]. It has been estimated that, worldwide, at least 100–200 women suffer annually from severe OHSS per 100 000 cycles of assisted reproductive technologies (ART); there are about 500 000 IVF/intracytoplasmic sperm injection (ICSI) cycles worldwide per year and probably as many if not more non-IVF cycles in which gonadotropins are used[3,4]. The largest cohort of OHSS cases was reported in Israel: the increase in incidence of the severe forms of OHSS surpassed the increase of total IVF activity during the same period (20-fold versus six-fold, respectively)[5]. Therefore, although the incidence of the severe form of OHSS is only about 1%, one should be aware of its recent, progressive increase. This constitutes a serious health hazard as well as a prophylactic challenge, since women treated with IVF/ICSI are *a priori* healthy young women. Moreover, there is a general unawareness of the syndrome among the lay public, which increases the risk for late or inappropriate diagnosis as well as its psychological impact on those who succumb to it.

Incidence of specific complications

Hemoconcentration has been found in 95.2% of patients affected by severe OHSS and in 71.1% of cases of mild or moderate forms of OHSS[6,7]. Approximately one-third of the patients affected by severe OHSS associated with clinical ascites suffered also from oliguria.

Electrolyte disorders were observed in 54.6% of patients with mild or moderate OHSS; 24.2% concerned potassium disorders only and 22.7% sodium disorders only[7].

Pulmonary manifestations were observed in 7.2% of severe OHSS forms: dyspnea was the most frequent respiratory symptom, affecting 92.3% of the cases, but 92% also suffered from tachypnea and in 80% a decrease of respiratory sounds was observed. A minority of patients presented some severe complications, such as lobar pneumonia (4%), adult respiratory distress syndrome (ARDS) (2%) and pulmonary embolism (2%)[6]. X-rays showed a raised diaphragm in 71% of cases and pleural effusion in 10–29%. These changes were predominantly found on the right side (51% on the right, 21% on the left and 27% bilateral) and about 4.5% of these patients required thoracentesis.

Abnormal liver tests were found in 26–40% (mean 27.5%) of OHSS patients[8].

Temperature above 38°C for at least 24 h was observed in 83.3% of severe OHSS cases and in one-third of them an infectious origin (most frequently urinary) was found, but in about two-thirds no infectious agent was found[9].

OHSS may cause adnexal torsion in 16% of pregnant patients and in 2.3% of non-pregnant women[10].

Thromboembolic accidents are the ultimate complication that, despite appropriate treatment, can lead to the death of the patient. Their incidence is difficult to estimate, because no systematic registration of OHSS cases or of their complications exists. Three large retrospective series of OHSS cases reported thromboembolic events. One case of cerebral thrombosis (0.8%) among 128 cases of OHSS (86.7% moderate and severe forms) was documented in Belgium during a period of 4 years. Similarly, in Israel, over a period of 10 years, an incidence of 2.4% of thromboembolic events was observed among 209 cases of severe forms of OHSS[6]. Serour and colleagues registered 10% of thromboembolic phenomena among 50 patients with severe OHSS[1]. We performed a systematic review of the literature and found 68 reported cases of thrombosis: 34.3% in arterial and 65.7% in venous sites; 83% were localized in the upper part of the body (60% venous and 40% arterial) and 17% in the lower part (81% venous and 18% arterial) and we recorded 11.8% of pulmonary embolisms. When thrombosis occurred, severe OHSS was present in 76.3% of cases and pregnancy in 85%. There were as many patients with early and late OHSS complicated by thrombosis and also as many singleton or multiple pregnancies complicated by thrombosis. One should always be cautious, after ovulation stimulation, since thromboses complicated about 12% of moderate OHSS, as well as about 12% mild OHSS. Moreover, thromboses could appear as late as 20 weeks' gestation even in the absence of hemoconcentration and, in several cases, the event occurred several weeks after total resolution of OHSS[8].

Thrombosis of the coronary arteries with myocardial infarction has also been described[11]. Two fatal cases were the consequence of a cerebral infarction occurring after a thromboembolic stroke[12,13].

The incidence of cerebral thromboembolism is probably far more common than was previously believed, as it may often be overlooked in patients who are asymptomatic or show only mild neurological signs. Finally, eight fatal cases have been reported: one in New Zealand, one in Japan, one in Israel, one in Egypt and four in the Netherlands[8]. It is highly likely that many fatal cases of OHSS have not been reported. Perhaps efforts to do so in a non-identifying discrete manner, e.g. in a central European Society for Human Reproduction and Embryology (ESHRE) Registry, should be taken up.

Factors influencing the incidence of OHSS

Age

Most studies have reported that women suffering from OHSS were significantly younger than those who were not. For instance, in a large retrospective Belgian study including 128 cases of OHSS and 256 controls, the mean age of OHSS patients was 30.2 ± 3.5 years versus 32.0 ± 4.5 years in controls. A similar difference was found in other prospective studies[7,14].

Body mass index

Only one author described a positive correlation between lean body mass and OHSS[15], whereas others did not find such a correlation[7,14]. Body mass index (BMI) does not appear to be a useful marker of increased risk for OHSS.

Allergies

Because the pathophysiological changes that occur in the ovaries during OHSS closely resemble an exuberant inflammatory response, some authors have hypothesized that differences in the immunological sensitivity of patients may be a predictive sign of OHSS[14]. In a prospective study, Enskog and colleagues observed a significant increase in the prevalence of allergies in the OHSS group (50% versus 21%). This observation should be studied through biological assessment on a larger cohort, but has not been used clinically as a predictor for the occurrence of OHSS.

Etiology of infertility

OHSS has been found as often in primary as in secondary infertility. The duration of infertility does not seem to influence the incidence of OHSS[15]. Women who have previously developed OHSS are at increased risk[16].

Polycystic ovary syndrome (PCOS) appears to be the major predisposing factor for OHSS in a large number of IVF studies. In one study, 63% of severe OHSS patients showed ultrasonically diagnosed PCOS[17]. Similarly, 37% of our own reported 128 OHSS patients suffered from PCOS, versus 15% among the 256 controls[7]. This could be explained by the fact that patients with PCOS are known to produce three times as many follicles and oocytes than normo-ovulatory patients who are stimulated using the same protocols. A higher incidence of OHSS is also observed in patients who have isolated characteristics of PCOS, but not from a 'complete' form (i.e. fulfilling clinical, echographic and biological criteria).

Finding ten follicles or more with a diameter of 4–8 mm in at least one ovary, i.e. a PCOS-like ultrasonographic image, in normo-ovulatory women was shown to be predictive of an exaggerated ovarian response and a risk factor for OHSS[18]. This concept has been subsequently described as the 'necklace sign' and suggests an increased risk for the occurrence of OHSS even in the absence of other clinical or biological signs of PCOS. Using three-dimensional ultrasonography, a significant correlation between the baseline ovarian volume and the risk of developing OHSS was observed in IVF patients[19].

A luteinizing hormone (LH)/follicle stimulating hormone (FSH) ratio of > 2 has also been considered as a risk factor for OHSS, even in the absence of other signs of PCOS[16]. LH dominance could lead to a disturbed androgen–estrogen conversion, leading to a higher propensity for OHSS[20].

Hyperandrogenic women with an increased ovarian contribution to circulating levels of androstenedione not related to PCOS, also constitute a group at risk for OHSS[20].

Type of stimulatory drugs

The incidence of OHSS is clearly related to the stimulation regimen used. Clomiphene citrate is only rarely associated with severe forms of OHSS and with only 8% of moderate OHSS. A much higher incidence has been observed when using urinary gonadotropins such as human menopausal gonadotropin (hMG) or purified FSH.

The LH/FSH ratio in gonadotropin preparations has no effect on the incidence of OHSS. A Cochrane database meta-analysis has shown that, only in clomiphene-resistant patients with PCOS, is the use of urinary purified forms of FSH advantageous in preventing the syndrome[21]. A systematic review and meta-analysis of 18 randomized, controlled trials, comparing recombinant FSH with urinary FSH confirmed that there was no difference in the incidence of OHSS[22].

Gonadotropin releasing hormone (GnRH) agonists have the effect of artificially inducing in all of the patients, even those with oligomenorrheic anovulation, a state of hypogonadotropic anovulation. A reduction of the OHSS incidence was thus expected. Neverthless, the introduction of GnRH agonists in 1986 resulted in a six-fold increase in the incidence of severe forms of OHSS as compared to the incidence in IVF cycles stimulated by clomiphene/hMG only[23]. This unfavorable effect of GnRH agonists may be due to the abolition of the spontaneous luteinization process which, in spontaneous cycles, is associated with the LH peak and may be a mechanism preventing excessive follicular growth. In addition, GnRH agonists increase the risk of OHSS regardless of being used in short or long protocols in IVF.

A meta-analysis of five randomized trials showed that there was no statistically significant reduction in incidence of severe OHSS using antagonist regimens as compared to the long GnRH agonist protocols[24]. Nevertheless, all but one study on antagonists showed a reduction in OHSS. All these studies were 'Company' phase II and III studies with a cancellation policy, which happens only in the agonist cycle. The cancelled patients were not exposed to human chorionic gonadotropin (hCG). The meta-analysis by Al-Inany and Aboulghar is not a definitive judgement. GnRH antagonists probably have a lower risk of OHSS but the low incidence of the disease makes statistical demonstration difficult. However, it should be kept in mind that the use of antagonists still allows the opportunity to trigger ovulation with an agonist instead of with hCG and this in itself may have a reductive effect on the incidence of OHSS.

Contradictory results have been published with respect to the incidence of OHSS in patients with PCOS in whom hyperinsulinemia has been documented. Drugs such as metformin and octreotide have been used to reduce insulin resistance in patients with PCOS but no reduction in the incidence of OHSS has been reported in IVF when these drugs were used[25].

In summary, to date no stimulation regimen can claim to avoid all risk of OHSS. A correct evaluation of the patient's clinical profile may allow the clinician to individualize the stimulation regimen in order to minimize the risk of OHSS. Close monitoring will be more effective in detecting risk situations and performing secondary prevention of OHSS, rather than relying on a particular medication regimen.

Dose of gonadotropins

Patients suffering from OHSS often receive much less gonadotropin preparation than other patients[7,14]. Ovarian hypersensitivity to gonadotropin stimulation, reflected by higher serum estradiol peak concentrations in response to low dosages of gonadotropin and by a steeper slope of the serum estradiol increment during stimulation, has been reported in several large cohorts[7].

Exogenous human chorionic gonadotropin to trigger ovulation

In most stimulation schemes used for infertility treatment, ovulation is triggered using hCG of urinary origin, which has been chosen for its LH-like effect. However, hCG is characterized by a longer half-life, a higher receptor affinity and a longer intracellular effect compared to endogenous LH. Consequently, hCG activity time lasts for up to 6 days.

hCG is a promotor of OHSS and seems to initiate the complex cascade that leads to the development of OHSS, whereas an endogenous LH surge rarely causes OHSS.

The pregnancy rate does not seem to increase when ovulation is triggered with hCG doses of > 5000 IU, and fewer OHSS cases were reported using 1000–5000 IU. Therefore, in the presence of risk factors for OHSS, the hCG dose should not exceed 5000 IU.

Since the administration of LH may reduce overstimulation of the ovary during the luteal phase, some authors examined the possibility of triggering ovulation using the flare-up effect of the GnRH agonists with rise of LH and FSH for only 34 h both in non-IVF patients and in IVF patients in combination with the use of a GnRH-antagonist[26,27]. This combination of initial gonadotropin 'flare-up' followed by pituitary down-regulation offers the unique advantage of minimizing the risk of OHSS. Only 0.1% of cases of severe OHSS was observed when women with extremely high levels of estradiol and PCOS were treated using this method[25]. Unfortunately, not enough controlled studies have been performed to validate this practice. The use of native GnRH to trigger ovulation has been observed to result in fewer subclinical signs of ovarian hyperstimulation[16].

A prospective randomized double-blind multicenter study assessed the safety of recombinant human LH (rhLH) in patients undergoing IVF in comparison with 5000 IU of hCG. This study concluded that a dose of between 5000 and 15 000 IU of rhLH induced significantly fewer moderate and severe cases of OHSS[28].

Response to ovulation stimulation

Serum estradiol level Many investigators have demonstrated that elevated levels of serum estradiol constitute a risk factor for OHSS[15]. Severe OHSS was observed in 38% of patients in whom serum estradiol level was > 6000 pg/ml and no OHSS was observed with serum estradiol levels of < 3500 pg/ml[29]. In another study, only 17% of OHSS cases were observed among patients with serum estradiol levels > 6000 pg/ml ($n = 34$)[30]. The sensitivity and specificity for different cut-off values of serum estradiol were calculated; a significant positive likelihood ratio of 6.37 was found for a serum estradiol level in excess of 2642 pg/ml and a significant negative likelihood ratio of 0.13 for a serum estradiol level below 1847 pg/ml[2]. These different results confirm that serum estradiol levels are significantly higher in OHSS patients when compared to control patients, but estradiol alone is not a sufficiently predictive factor, owing to the overlap of estradiol values between the two populations[7]. Using a mathematical model, which included the increase in serum estradiol levels (expressed after logarithmic transformation), we were able to show that the slope of estradiol during the stimulation is also a risk factor[16].

Number and size of follicles during stimulation Most studies have found that a large number of pre-ovulatory follicles constitute a risk factor for OHSS. The size of the follicles that should be considered to assess the risk varies from one author to another. This debate is now largely obsolete, because of a substantial error in follicle measurement and counting and the relationship between this error and the number of follicles[14,15,29]. Therefore, it is more useful to relate the risk for OHSS to the total number of developing follicles irrespective of their size and to the number of collected oocytes[29]. In this study no patient developed severe OHSS when < 20 oocytes were collected, whereas retrieval of > 30 oocytes was associated with 22.7% of OHSS. Others observed 14% of OHSS among IVF patients who yielded > 30 oocytes[30].

The considerable overlap of the distribution of values for different parameters between control and OHSS patient populations makes any single variable inefficient for a reliable risk prediction. Combinations of variables were studied in a discriminant function in order to increase predictive power and decrease the false-negative prediction among 128 OHSS patients and 256 controls. A prediction of 78.5% with a corresponding false-negative rate of 18.1% was obtained for OHSS under post-retrieval conditions using log estradiol concentration, slope of log estradiol increment, gonadotropin dosage, number of oocytes retrieved and ratio of LH/FSH in the formula. However, effective prevention of OHSS implies the ability to withhold hCG injection. Therefore, a formula for pre-oocyte retrieval conditions was established, yielding a prediction rate of 76.1% with a false-negative rate of 18.1%[7].

Pregnancy rate

The risk of developing OHSS is 2–5 times higher when pregnancy occurs in IVF[25]. The incidence of OHSS was assessed among oocyte donors and classical IVF patients who presented risk factors for OHSS. OHSS was not observed among the donor patients while there were OHSS cases in the series of classical IVF patients ($p < 0.05$). The relative risk for OHSS followed by a pregnancy was 12 (95% CI 2.2–66.1, $p < 0.01$)[30].

The incidence of OHSS seems to be directly related to hCG levels: the number of gestational sacs is predictive of the incidence of late OHSS[2]. In addition, it has been suggested that undiagnosed biochemical pregnancies (defined as a transient serum hCG increase of > 10 U/l) occurring during the first 2 weeks following hCG administration, may also play a causative role in cases of severe OHSS not followed by a clinical pregnancy[30]. We also emphasized the role of biochemical pregnancy in unpredictable cases of OHSS[25].

PATHOPHYSIOLOGY

The ovarian hyperstimulation syndrome is characterized by an increase in the size of the ovaries, with the appearance of multiple cysts, and by an increase in the vascular permeability of ovarian vessels causing ascites, pleural effusion and sometimes pericardiac effusion. The severe form is also accompanied by electrolyte disturbances, as well as by cardiopulmonary, hepatic, renal and hemodynamic disturbances leading to an increased thromboembolic risk. The dominant finding is the bilateral multicystic enlargement of the ovaries. Morphological examination of these ovaries reveals multiple corpora lutea, follicle cysts and massive edema of the ovarian stroma. It has been suggested that the formation of the cysts is a direct reaction to the stimulation with gonadotropins, since similar ovarian observations exist in other conditions associated with high levels of endogenous gonadotropins such as hydatidiform mole, choriocarcinoma and multiple pregnancy.

Animal experiments have shown that the main pathological feature of OHSS is the increase in capillary permeability, as demonstrated in the rabbit experimental model using intravenous dyes[31]. Furthermore, angiogenesis is also enhanced in OHSS. It has been demonstrated in animals that the amount of fluid shifting from the intravascular space into the abdominal cavity depends on the presence of the ovaries. The latter, however, do not have to be in the peritoneal cavity[32]. Neither estrogen nor progestin in excessive amounts could cause ascites in female rabbits[31]. Moreover, OHSS cannot be induced in male animals or in men treated with large doses of gonadotropins.

Consequently, the following principles can be considered established: first, the presence of an ovary is a compulsory condition for OHSS; and second, a vasoactive mediator secreted by the ovaries plays a major role in the development of OHSS, after ovarian stimulation. This factor is probably secreted into the peritoneal cavity and liberated in the systemic circulation, where it can exert its action (Figure 1).

Some investigators have hypothesized that ascites of women with OHSS contains this chemical ovarian product responsible for OHSS. This hypothesis has been confirmed by *in vitro* permeability experiments, using follicular fluid and ascites of patients suffering from OHSS[33]. Subsequently, much research has been directed towards identifying this mediator either in blood or in ascites of patients with OHSS, and these studies are presented in this review[34].

Potential biochemical mediators

Estrogens, prolactin and prostaglandins

Estrogen is a marker of ovarian response but is not the causative agent of OHSS, since the administra-

tion of estradiol does not induce OHSS. Some authors have suggested other causal candidates such as prolactin and prostaglandins, but no evidence of a directly causative role of these substances has been demonstrated to date[34].

Activation of the ovarian prorenin–renin–angiotensin system

The ovary possesses an independent prorenin–renin–angiotensin system (RAS). Angiotensin II is involved in the autocrine and paracrine modulation of ovulation and could be a major contributor to the neovascularization required in luteinization. Active renin levels in follicular fluid increase in the follicular phase, reaching peak levels in the periovulatory period. The RAS is activated by the LH surge as well as by exogenous and endogenous hCG leading to an increase of the conversion of inactive angiotensin I into active angiotensin II.

These observations suggest that the local active RAS, through induction of new vessel formation with increased permeability, could play a causal role in the ovarian enlargement and extracellular fluid accumulation that are the hallmarks of OHSS[35]. Navot and associates compared the RAS in OHSS patients and normal ovulatory women. In OHSS patients, elevation of the midluteal prorenin–renin–

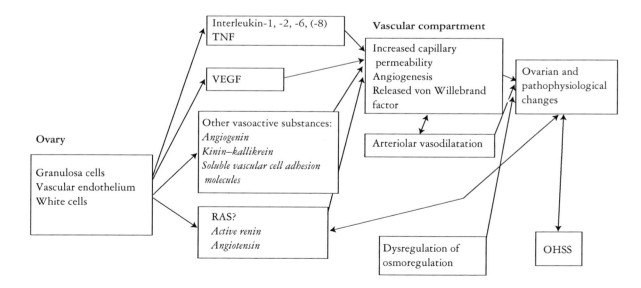

Figure 1 Pathophysiology of ovarian hyperstimulation syndrome (OHSS). TNF, tumor necrosis factor; VEGF, vascular endothelial growth factor; RAS, renin–angiotensin system

angiotensin levels was proportional to the severity of OHSS and correlated with both progesterone and estradiol serum levels. Moreover, the very high plasma levels of total and active renin and aldosterone in case of OHSS did not fall when the extravascular compartment was expanded, suggesting a non-renal origin of the renin[35].

Delbaere and colleagues[36] studied the RAS by evaluating the renin-like activity and angiotensin II immunoreactivity in ascites fluid and serum of OHSS patients and controls. Angiotensin II was higher in the ascites and peritoneal fluid than in the corresponding plasma, suggesting an ovarian origin of angiotensin II. The highest levels of renin-like activity and angiotensin II are found in ascites fluid of OHSS patients who are pregnant suggesting a stimulatory role of hCG on the ovarian RAS. The authors concluded that angiotensin II may contribute to the maintenance of the ascites in severe OHSS, but is probably not responsible for the initial formation of ascites, since high levels of angiotensin II in peritoneal fluid of some control patients did not necessarily lead to the formation of ascites. Probably, angiotensin II is produced in extremely large amounts together with ascites fluid when OHSS develops. In huge quantities it could maintain the shift of fluid to the extravascular space and thereby contribute, at least partially, to the hemodynamic changes present in OHSS. The same authors measured prorenin, total renin, active renin, renin activity and aldosterone in plasma and in ascites fluid in patients with severe OHSS. Total renin and prorenin concentrations were significantly higher in the ascites fluid than in plasma. Conversely, active renin and renin activity concentrations tended to be lower in ascites fluid than in plasma. Aldosterone concentrations were significantly higher in serum than in ascites fluid. This suggests stimulation of both ovarian and renal RAS during OHSS[37].

Finally, inhibition by the ovarian-derived prorenin of the angiotensin cascade has been studied in the rabbit model. Using the angiotensin-converting enzyme inhibitors enapril and captopril has produced a decrease in the incidence of OHSS by 40% and 30%, respectively, suggesting a role for angiotensin II in the OHSS process. Nevertheless, the rabbit model is not a perfect model to study severe OHSS in women, because OHSS in the rabbit induces hypertension and not hypotension, as it does in women[34].

In addition, there is a correlation between plasma renin activity and the plasma levels of other volume-dependent endogenous vasoactive substances, such as norepinephrine and the antidiuretic hormone (ADH), which are markedly increased in OHSS. This strongly suggests that activation of the RAS in severe OHSS is a secondary rather than a primary event[38].

In conclusion, there is a proven contribution of the RAS to the process of OHSS. It has been established that some activators of the RAS are secreted by the ovary and that the RAS process can be influenced by some well-known risk factors of OHSS such as hCG. The systemic activation of the RAS during the hemodynamic perturbations related to OHSS has also been documented. What remains to be established is whether an imbalance in the RAS is a 'primum movens' in the pathogenesis of OHSS or whether it is a catalyzer of the hemodynamic degradation that occurs in OHSS. Alternatively, the activation of the RAS may be a homeostatic response to hypovolemia during OHSS.

Cytokines

Cytokines are known mediators of increased vascular permeability, leukocyte mobilization and shock. Interleukin (IL)-6 and probably IL-1β are produced during normal ovarian function and participate in the process of neovascularization and angiogenesis, which is required for the development of ovarian follicles. Considering the biological activity of cytokines and their implication in folliculogenesis, some authors suggested that cytokines may have an etiological role in the OHSS process. In particular, the following cytokines have been studied: IL-1, IL-2, IL-6, IL-8, tumor necrosis factor (TNF)-α and vascular endothelial growth factor (VEGF). VEGF is discussed separately later on.

Among the interleukin family, IL-6 has been most studied. Elevated concentrations of IL-6 have been reported in blood, ascites and follicular fluid in OHSS patients[39–42]. These concentrations were ten-fold higher in follicular fluid compared to the serum, suggesting an ovarian origin[44]. Moreover, gonadotropin administration stimulated the production of IL-6[40]. For some authors, IL-6 in follicular fluid at the time of oocyte retrieval may be used as an early predictor for the development of OHSS in high responders[43].

Nevertheless, the etiological role of IL-6 remains questionable, since IL-6 has not been shown to cause vasodilatation and hypotension independently of IL-1 and TNF, and controversial data have been published concerning IL-1, IL-8 and TNF during OHSS[39,41–46].

A particular interest in IL-2 has also been raised because of the previously reported association between the intravenous administration of IL-2 with the 'vascular leak syndrome', which resembles OHSS[48]. Nevertheless, although some authors observed elevated concentrations of IL-2 in the three media (blood, ascites and follicular fluid) in OHSS cases, these findings have not been constant[41,43,45,47,48]. These conflicting results regarding IL-2 measurements may be due to the short half-life of this cytokine.

Finally, the kinetics of certain cytokines measured in blood (IL-1, IL-6, TNF) and/or in ascites fluid (VEGF, IL-6) mimic the OHSS evolution, with a significant drop occurring with clinical improvement and reaching minimal values after complete resolution of the syndrome. Moreover, IL-1, IL-6 and TNF levels were correlated with different hemoconcentration factors[42].

Finally, IL-4, IL-10 and IL-13 are immunosuppressive cytokines involved in the down-regulation of inflammatory processes that control and restrict the process in both a time- and site-specific way. Enskog and co-workers observed significantly lower levels of IL-10 at the start of gonadotropins stimulation in OHSS patients[49,50]. These authors suggested a link between an aberrant immune response and OHSS, and speculated that the expression of immunosuppressive cytokines might be affected in patients developing OHSS. IL-10 may have a physiopathological role on the inflammatory reaction and generalizing of OHSS. In this respect, one may view the increase in IL-10 serum and ascites fluid as a systemic attempt to suppress the inflammation of OHSS[43].

In summary, studies of cytokines produce contradictory results even in apparently similar populations affected by OHSS for different reasons.

These low-molecular-weight proteins are active in extremely low concentrations and can be affected in an autocrine, paracrine or endocrine fashion.

Cytokine activity is influenced by the functional status of the cytokine receptors, the presence of cytokine inhibitors, soluble receptors and binding proteins. Nevertheless, most data converge to show that positive modulators of the early phase of inflammation (IL-1, IL-2, IL-6, IL-8, TNF and VEGF) are increased during the early stage of OHSS and that immunosuppressive and anti-inflammatory cytokines (IL-10) tend to be lower in OHSS patients before treatment. One may hypothesize that patients with OHSS suffer from an intrinsic deficiency in their immune response and that this differentiates them from those high-risk OHSS patients who do not develop OHSS.

Allergy, cytokines and histamine

Because the pathophysiological changes during OHSS resemble an excessive inflammatory response, the possibility of hyper-reactivity of the ovarian mast cells in patients suffering OHSS has been suggested. With regard to allergy, histamine and histamine blockade have been studied. Histamine blockade has been shown to prevent the occurrence of OHSS in the rabbit model. However, OHSS in these rabbits did not involve antigen–antibody complexes, suggesting that antihistamine blockade of OHSS could take place directly at the ovarian level. Another rabbit study showed no difference in either histamine levels or ovarian mast-cell contents between OHSS and controls. Conflicting results were obtained for the inhibition of ascites fluid formation and ovarian enlargement using H-1 receptor blockers[34].

Vascular endothelial growth factor

VEGF is a dimeric glycoprotein that stimulates cell mitosis and renders capillaries highly permeable to high-molecular-weight proteins. VEGF expression has been identified during the early follicular and luteal phases and is produced by the theca interna and by the granulosa cells of the human ovaries. Gonadotropins influence VEGF mRNA expression, LH and hCG having a prominent effect in this respect in granulosa cells. High concentrations of VEGF, in the presence of a tumor, increase vascular permeability and lead to extravasation of plasma followed by ascites formation and hemoconcentration. For these reasons, VEGF, overproduced by multiple corpora lutea resulting from hyperstimulation, could be the ovarian mediator responsible for the increase in vascular permeability in OHSS.

McClure and colleagues were the first to provide evidence that the major capillary permeability agent in OHSS fluid is VEGF[51]. These authors studied the vascular permeability in guinea pigs exposed to ascites fluid collected from OHSS patients and from patients with non-malignant chronic liver failure. They further assessed the effect of recombinant human VEGF and recombinant human VEGF antiserum with respect to permeability activity. Their observations were confirmed in 1998 by Levin and co-workers using VEGF antibodies to conclude that the follicular fluid factor responsible for increased endothelial cell permeability is VEGF[52].

VEGF was prospectively measured in serum, peritoneal fluid and follicular fluid in patients at high risk for OHSS. After hCG administration, the VEGF concentrations of follicular fluid were approximately 100 times greater than in serum or peritoneal fluid, suggesting that the ovary may be the possible source of VEGF. Serum VEGF was higher in OHSS patients at 14 days following hCG administration, but no difference in VEGF concentrations was detected in follicular fluid or in serum earlier in the cycle. Nevertheless, other observations confirmed a significant increase in serum VEGF from the time of hCG administration onwards until the time of oocyte retrieval in OHSS patients. Even when only free serum VEGF was evaluated in a prospective study, the concentration of free VEGF was significantly higher both on the day of hCG administration and on the day of embryo transfer in the OHSS group[34].

Aboulghar and associates observed higher VEGF plasma levels in patients hospitalized for OHSS than in controls and a significant correlation with white blood cell count and with the hematocrit[45]. These high VEGF values dropped significantly with clinical improvement, reaching minimum values after complete resolution.

Follicular fluid VEGF concentrations are 3–10-fold higher than serum levels. On the day of egg retrieval, follicular fluid VEGF was correlated with serum and follicular fluid progesterone concentrations but not with estradiol concentration or the number of collected oocytes, suggesting that periovulatory luteinizing follicles produce significant

amounts of VEGF and that VEGF production is determined by the degree of follicular luteinization. Moreover, serum VEGF level was correlated only with estradiol level, and may provide an important non-steroidal marker of the ovarian response[34].

Controlled studies in patients at risk of OHSS found that plasma VEGF increased only after hCG had been given in case of OHSS and on the day of oocyte retrieval for the patients at risk who did develop OHSS. That suggested a progressive sensitivity to hCG proportional to the superovulation response. Among high-risk patients, only those in whom the LH surge was able to induce a marked increase in plasma VEGF concentration would ultimately develop OHSS. The increased expression of VEGF mRNA within the hyperthecal stroma of women with PCOS helps to clarify the higher risk of OHSS in PCOS patients[34].

Others have reported contradictory results with no difference in serum, plasma and follicular fluid VEGF concentrations in the OHSS group and between VEGF concentration in serum and peritoneal fluid[53–55].

In conclusion, the vascular permeability and the subsequent development of ascites fluid are thought to be induced by follicular fluid. The ovarian production of VEGF is demonstrated by the fact that, in most studies, higher concentrations are found in the follicular fluid than in the serum. Most, but not all, observations report an increase in plasma or serum VEGF concentrations in OHSS patients at the time of ovulation. In addition, hCG administration enhances the mRNA expression of VEGF by luteinized granulosa cells in a dose-dependent manner, explaining why the use of hCG in IVF protocols is often a critical step in the development of OHSS. The increased expression of VEGF mRNA has been described in high-risk women with PCOS.

Nevertheless, many questions about the ovarian production and action of VEGF remain unanswered, and certain observations are contradictory. These contradictory results can be at least partially attributed to the method of VEGF assessment:

(1)   VEGF can be measured in plasma or in serum, but the clotting process increases VEGF levels 8–10-fold in serum, and degranulation or hemoconcentration occurring in OHSS may

entail misinterpretation of true levels of free active VEGF.

(2)   In OHSS, ovarian-derived VEGF could be trapped in the ascites fluid and large cystic corporea lutea.

(3)   Immunoassays cannot differentiate the four isoforms of VEGF.

(4)   The biologically active isoform of VEGF in the circulation has not been determined.

(5)   The relationship between soluble VEGF receptors and VEGF in the follicular fluid may influence the biological activity of VEGF, and a different biological affinity of VEGF for receptors may exist[34].

Moreover, the studied populations are heterogeneous and the control group may influence the results, particularly whether OHSS and control patients were or were not matched for the number of follicles.

VEGF is thus certainly a mediator of the OHSS cascade, but it remains unknown whether the disruption of the normal controlled follicular expression of VEGF constitutes a 'primum movens' of OHSS.

Miscellaneous substances that may play a role in OHSS

Angiogenin has been found in significantly higher levels in blood and in ascites fluid of OHSS patients, suggesting that angiogenin may be associated with neovascularization in OHSS.

The kinin–kallikrein system has been studied in the rat model. The results suggest that the kinin–kallikrein system plays an intermediate role in capillarity permeability during OHSS.

Soluble vascular cell adhesion molecule 1 (sVCAM-1) and soluble intercellular adhesion molecule-1 (sICAM-1) belong to the immunoglobulin superfamily and are major mediators of white blood cell adhesion, interaction and extravasation during inflammatory and immune reactions. A case–control study of peritoneal fluid and plasma levels of sVCAM-1 and sICAM-1 has suggested that soluble cell adhesion molecules may play a role in the pathogenesis and evolution of OHSS.

The serum and ascites concentrations of sICAM-1 and of soluble E-selectin, another endothelial cell adhesion molecule, were followed in a controlled study. Higher levels of sICAM-1 and lower levels of E-selectin were observed in serum and ascites fluid. More studies are needed to understand the kinetics and the cause–effect relationship between OHSS and these adhesion molecules. However, they seem to be implicated in the pathophysiological process leading to capillary hyperpermeability in severe OHSS.

The von Willebrand Factor (vWF) is considered to be a marker of endothelial cell activation. Excessive endothelial cell VEGF production enhances vWF concentrations. The increased vWF concentration on the day of embryo transfer has been shown to be related to the severity of OHSS, and an elevation of the level of vWF precedes the clinical manifestations in severe OHSS. This increase was not observed in follicular fluid, suggesting that vWF is not produced by the ovary. vWF may be of endothelial origin and influenced by vasoactive ovarian factors. Higher plasma levels of vWF in OHSS patients compared with high responders on the day preceding oocyte retrieval lasted until after embryo transfer and were maintained well into the late luteal phase. In high responders without OHSS, the levels of vWF also increased during the pre-ovulatory phase, but decreased from the day of oocyte retrieval onwards. Subsiding levels of vWF in patients with severe OHSS indicate improvement of the disease. This test might become clinically useful as an additional 'discriminating parameter' or 'prognostic marker'. It is likely that vWF plays a role in the cascade that leads to OHSS but rather as a consequence of the activation of endothelial cells by a causal factor of ovarian origin than as its causal factor.

Endothelin-1, another vasoconstrictor that increases capillary permeability, was found to be 100–300-fold higher in follicular fluid than in plasma. In OHSS patients, the serum endothelin-1 level is elevated, but in parallel with other neurohormonal vasoactive factors and without correlation with the OHSS grading, suggesting a homeostatic response rather than an initiating role in OHSS[38].

Contribution of neurohormonal and hemodynamic changes to arteriolar vasodilatation

Balasch and colleagues evaluated systemic, endogenous vasoactive neurohormonal factors in severe

OHSS during the appearance of the syndrome for a period of 4–5 weeks[38]. The authors recorded an increased hematocrit, decreased mean arterial pressure, increased cardiac output and reduced peripheral vascular resistance. This was accompanied by marked increases in plasma renin, norepinephrine, ADH and atrial natriuretic peptide levels. The authors compared the previous results in women with and without hemoconcentration: similar values were observed except for renin, norepinephrine and ADH, which were found to be higher in OHSS patients. These observations suggest that OHSS is associated with arteriolar vasodilatation. Indeed, if circulatory dysfunction were due solely to an extravascular shift, the contraction of the circulating blood volume should induce a reduction in cardiac output, an increase in peripheral vascular resistance and a decrease in atrial natriuretic peptide. In contrast, cardiac output and atrial natriuretic peptide are increased and peripheral vascular resistance is markedly reduced, indicating a marked peripheral arteriolar vasodilatation. The simultaneous occurrence of these disorders leads to hyperdynamic circulatory dysfunction with marked stimulation of the sympathetic nervous system, renin–angiotensin system and ADH.

Evbuomwan and co-workers observed an alteration of osmoregulation during OHSS, with an osmotic threshold for arginine vasopressin secretion that is reset to lower plasma osmolality during superovulation[56]. This new lower body tonicity is maintained in OHSS patients until at least 10 days after administration of hCG. These authors suggest that a decrease in plasma osmolality and plasma sodium levels is due to altered osmoregulation rather than to electrolyte losses.

CONCLUSION

The main hypothesis concerning the development of OHSS is that regulation of the inflammation-like ovulation process is disturbed. This leads to overproduction of local pro-inflammatory factors in the ovary, resulting in secondarily increased capillary leakage and in transmission of inflammatory mediators to other compartments. In the most severe form of OHSS this process also leads to systemic manifestations.

In addition to the shift of fluid to extravascular spaces, OHSS is consistently associated with marked arteriolar vasodilatation.

The site and mechanism of arterial vasodilatation and increased permeability has not yet been elucidated. A link between arterial vasodilatation and capillary leakage may exist, because arteriolar dilatation induces the formation of interstitial edema by increasing the capillary surface area and capillary hydrostatic pressure[35].

REFERENCES

1. Serour GI, Aboulghar M, Mansour R, et al. Complications of medically assisted conception in 3,500 cycles. Fertil Steril 1998;70:638–42

2. Mathur RS, Akande AV, Keay SD, et al. Distinction between early and late ovarian hyperstimulation syndrome. Fertil Steril 2000;73:901–7

3. Schenker JG, Ezra Y. Complications of assisted reproductive techniques. Fertil Steril 1994;61:411–22

4. Nygren KG, Nyboe-Andersen A. Assisted reproductive technology in Europe; results generated from European registers by ESHRE. Hum Reprod 1999;12:3260–74

5. Abramov Y, Elchalal U, Schenker JG. Severe OHSS. An 'epidemic' of severe OHSS: a price to pay? Hum Reprod 1999;14:2181–5

6. Abramov Y, Elchalal U, Schenker JG. Pulmonary manifestations of severe ovarian hyperstimulation syndrome: a multicenter study. Fertil Steril 1999;71:645–51

7. Delvigne A, Demoulin A, Smitz J, et al. The ovarian hyperstimulation syndrome in in-vitro fertilization: a Belgian multicentric study. I. Clinical and biological features. Hum Reprod 1993;8:1353–60

8. Delvigne A, Rozenberg S. Review of clinical course and treatment of ovarian hyperstimulation syndrome (OHSS). *Hum Reprod Update* 2003;9:77–96

9. Abramov Y, Elchalal U, Schenker JG. Febrile morbidity in severe and critical ovarian hyperstimulation syndrome: a multicentre study. *Hum Reprod* 1998;13:3128–31

10. Mashiach S, Bider D, Moran O, *et al.* Adnexal torsion of hyperstimulated ovaries in pregnancies after gonadotrophin therapy. *Fertil Steril* 1990;53:76–80

11. Ludwig M, Tolg R, Richardt G, *et al.* Myocardial infarction associated with ovarian hyperstimulation syndrome. *J Am Med Assoc* 1999;282:632–3

12. Mozes M, Bogokowsky H, Antebi E, *et al.* Thromboembolic phenomena after ovarian stimulation with human gonadotrophins. *Lancet* 1965;2:1213–15

13. Cluroe AD, Synek BJ. A fatal case of ovarian hyperstimulation syndrome with cerebral infarction. *Pathology* 1995;27:344–6

14. Enskog A, Henriksson M, Unander M, *et al.* Prospective study of the clinical and laboratory parameters of patients in whom ovarian hyperstimulation syndrome developed during controlled ovarian hyperstimulation for *in vitro* fertilization. *Fertil Steril* 1999;71:808–14

15. Navot D, Relou A, Birkenfeld A, *et al.* Risk factors and prognostic variables in the ovarian hyperstimulation syndrome. *Am J Obstet Gynecol* 1988;159:210–15

16. Delvigne A, Dubois M, Battheu B, *et al.* The ovarian hyperstimulation syndrome in *in-vitro* fertilization: a Belgian multicentric study. II. Multiple discriminant analysis for risk prediction. *Hum Reprod* 1993;8:1361–6

17. MacDougall MJ, Tan SL, Jacobs HS. *In-vitro* fertilization and the ovarian hyperstimulation syndrome. *Hum Reprod* 1992;7:597–600

18. Tibi C, Alvarez S, Cornet D, *et al.* Prédiction des hyperstimulations ovariennes. *Contra-Fertil-Sex* 1989;17:751–2

19. Danninger B, Brunner M, Obruca A, *et al.* Prediction of ovarian hyperstimulation syndrome by ultrasound volumetric assessment of baseline ovarian volume prior to stimulation. *Hum Reprod* 1996;11:1597–9

20. Bodis J, Török A, Tinneberg HR. LH/FSH ratio as a predictor of ovarian hyperstimulation syndrome. *Hum Reprod* 1996;11:1597–9

21. Hughes E, Collins J, Vandekerckhove P. Ovulation induction with urinary follicle stimulating hormone versus human menopausal gonadotrophin for clomiphene-resistant polycystic ovary syndrome. *Cochrane Database Syst Rev* 2000;2:CD000087

22. Daya S. Updated meta-analysis of recombinant follicle-stimulating hormone (FSH) versus urinary FSH for ovarian stimulation in assisted reproduction. *Fertil Steril* 2002;77:711–14

23. Delvigne A, Rozenberg S. Epidemiology and prevention of ovarian hyperstimulation syndrome (OHSS): a review. *Hum Reprod* 2002;8:559–77

24. Al-Inany H, Aboulghar M. GnRH antagonist in assisted reproduction: a Cochrane review. *Hum Reprod* 2002;17:874–85

25. Delvigne A, Kostyla K, De Leener A, *et al.* Metabolic characteristics of women who developed ovarian hyperstimulation syndrome. *Hum Reprod* 2002;17:1994–6

26. Gerris J, De Vits A, Joostens M, *et al.* Triggering of ovulation in human menopausal gonadotrophin-stimulated cycles: comparison between intravenously administered

gonadotrophin-releasing hormone (100 and 500 micrograms), GnRH agonist (buserelin, 500 micrograms) and human chorionic gonadotrophin (10,000 IU). *Hum Reprod* 1995;10:56–62

27. Fauser BC, de Jong D, Olivennes F, *et al*. Endocrine profiles after triggering of final oocyte maturation with GnRH agonist after cotreatment with the GnRH antagonist ganirelix during ovarian hyperstimulation for *in vitro* fertilization. *J Clin Endocrinol Metab* 2002;87:709–15

28. The European recombinant LH study group. Recombinant human luteinizing hormone is as effective as, but safer than, urinary human chorionic gonadotrophin in inducing final follicular maturation and ovulation in *in vitro* fertilization procedures: results of a multicenter double-blind study. *J Clin Endocrinol* 2001;86:2607–16

29. Asch RH, Li HP, Balmaceda JP, *et al*. Severe ovarian hyperstimulation syndrome in assisted reproductive technology: definition of high risk groups. *Hum Reprod* 1991;6:1395–9

30. Morris RS, Paulson RJ, Sauer MV, *et al*. Predictive value of serum oestradiol concentrations and oocyte number in severe ovarian hyperstimulation syndrome. *Hum Reprod* 1995;10:811–14

31. Polishuk WZ, Schenker JG. Ovarian overstimulation syndrome. *Fertil Steril* 1969;20:443–50

32. Yarali H, Fleige-Zahradka BG, Yuen BH, *et al*. The ascites in the ovarian hyperstimulation syndrome does not originate from the ovary. *Fertil Steril* 1993;59:657–61

33. Goldsman MP, Pedram A, Dominguez CE, *et al*. Increased capillary permeability induced by human follicular fluid: a hypothesis for an ovarian origin of the hyperstimulation syndrome. *Fertil Steril* 1995;63:268–72

34. Delvigne A, Rozenberg S. Systematic review of data concerning etiopathology of ovarian hyperstimulation syndrome. *Int J Fertil Wom Med* 2002;47:211

35. Navot D, Margalioth EJ, Laufer N, *et al*. Direct correlation between plasma renin activity and severity of the ovarian hyperstimulation syndrome. *Fertil Steril* 1987;48:57–61

36. Delbaere A, Bergmann PJ, Gervy-Decoster C, *et al*. Angiotensin II immunoreactivity is elevated in ascites during severe ovarian hyperstimulation syndrome: implications for pathophysiology and clinical management. *Fertil Steril* 1994;62:731–7

37. Delbaere A, Bergmann PJ, Gervy-Decoster C, *et al*. Prorenin and active renin concentrations in plasma and ascites during severe ovarian hyperstimulation syndrome. *Hum Reprod* 1997;12:236–40

38. Balasch J, Arroyo V, Fabregues F, *et al*. Neurohormonal and hemodynamic changes in severe cases of the ovarian hyperstimulation syndrome. *Ann Intern Med* 1994;121:27–33

39. Friedlander MA, Loret de Mola JR, Goldfarb JM. Elevated levels of interleukin-6 in ascites and serum from women with ovarian hyperstimulation syndrome. *Fertil Steril* 1993;60:826–33

40. Loret de Mola JR, Flores JP, Baumgardner GP, *et al*. Elevated interleukin-6 levels in the ovarian hyperstimulation syndrome: ovarian immunohistochemical localization of interleukin-6 signal. *Obstet Gynecol* 1996;87:581–7

41. Revel A, Barak V, Lavy Y, *et al*. Characterization of intraperitoneal cytokines and nitrites in women with severe ovarian hyperstimulation syndrome. *Fertil Steril* 1996;66:66–71

42. Abramov Y, Schenker JG, Lewin A, *et al*. Plasma inflammatory cytokines correlate to

the ovarian hyperstimulation syndrome. *Hum Reprod* 1996;11:1381–6

43. Geva E, Lessing JB, Lerner-Geva L, *et al.* Elevated levels of interleukin-6 in the follicular fluid at the time of oocyte retrieval for *in vitro* fertilization may predict the development of early-form ovarian hyperstimulation syndrome. *Fertil Steril* 1997;68:133–7

44. Pellicer A, Albert C, Mercader A, *et al.* The pathogenesis of ovarian hyperstimulation syndrome: *in vivo* studies investigating the role of interleukin-1beta, interleukin-6, and vascular endothelial growth factor. *Fertil Steril* 1999;71:482–9

45. Aboulghar MA, Mansour RT, Serour GI, *et al.* Elevated levels of interleukin-2, soluble interleukin-2 receptor alpha, interleukin-6, soluble interleukin-6 receptor and vascular endothelial growth factor in serum and ascitic fluid of patients with severe ovarian hyperstimulation syndrome. *Eur J Obstet Gynecol Reprod Biol* 1999;87:81–5

46. Chen CD, Chen HF, Lu HF, *et al.* Value of serum and follicular fluid cytokine profile in the prediction of moderate to severe ovarian hyperstimulation syndrome. *Hum Reprod* 2000;15:1037–42

47. Artini PG, Monti M, Fasciani A, *et al.* Vascular endothelial growth factor, interleukin-6 and interleukin-2 in serum and follicular fluid of patients with ovarian hyperstimulation syndrome. *Eur J Obstet Gynecol Reprod Biol* 2002;101:169–74

48. Orvieto R, Voliovitch I, Fushman P, Ben-Rafael Z. Interleukin-2 and ovarian hyperstimulation syndrome: a pilot study. *Hum Reprod* 1995;10:24–7

49. Enskog A, Nilsson L, Brannstrom M. Low peripheral blood levels of the immunosuppressive cytokine interleukin 10 (IL-10) at the start of gonadotrophin stimulation indicates increased risk for development of ovarian

hyperstimulation syndrome (OHSS). *J Reprod Immunol* 2001;49:71–85

50. Manolopoulos K, Lang U, Gips H, Braems GA. Elevated interleukin-10 and sex steroid levels in peritoneal fluid of patients with ovarian hyperstimulation syndrome. *Eur J Obstet Gynecol Reprod Biol* 2001;99:226–31

51. McClure N, Healy DL, Rogers PA, *et al.* Vascular endothelial growth factor as capillary permeability agent in ovarian hyperstimulation syndrome. *Lancet* 1994;344:235–6

52. Levin ER, Rosen GF, Cassidenti DL, *et al.* Role of vascular endothelial cell growth factor in ovarian hyperstimulation syndrome. *J Clin Invest* 1998;102:1978–85

53. Geva E, Amit A, Lessing JB, *et al.* Follicular fluid levels of vascular endothelial growth factor. Are they predictive markers for ovarian hyperstimulation syndrome? *J Reprod Med* 1999;44:91–6

54. D'Ambroglio G, Fasciani A, Monti M, *et al.* Serum vascular endothelial growth factor levels before starting gonadotrophin treatment in women who have developed moderate forms of ovarian hyperstimulation syndrome. *Gynecol Endocrinol* 1999;13:311–15

55. Enskog A, Nilsson L, Brannstrom M. Plasma levels of free vascular endothelial growth factor (165) (VEGF(165)) are not elevated during gonadotrophin stimulation in *in vitro* fertilization (IVF) patients developing ovarian hyperstimulation syndrome (OHSS): results of a prospective cohort study with matched controls. *Eur J Obstet Gynecol Reprod Biol* 2001;96:196–201

56. Evbuomwan IO, Davison JM, Baylis PM, Murdoch AM. Altered osmotic thresholds for arginine vasopressin secretion and thirst during superovulation and in the ovarian hyperstimulation syndrome (OHSS): relevance to the pathophysiology of OHSS. *Fertil Steril* 2001;75:933–41

13

Clinical management and therapy of ovarian hyperstimulation syndrome

P. A. van Dop

INTRODUCTION

In Chapter 12, it was made clear that the fundamental cause of ovarian hyperstimulation syndrome (OHSS) is not known with certainty and that the pathophysiology is only partly understood. The hallmark of the syndrome is the pathological shift of fluid between body compartments, essentially resulting in the unnatural relocation of water due to leakage of existent and newly formed capillaries (angioneogenesis). Since the cause of OHSS is not exactly known, therapy of OHSS is not the correct connotation. A better term is management of OHSS, in particular management of its consequences, which can dangerously derange the interior milieu.

In the management of OHSS there is no sharp border between intervention and prevention. Many studies of intervention and prevention of OHSS lack a proper design, and randomized clinical trials are scarce. Outcomes are mainly based on clinical observations and experience. For these reasons the conclusions of many studies have to be read with attention and caution.

For a good clinical understanding, it should be stressed that there is a large group of patients who will not develop OHSS during ovarian hyperstimulation, although some primary and/or secondary risk factors are clearly present. Once again, since the cause of OHSS is not known, it is not understood why these patients under entirely non-physiological conditions of ovarian hyperstimulation do *not* develop OHSS, whereas a much smaller group of patients under the same conditions do develop OHSS. In other words, the possible development of

OHSS is at present mainly to be considered as a risk factor. In risk assessment (of OHSS as of other risks), the best method would be the calculation of likelihood ratios. Apart from relatively rough estimates with wide confidence intervals, differing from one population of patients to another, this has seldom been done. Moreover, even when likelihood ratios were known, this did not mean that this knowledge would allow us to rule out OHSS.

RISK REDUCTION AT STIMULATION AND EGG RETRIEVAL

The first step in the management of OHSS is the identification of patients at risk. The main risk factors before the start of controlled ovarian hyperstimulation are young or lean women, the presence of polycystic ovary syndrome and a history of previous (threatening) OHSS. Women with these risk factors should be actively informed of the existence and meaning of OHSS, stimulated with individualized low-dose (step-up) regimens and subjected to very careful monitoring[1]. During controlled ovarian hyperstimulation other (secondary) predictors for OHSS are the number of follicles and high levels of serum estradiol[2,3]. Not only are the absolute numbers of follicles and serum levels of estradiol important, but so is the time at which these are reached (slope of increment). The European Society for Human Reproduction and Embryology (ESHRE) Capri Workshop as well as a recent review on this issue consider serum estradiol levels of ≥ 10 nmol/l (≥ 2500 pg/ml) and > 35 follicles to represent an increased risk for developing OHSS[4,5].

Estradiol levels exceeding 12.8 nmol/l (4000 pg/ml) are considered a high risk for a severe form of OHSS. Although, owing to local differences in laboratory assessments, these cut-off values should be interpreted with some flexibility, each assisted reproduction program should employ a written and ratified protocol in which the criteria for cancellation of the stimulation phase in controlled ovarian stimulation both in *in vitro* fertilization (IVF)/intra-cytoplasmic sperm injection (ICSI) and in non-IVF/ICSI treatment cycles are notified. It should be realized both by the physician and by the patient that not cancelling stimulation under such circumstances means that controlled ovarian stimulation may become uncontrolled in such a way that it may become life threatening.

In a systematic review on the use of recombinant (r) versus urinary (u) follicle stimulating hormone (FSH) for ovarian stimulation in assisted reproduction no significant differences were demonstrated between rFSH and uFSH in the rates of OHSS[6]. In a meta-analysis, Ludwig and co-workers showed a decrease in the rate of OHSS for the gonadotropin releasing hormone (GnRH)-antagonist cetrorelix, but not for ganirelix[7]. Al-Inany and Aboulghar studied the difference between GnRH-agonists and GnRH-antagonists. Their conclusion was that the new fixed GnRH-antagonist protocol (i.e. with antagonist started on day 6 of gonadotropin stimulation) is a short and simple protocol with a significant reduction in incidence of severe OHSS, but with a lower pregnancy rate compared to the GnRH-agonist long protocol[8].

In contrast with animal studies, there is in humans still no clarity about the relationship between the dose of gonadotropins and the severity of OHSS[9–12].

Asch and colleagues were the first to administer intravenous human albumin during follicular aspiration and immediately thereafter[13]. Subsequently, some authors agreed with them[14,15] whereas others disagreed[16–18]. For the time being the argument has been decided in favor of albumin in a Cochrane study[19].

At present 14 papers can be found in Medline with 'coasting' in the title. Only one paper reports on a randomized trial, and even in this paper randomization did not take place between coasting and not coasting, but between coasting and early unilateral follicular aspiration[20]. The conclusions of all these papers are that coasting is a successful approach. However, the design of these studies (no randomized clinical trials) does not warrant these conclusions to be drawn. Coasting may seem a logical approach in the prevention of OHSS and can be applied, but it has no scientific basis for its effectiveness.

THE LUTEAL PHASE

OHSS is a syndrome of the luteal phase. Without luteinizing hormone (LH) or its imitator human chorionic gonadotropin (hCG) the luteal phase will not occur and OHSS will not develop. Since nearly all IVF programs use GnRH-agonists or GnRH-antagonists the abstinence from hCG (or LH) during ovarian hyperstimulation offers the opportunity to avoid OHSS in high-risk patients. However, cycle cancellation does not present only medical and risk analysis aspects. The financial consequences (reimbursement), expectations and possibilities of the patient as well as previous experience with laborious ovarian stimulations, among others, play a role in the decision to cancel a cycle. In patients at risk for OHSS, secondary prevention may be helpful by reducing the dose of hCG from the usual 10 000 IU to 5000 IU[21]. Similarly, rigorous puncture of as many follicles as possible may be helpful[22], but no randomized trial has been performed to confirm this in a methodologically correct way. When GnRH-agonists during the gonadotropin stimulation phase and hCG for luteal support have been used, progesterone can replace hCG[23]. Stopping luteal support and cryopreservation of the appropriate embryos for later embryo transfer is nearly always preventive[24], since at the time of embryo transfer OHSS will be a threat and will not yet have developed.

OUT-PATIENT MANAGEMENT OF MILD TO MODERATE OHSS

Important issues are the information and instructions given to the patient. The patient must know the symptoms of OHSS and, particularly if abdominal complaints develop, she must turn to the gynecologist who provides the IVF treatment. This may avoid incorrect diagnoses and interventions by physicians in emergency departments not familiar with the symptoms and signs of OHSS.

Useful advice is daily weighing under standardized conditions after waking up and voiding morning urine. Weight gain of more than 1 kg (> 2 lb) within a day may point to intraperitoneal fluid collection and is a reason for contacting the gynecologist in attendance.

The most reliable symptoms are abdominal bloating, abdominal discomfort, nausea and vomiting. Other important signs are abdominal distention, weight gain and ovaries enlarged between 5 and 12 cm on ultrasound. In this stage of OHSS laboratory investigation shows an increased hematocrit (< 45%), normal to slightly reduced serum albumin, < 15 million/ml leukocytes, and normal kidney function and liver enzymes. The advice to the patient must be light physical activity, ample intake of fluid (continuing daily weighing is probably more accurate for assessing the accumulation of extravascular fluid than recording fluid intake and output) and medical consultation if weight gain is more than 1 kg/day (2 lb/day). Bed rest may increase the risk for thromboembolic events. If hCG has been used for luteal support, it should be discontinued and changed to progesterone. Paracetamol can be used for pain relief. If necessary, anti-emetics may be prescribed. Depending on the clinical signs and symptoms, frequent to daily consultations (preferably by the same physician) are provided with assessment of hematocrit, leukocytes, thrombocytes, albumin, sodium, potassium, and kidney and liver functions. Admission is indicated on deterioration of the clinical picture and when the hematocrit exceeds 45%.

HOSPITAL MANAGEMENT OF SEVERE OHSS

Fortunately severe or critical OHSS is not common, although quite dangerous[25]. Those who have no experience of the management of severe and critical OHSS should confer with an experienced colleague in a large IVF center or, depending on transportation and distance, have the patient transferred to a center where such expertise with these stages of OHSS exists. This advice is not excessive, since severe and critical forms of OHSS are potentially lethal disorders. In the worst case scenario there is an increased risk for thromboembolism due to circulatory impairment, blood concentration and high levels of serum estradiol; circulatory failure; breathing difficulties; liver and renal failure with oliguria or anuria; adult respiratory distress syndrome (ARDS); multi-organ failure and possibly death.

History taking and physical examination are paramount on admission. Most clinical situations require bed rest. Daily physical examination including the measuring of weight and abdominal girth are mandatory. The frequency of checking of vital signs depends on the clinical situation. Tabulation of fluid balance every 4 h is mandatory.

Laboratory monitoring comprises leukocyte count, hemoglobin and hematocrit measurements, serum electrolytes, and liver and kidney function tests. Prothrombin time and partial prothrombin time are initially measured. Leukocyte count is related to the seriousness of OHSS and the risk of thromboembolism.

The main intervention is fluid management, since the patient with a severe form of OHSS will be hypovolemic. An initial immediate (within 1 h of admission) intravenous administration of normal saline is begun. If urine production is restored or improved, a maintenance protocol is initiated. Normal saline, or dextrose 5% in normal saline, is infused at 125–150 ml/h under 4-hourly tabulation of urine production. Clinical examination with special interest in pulmonary function (to diagnose potential overhydration) is necessary. If urine output is unsatisfactory after the first fast intravenous fluid bolus, hyperosmolar intravenous therapy is indicated. An intravenous drip of 200 ml 25% human albumin is given in about 4 h. Too fast an infusion of albumin may result in hemodilution with a deterioration of the clinical situation. The use of diuretics in low urine production together with a hypovolemic state is counter-productive and dangerous. Close surveillance of fluid management is mandatory for it not to be excessive. Intravenous fluid management is based on urine production and clinical improvement, shown by an increase in appetite and interest in drinking. In the resolution phase of severe OHSS, fluid intake should be restricted to avoid having to repeat the whole procedure, owing to renewed hemodilution.

Subcutaneous heparin 5000–7500 U daily to prevent thrombosis is given from the first day of admission and can be stopped after adequate mobilization.

ASCITES MANAGEMENT

Ultrasound-guided vaginal paracentesis is indicated in the presence of severe discomfort or pain, or pulmonary or renal compromise[26]. For this procedure the same set-up is used as for transvaginal follicular puncture. Whelan and Vlahos advise assistance by an anesthesiologist to provide intravenous sedation and to monitor cardiopulmonary and hemodynamic status[27]. After fluid management, tapping the excessive intraperitoneal fluid is the most important measure of intervention. Tapping gives immediate relief and clinical improvement. Depending on the clinical situation it may be necessary to repeat paracentesis. Transvaginal paracentesis is an easy procedure and should not be withheld in severe situations.

HOSPITAL MANAGEMENT OF CRITICAL OHSS

Despite all steps taken in the management of severe OHSS the situation can proceed unpredictably to the critical stage of OHSS. In the worst situation renal failure, hepatic damage, thromboembolic phenomena, ARDS and multi-organ failure may develop. In such cases admission into an intensive care ward and medical expertise in intensive care are mandatory. Invasive monitoring of the circulation, venous pressure, pulmonary capillary wedge pressure and oxygenation might be additional necessities. Renal failure should be treated with an intravenous dopamine regimen of 0.18 mg/kg per h. Thromboembolism needs therapeutic doses of anticoagulants. Pulmonary failure may need assisted ventilation and/or thoracocentesis in the case of severe hydrothorax. If a pregnancy maintains critical (i.e. life-threatening) OHSS, therapeutic abortion must be considered.

CONCLUSIONS

OHSS is an unintentional, iatrogenic, potentially life-threatening syndrome, composed of a combination of ovarian enlargement and an acute fluid shift out of the intravascular space. The enlargement is caused by ovarian cyst formation and the fluid shift

may result in ascites, hydrothorax, or generalized edema.

Many causes and/or mechanisms for OHSS have been suggested, but are not known with certainty. For that reason specific etiological therapy for OHSS is not available. The main objectives are prevention and management of the sequelae of OHSS. Unfortunately, studies on prevention and management do not fulfil the criteria of a randomized clinical trial. Management of OHSS at present requires clinical experience with the syndrome, a keen clinical eye and understanding of the laboratory results. One can not visit a patient too often if she has severe or worsening forms of OHSS. Fluid management and tapping of excess intraperitoneal fluid are the keys in the management of OHSS. The gynecologist involved in assisted reproduction technologies must be on the alert for OHSS, try to prevent it and be able to manage the sequelae. For any co-worker in an IVF program, a written protocol referring to the recognition, prevention and management of OHSS is indispensable. Abramov and colleagues have wondered whether (severe) OHSS is the price we have to pay for assisted reproduction technologies[28]. If so, the price should be kept as low as possible.

REFERENCES

1. Golan A, Ron-El R, Herman A, et al. Ovarian hyperstimulation syndrome: an update review. *Obstet Gynecol Surv* 1989;44:430–40

2. Haning RV, Austin CW, Carlson IH, et al. Plasma estradiol is superior to ultrasound and urinary estriol glucuronide as a predictor of ovarian hyperstimulation during induction of ovulation with menotropins. *Fertil Steril* 1983;40:31–6

3. Delvigne A, Dubois M, Battheu B, et al. The ovarian hyperstimulation syndrome in *in-vitro* fertilization: a Belgian multicentric study. *Hum Reprod* 1993;8:1361–6

4. The ESHRE Capri Workshop. Infertility revisited: the state of the art today and tomorrow.

Risks of ovarian hyperstimulation. *Hum Reprod* 1996;11:1785–7

5. Aboulghar MA, Mansour RT. Ovarian hyperstimulation syndrome: classifications and critical analysis of preventive measures. *Hum Reprod Update* 2003;9:275–89

6. Daya S, Gunby J. Recombinant versus urinary follicle stimulating hormone for ovarian stimulation in assisted reproduction cycles. *Cochrane Database Syst Rev* 2000;4:CD002810

7. Ludwig M, Katalinic A, Diedrich K. Use of GnRH antagonists in ovarian stimulation for assisted reproductive technologies compared to the long protocol. *Arch Gynecol Obstet* 2001;265:175–82

8. Al-Inany H, Aboulghar M. Gonadotrophin-releasing hormone antagonists for assisted conception (Cochrane Review). *Cochrane Database Syst Rev* 2001;4:CD001750

9. Schenker JG, Weinstein D. Ovarian hyperstimulation syndrome: a current survey. *Fertil Steril* 1978;30:255–68

10. Polishuk WZ, Schenker JG. Ovarian hyperstimulation syndrome. *Fertil Steril* 1969;20: 443–50

11. Rabau E, David A, Serr DM. Human menopausal gonadotrophins for anovulation and sterility. *Am J Obstet Gynecol* 1967;98:92–8

12. Aboulghar MA, Mansour RT, Serour GI, *et al.* Follicular aspiration does not protect against development of ovarian hyperstimulation syndrome. *J Assist Reprod Genet* 1992;9: 238–43

13. Asch RH, Ivery G, Goldsman M, *et al.* The use of intravenous albumin in patients at high risk for severe ovarian hyperstimulation syndrome. *Hum Reprod* 1993;8:1015–20

14. Shalev E, Giladi Y, Matilsky M, Ben-Ami M. Decreased incidence of severe ovarian hyperstimulation syndrome in high risk *in-vitro* fertilization patients receiving intravenous albumin: a prospective study. *Hum Reprod* 1995;10:1373–6

15. Shoham Z, Weissman A, Barash A, *et al.* Intravenous albumin for the prevention of severe ovarian hyperstimulation syndrome in an *in vitro* fertilization program: a prospective, randomized, placebo-controlled study. *Fertil Steril* 1994;62:137–42

16. Shaker AG, Zosmer A, Dean N, *et al.* Comparison of intravenous albumin and transfer of fresh embryos with cryopreservation of all embryos for subsequent transfer in prevention of ovarian hyperstimulation syndrome. *Fertil Steril* 1996;65:992–6

17. Lewit N, Kol S, Ronene N, Iskovitz-Eldor J. Does intravenous administration of human albumin prevent severe ovarian hyperstimulation syndrome? *Fertil Steril* 1996;66:656

18. Ng E, Leader A, Claman P, *et al.* Intravenous albumin does not prevent the development of severe ovarian hyperstimulation syndrome in an *in-vitro* fertilization programme. *Hum Reprod* 1995;10:807–10

19. Aboulghar M, Evers JH, Al-Inany H. Intravenous albumin for preventing severe ovarian hyperstimulation syndrome. *Cochrane Database Syst Rev* 2000;2:CD001302

20. Egbase PE, Sharhan MA, Grudzinskas JG. Early unilateral follicular aspiration compared with coasting for the prevention of severe ovarian hyperstimulation syndrome: a prospective randomized study. *Hum Reprod* 1999;14:1421–5

21. Abdallah HI, Howe DL, Ah-Moye M, *et al.* The effect of the dose of hCG and the type of gonadotropins stimulation on oocytes recovery rates in an IVF program. *Fertil Steril* 1987;48:958–63

22. Navot D, Margalioth DJ, Laufer N, *et al.* Direct correlation between plasma renin activity and severity of the ovarian hyperstimulation syndrome. *Fertil Steril* 1987;48:57–61

23. McClure N, Leya J, Radwanska E, *et al.* Luteal phase support and severe ovarian hyperstimulation syndrome. *Hum Reprod* 1992;7:758–64

24. Wada I, Matson PL, Troup SA, *et al.* Does elective cryopreservation of all embryos from women at risk of ovarian hyperstimulation syndrome reduce the incidence of the condition? *Br J Obstet Gynaecol* 1993;100:265–9

25. Navot D, Bergh PH, Laufer N. Ovarian hyperstimulation syndrome in novel reproductive technologies: prevention and treatment. *Fertil Steril* 1992;58:249–61

26. Aboulghar MA, Mansour RT, Serour GI, Amin Y. Ultrasonically guided vaginal aspiration of ascites in the treatment of severe ovarian hyperstimulation syndrome. *Fertil Steril* 1990;53:933–5

27. Whelan JG III, Vlahos NF. The ovarian hyperstimulation syndrome. *Fertil Steril* 2000;73:883–96

28. Abramov Y, Elchalal U, Schenker JG. Severe OHSS: An 'epidemic' of severe OHSS: a price we have to pay? *Hum Reprod* 1999;14:2181–3

14

Ovarian hyperstimulation syndrome: prevention in IVF and non-IVF treatment

J. Guibert and F. Olivennes

INTRODUCTION

Since the treatment of infertility represents non-vital care offered to young and healthy patients, avoiding major somatic complications of *in vitro* fertilization (IVF) or non-IVF procedures remains an important challenge for the physicians involved in their management. Among these complications, ovarian hyperstimulation syndrome (OHSS) is one of the most severe. Although fortunately rare, it entails potentially serious or even life-threatening medical damage. OHSS is not frequent, its patho-physiology remains unclear and there are few criteria of reliable predictive value for its occurrence. For these reasons, its prevention remains an unresolved problem for reproductive specialists, who are without a sufficient scientific or clinical basis to develop methods to guarantee complete safety.

Nevertheless, prevention of OHSS should in principle be possible at different steps of the management of infertility:

1. *Primary prevention* could be proposed *before the treatment*, by identifying known risk factors, in order to target a high-risk group of patients for specific preventive strategies. These include systematic interrogation about the necessity of ovarian stimulation, the duration of infertility, the timeliness of the treatment and the development of minimal-risk management procedures, with consideration for the alternative treatments of infertility, e.g. tubal surgery, ovarian drilling by electrocautery or laser vaporization, insulin-resistance-reducing drugs,

culture of immature oocytes and natural-cycle IVF.

2. *Primary prevention during the treatment*, by respecting minimal safety rules of stimulation for all patients and especially for those with an identified high risk. These rules concern the choice of the stimulation regimen (drug, dose, protocol), the adjustment of the dose of gonadotropin according to the ovarian response (monitoring of the cycle), the way to trigger ovulation and the reduced exposure to human chorionic gonadotropin (hCG) in the luteal phase.

3. *Secondary prevention* can be proposed during the treatment, by applying preventive measures when an exaggerated ovarian response occurs. These measures include the cancellation of the cycle, the coasting approach with postponement of hCG administration, early unilateral follicular aspiration, the use of gonadotropin releasing hormone (GnRH) agonists instead of hCG to trigger ovulation, the use of steroids, macromolecules and progesterone, and the postponement of embryo transfer by the cryopreservation of all embryos. The major difficulty in secondary prevention is the accurate recognition of the pre-ovulatory indices of the probable onset of OHSS, because the main signs usually described are relevant for the early onset of the syndrome, but not for its occurrence in the late luteal phase. All secondary preventive measures are available only in the periovulatory period, when a significant proportion of patients who will later develop

severe OHSS show no risk factor and no evidence of an excessive ovarian response. Another important difficulty in the validation of preventive measures of OHSS is the extremely low incidence of severe cases, which results in the need for large randomized multi-center studies to validate the methods of prevention with sufficient statistical power. The wide variability of possible prophylactic strategies between centers results in difficulties in establishing a reliable meta-analysis. We review the different methods most commonly proposed and used by physicians to avoid the occurrence of severe OHSS, with a specific interest in their documented validity, as can be deduced from the literature.

PRIMARY PREVENTION BEFORE THE TREATMENT

Identification of factors influencing the incidence of OHSS

Young patients, patients with polycystic ovary syndrome (PCOS) or showing isolated characteristics (clinical, ultrasonographic, or biological) of PCOS, should be considered at high risk of developing OHSS[1]. No stimulation should be performed without a day-3 evaluation of the luteinizing hormone (LH)/follicle stimulating hormone (FSH) ratio and of the number of resting follicles observed on ultrasound. Previous ovarian responses need to be considered, as they are useful in predicting individual (hyper)sensitivity to gonadotropin stimulation[2]. The previous occurrence of OHSS in a mild or severe form is highly predictive of a high-risk situation in subsequent treatment cycles. It has also been reported that patients showing allergic dispositions may be more likely to develop OHSS[1]. Such criteria should therefore lead physicians to consider a preventive strategy for avoiding OHSS.

Initiation of the treatment

The severity of the medical damage caused by OHSS has to be weighed against the necessity of ovarian stimulation. It is likely that most IVF procedures are initiated with good evidence for their

medical justification. However, in many situations IVF is not performed for any gynecological pathology. Examples are intracytoplasmic sperm injection (ICSI) for male-related infertility, oocyte donors and HIV-serodifferent couples asking for virus-safe procreation. It is noteworthy that patients with these indications for treatment frequently undergo strong ovarian stimulation despite the fact that these women usually do not show any reproductive disability. Complications following such treatments are particularly undesirable, and should be carefully explained to the women concerned.

In non-IVF procedures, the correct moment to initiate treatment is not easy to determine. It appears that OHSS does not occur in more severe forms in normo-ovulatory patients, but obviously the occurrence of a serious complication with no medical evidence of the necessity for such treatment is unjustifiable. This is particularly important for couples requiring donor sperm insemination, if no gynecological abnormality is present, and for couples requiring assisted reproduction treatments despite a short duration of infertility, e.g. because of advanced female age or because of recurrent miscarriage. In these patients, the safety rules of ovarian stimulation have to be strictly followed, including information given to the patients about possible medical consequences and about the benefits of the particular choice of stimulation that has been made[3].

Development of minimal-risk procedures

With respect to non-IVF procedures, alternative approaches exist for the pharmacological induction of ovulation for patients with PCOS. Benefits and risks of such treatments have to be balanced against the risk of OHSS. Diet and weight loss have been demonstrated to restore ovulation in some obese anovulatory women with PCOS, with beneficial effects on the incidence of diabetes mellitus and on cardiovascular risk. Insulin-sensitizing drugs (e.g. metformin) have been shown to be beneficial in facilitating normal menses and pregnancy, and in preventing type-2 diabetes mellitus[4]. Ovarian drilling (either by laparoscopic electrocauterization or by laser vaporization) is also able to restore spontaneous menses and ovulation and induce pregnancy, with a very low risk of multiple pregnancy, OHSS and miscarriage, even though the procedure remains somewhat controversial[5].

Preliminary weight loss prior to both non-IVF and IVF treatment and the administration of metformin or octreotide has been shown to normalize the ovarian response to exogenous gonadotropin in women with PCOS resistant to clomiphene citrate (CC), with a significant reduction of the serum estradiol level, the number of follicles and the cancellation rate, and with a similar pregnancy rate[6,7]. A statistically significant effect on prevention of OHSS could not be demonstrated in non-IVF patients, probably because of its very low incidence[6]. Ovarian drilling before stimulation for IVF in women with a high risk due to PCOS or with a previous experience of OHSS may help to avoid severe complications or the cancellation of the cycle, but it has to be balanced against the risk of the operation[8].

In high-risk patients, new approaches in IVF should be considered. The debate about natural IVF, conducted in a natural unstimulated cycle, has recently re-emerged, since the use of GnRH antagonists permits delay of the LH surge while a single follicle is spontaneously growing[9]. Further studies have to be conducted to compare the results between several 'natural' IVF cycles and a single hyperstimulated cycle. Obviously, multiple pregnancy and OHSS rates would be reduced, but relatively little information is available regarding the pregnancy rate from this procedure.

The development of the culture of immature oocytes may lead in the near future to abandonment of ovarian controlled hyperstimulation and the administration of hCG in IVF procedures, at least in high-risk groups of patients, e.g. women with PCOS or with previous severe OHSS[10].

PRIMARY PREVENTION WHILE CONDUCTING THE TREATMENT

Effective prevention of OHSS is also possible through an appropriate choice and application of drugs during the treatment.

Choice of the stimulation regimen

Clomiphene citrate

In non-IVF procedures, induction of ovulation by CC is rarely associated with severe OHSS. Therefore, CC remains the treatment of choice for induction of ovulation rather than gonadotropins (urinary or recombinant), which increase the incidence of OHSS. However, in the rare patients who have experienced previous OHSS after the use of CC, gonadotropin stimulation allows modulation of the therapy throughout the cycle, which is impossible with CC. In high-risk patients, the initial dose of CC has to be increased carefully to find the ovulatory threshold, and gonadotropins are recommended for CC-resistant patients[11]. CC resistance is defined as failure to ovulate after a dose of 150 mg of CC for three cycles, even though higher doses have been proposed with variable success.

Gonadotropins

When gonadotropins are used, the low step-up regimen in ovarian induction or the low-dose stimulation protocol in IVF seem to reduce the incidence of OHSS. In IVF, halving of the initial dosage of gonadotropins also appears to prevent OHSS in high-risk patients[12]. Likewise, the use of limited ovarian stimulation in PCOS patients with previous OHSS avoids OHSS recurrence by triggering ovulation when the leading follicle reaches a diameter of 12 mm[13]. The choice of urinary or recombinant human menopausal gonadotropin (hMG) or FSH does not seem to influence the incidence of OHSS[14].

Gonadotropin releasing hormone agonists and antagonists

A reduction in the incidence of OHSS is observed in the majority of prospective randomized studies using GnRH antagonists[15]. Patients receiving antagonist treatment have lower serum estradiol levels at the time of hCG administration, probably because of a lower number of follicles, which could explain the lower incidence of OHSS. However, recent meta-analyses failed to find a significant reduction in OHSS[16]. The use of GnRH antagonists could further decrease the incidence of OHSS in high-risk patients by replacing hCG by a GnRH analog to trigger ovulation. Several authors[17] have proposed triggering ovulation with a GnRH analog to decrease the risk of OHSS. However, this approach cannot be proposed in patients previously desensitized with a GnRH agonist, but GnRH analogs can be used to induce an endogenous LH surge during an ovarian stimulation cycle in which a GnRH antagonist is used to prevent LH surges. A recent study, comparing hCG (5000 IU), leuprolide (0.2 mg) and triptorelin (0.1 mg) to trigger ovulation in IVF patients treated with ganirelix (0.25 mg), found similar results between the three groups of patients[18]. A small group of high responders was treated with a combination of a GnRH antagonist and agonists and no OHSS was observed in this preliminary report. Patients with an increased risk for OHSS can be managed with this simple and effective approach during controlled ovarian hyperstimulation consisting of the combination of a GnRH antagonist and an agonist. Overall, GnRH antagonists could offer a good alternative to current stimulation protocols with a reduced incidence of OHSS[19].

Monitoring the cycle

A careful adaptation of the daily dose of gonadotropin administered for ovarian stimulation to the ovarian response results, in non-IVF and IVF procedures, resulted in a decreased incidence of OHSS. This necessary adaptation is possible by monitoring of the cycle, using a combination of frequent serum estradiol measurements and ultrasonographic assessments of follicular growth. Some studies report a similar efficacy in preventing OHSS when using ultrasound assessment alone, but this point remains controversial[20]. Nevertheless, strict observance of monitoring rules by itself does not avoid all severe forms of OHSS. It merely allows tracking of the biological and ultrasonographic clues which compel use of preventive measures (see Secondary prevention). Conducting ovarian stimulation without any monitoring cannot be considered good clinical practice, even when using CC.

Triggering of ovulation

An endogenous LH surge rarely results in symptomatic hyperstimulation, which is essentially caused by the administration of hCG. Therefore, prevention of OHSS by using either a GnRH agonist-induced LH surge or recombinant human LH (rhLH) has been proposed. The clinical potential of these alternative approaches in comparison with urinary hCG for reducing the incidence of OHSS has been studied specifically in patients with an exaggerated ovarian response (compare with Secondary prevention), and not with the systematic objective of avoiding OHSS in all patients. Only one study prospectively assessed the safety of rhLH administration in unselected patients undergoing IVF in comparison with intramuscular administration of 5000 IU of urinary hCG. The rhLH group developed significantly less OHSS than the hCG group[21]. This observed effect can be expected to be even more significant if compared with the widespread use of 10 000 IU of hCG to trigger ovulation in most IVF programs.

Luteal support

Many studies report a significant reduction in the incidence of OHSS when progesterone instead of hCG is used for luteal support[22]. As the vaginal or intramuscular administration of progesterone preparations has been reported to result in similar pregnancy rates after IVF, it is recommended not to use hCG for luteal support in all patients[23].

The incidence of OHSS is directly related to serum hCG levels, which are also increased in multiple pregnancies. The severity of OHSS has been shown to be enhanced by the number of gestational sacs[24]. Avoiding multiple pregnancies is therefore an indirect way to prevent late severe OHSS, and this objective could be theoretically reached by reducing the number of embryos to transfer and by applying single-embryo transfer. This hypothesis has to be assessed by studies comparing the occurrence of OHSS after single-embryo transfer and usual procedures.

SECONDARY PREVENTION IN CASE OF EXCESSIVE OVARIAN RESPONSE

All preventive methods that are discussed in this section are summarized in Table 1.

Table 1   Methods for secondary prevention of ovarian hyperstimulation syndrome: level and timing of action

	Method
Follicular phase	
All levels	cycle cancellation
Enhancing luteolysis	coasting; follicular aspiration
Periovulatory period	
Fighting vascular effects	macromolecules; albumin or hydroxyaethyl starch solution; steroids
Reducing hCG levels	GnRH analog triggering; progesterone
Luteal phase	
Reducing hCG levels	cryopreservation of all embryos, with or without GnRH analog administration

hCG, human chorionic gonadotropin; GnRH, gonadotropin releasing hormone

Cancelling the cycle

Severe OHSS is very rare in cycles without hCG administration, although it has been reported in spontaneous cycles[25]. Therefore, withholding hCG has been proposed to prevent OHSS, at the expense of cycle cancellation. This method has been shown to be efficient, but both physicians and patients are often reluctant to propose or accept it[26]. The main problem is to determine the criteria on which to decide to withhold hCG, and to establish a danger threshold. Several studies have attempted to determine laboratory or clinical variables for the early precise diagnosis of threatening OHSS. Most of the studies reported have used serum estradiol levels to determine when to withhold hCG, but serum estradiol cut-off levels vary widely between IVF centers, from 800 pg/ml to 4000 pg/ml[27]. There seems to be some agreement that it is more accurate to take into account the number of follicles as well. The association of high serum estradiol values (> 3000 pg/ml) and a large number of intermediate-sized follicles of > 12 mm puts the patient at high risk of developing OHSS[27]. Cancelling the cycle is the only method available for absolute prevention of OHSS in non-IVF or in IVF treatment. All other procedures succeed in decreasing either the severity or the incidence of the syndrome, or both, but never totally prevent it[28].

Coasting

Since serum estradiol levels at the time of ovulation triggering have been described to be predictive of the risk of developing OHSS, some authors have proposed to postpone hCG administration to allow serum estradiol levels to fall below a certain preset lower threshold, e.g. 3000 pg/ml. It has been proposed to apply a controlled drift period ('coasting') and wait until serum estradiol concentrations drop to lower and safer levels, owing to the atresia of granulosa cells. It should be remembered, however, that the estradiol level may continue to rise for a few days despite discontinuation of stimulation. Serum estradiol level reaches a plateau after 1–3 days, and then starts to decrease.

Since this method avoids cycle cancellation, allows fresh embryo transfer and involves no supplementary therapy, it has become the most popular method among physicians for preventing OHSS[29].

Two recent reviews have reported the results of all studies conducted between 1995 and 2002 assessing the coasting approach in IVF, with regard to both its efficacy in preventing OHSS and its effect on the pregnancy rate[30,31]. Thirteen studies were identified, of which only one trial had a randomized controlled design comparing the coasting approach with early unilateral follicular aspiration (EUFA)[32]. The main obstacle to match the results of all these studies is their heterogeneity regarding several parameters: number of patients

(5–120), mean age of patients (29.9–37.3 years), causes of infertility, protocols used for ovarian stimulation (long-term scheme with pituitary desensitization by GnRH analogs, short-term scheme with GnRH analogs and GnRH-analog-free protocols), selection criteria to determine the decision to prevent OHSS (serum estradiol levels of > 3000 to 6000 pg/ml, estradiol slope, number of follicles > 20), initial dose of gonadotropins used, later adjustments for coasting, criteria for coasting duration and classification of OHSS. This heterogeneity makes it difficult to synthesize all data. Surprisingly, OHSS rates seem to be reduced in patients showing high-risk criteria (serum estradiol level > 6000 pg/ml, number of follicles > 30), but

with no additional benefit in comparison with EUFA. Results are summarized in Table 2[32–44].

IVF outcome in terms of pregnancy rates in the coasted cycles has been reported to be good, but seems to be lowered either by a duration of coasting of > 4 days, or by a marked drop in serum estradiol levels (< 20% below the maximum value). Most authors have described a reduced oocyte collection rate in coasted cycles. The effect of coasting on embryo quality remains controversial, but a recent study has described a good embryological and clinical outcome after a fixed coasting duration of 3 days in high-risk patients (obese patients with polycystic ovaries showing an excessive ovarian follicular response)[44].

Table 2   The 'coasting' approach: studies between 1995 and 2002

Authors	Year	Design	n	Coasting duration	Result: moderate/ severe OHSS
Sher et al.[33]	1995	descriptive	51	6.1	12/0 (0)
Benadiva et al.[34]	1997	retrospective	22	1.9 ± 0.9	1/0 (0)
Tortoriello et al.[35]	1998	retrospective	44	2.6 ± 0.3	6/3 (6.8)
Dhont et al.[36]	1998	retrospective	120	1.94 ± 0.8	7/1 (0.8)
Lee et al.[37]	1998	retrospective	20	2.8 ± 1.3	—/4 (20)
Fluker et al.[38]	1999	descriptive	63	5.3 ± 0.2	11/1 (1.6)
Waldenström et al.[39]	1999	descriptive	65	4.3	11/2 (3.1)
Egbase et al.[32]	1999	prospective randomized	15	4.9 ± 1.6	3/0 (0)
Dechaud et al.[40]	2000	descriptive	14	1.6	—/0 (0)
Ohata et al.[41]	2000	descriptive	5	4	5/0 (0)
Aboulghar et al.[42]	2000	retrospective	24	2.92 ± 0.92	4/0 (0)
Al-Shawaf et al.[43]	2001	prospective	50	3.4 ± 1.6	2/0 (0)
Egbase et al.[44]	2002	descriptive	102	3 (fixed)	0 (0)

OHSS, ovarian hyperstimulation syndrome
Percentages of severe OHSS in parentheses

More reliable conclusions about the benefit of coasting should be provided by larger randomized controlled studies, with standardized protocols for ovarian stimulation, in which either coasting or cycle cancellation would be proposed to high-risk patients.

Early unilateral follicular aspiration

Aspiration of growing follicles has been proposed as a method of preventing OHSS. This method is based on the assumption that withdrawal of the follicular contents, mainly granulosa cells, may significantly interfere with follicular maturation and modify the intraovarian mechanisms responsible for OHSS. Different procedures have been proposed, differing as to the timing of hCG administration (6–8 h before hCG, 12 h after hCG) with respect to the follicular aspiration[45]. Unilateral ovarian aspiration, 10–12 h after hCG administration, followed by regular oocyte retrieval 36 h later in the contralateral ovary, was shown in patients at risk of OHSS (excessive estradiol values, multiple follicles) to prevent the development of OHSS without cancellation of the cycle, and with similar pregnancy rates. A prospective randomized study compared this method with the coasting approach for high-risk patients, defined by estradiol levels of > 6000 pg/ml and > 15 follicles of > 18 mm per ovary, with similar results in both groups[32]. However, EUFA remains an invasive method which is not more efficient than coasting in completely preventing OHSS.

Alternatives to human chorionic gonadotropin in triggering ovulation

This alternative approach is based on the assumption that the longer half-life of hCG compared with endogenous or exogenous LH leads to the development of multiple corpora lutea and a sustained luteotropic effect, which is thought to boost the development of OHSS in patients with a high number of follicles.

Many studies have reported efficacy of this method in avoiding severe OHSS[46], in association with the use of a GnRH antagonist during the controlled ovarian hyperstimulation (see Primary prevention). A recent controlled trial confirms previous results in terms of pregnancy rates and the prevention of OHSS[46]. The main problem is that most IVF cycles are still conducted with so-called long protocols, implying previous pituitary desensitization, and are therefore not good candidates for this method of prevention.

Steroids

The physiopathology of OHSS remains unclear, but some data are available suggesting a possible involvement of inflammatory mechanisms in the pathological pathway[47]. On this basis, some authors have assumed that corticosteroids could prevent OHSS when the ovarian response becomes excessive. One controlled study failed to demonstrate, in 17 patients at high risk of OHSS, any efficacy of the administration of intravenous hydrocortisone immediately after oocyte retrieval, followed by a decreasing oral treatment for 10 days[48]. Since no data are available regarding more patients, this method has no validated value for the prevention of OHSS.

Macromolecules

Intravenous albumin

Intravenous administration of albumin has been proposed to oppose vasoactive substances and other active substances in OHSS, by maintaining the intravascular volume. Albumin can also prevent hypovolemia, hemoconcentration and ascites. A review of the use of albumin shows a clear benefit of the administration of intravenous albumin at the time of oocyte retrieval for the prevention of severe OHSS in high-risk patients[28]. The dose used in these studies varied from 10 to 125 g given in one or five administrations, also with a variable duration after oocyte retrieval (1 day before to 5 days after). These studies failed to demonstrate a preventive effect of late severe OHSS, caused by early pregnancy, but albumin could well be efficient in preventing early severe OHSS, beginning in the periovulatory period. The main problem is the possible adverse effect of albumin on implantation rates[49], and the possibility of virus transmission through the administration of a human serum product.

These risks have to be balanced against the expected severity of OHSS and the uncertain efficacy of albumin in preventing its late severe form, since severe OHSS cases have been reported despite the use of albumin.

Hydroxyaethyl starch solution

Synthetic macromolecules can be used, instead of albumin, to prevent OHSS without the risk of using potentially unsafe human products. Hydroxyaethyl starch solution (HAES) increases intravascular volume with comparable physical properties to those of human albumin. One retrospective study, one placebo-controlled study and one controlled study provide concordant results and suggest that HAES decreases the incidence of OHSS when administered at the time of oocyte retrieval in high-risk patients showing an excessive ovarian response[50–52]. No data are available about pregnancy rates and about a possible adverse effect of HAES on implantation. Further studies are necessary to validate this method of OHSS prevention.

Intramuscular progesterone

Only one controlled study has assessed the efficacy of intramuscular progesterone administration, in comparison with intravenous albumin in patients showing an excessive ovarian response. Progesterone was administered at the time of oocyte retrieval, and was continued throughout the luteal phase. OHSS rates in this study do not permit conclusions to be drawn on the superiority of either method in preventing severe OHSS, but progesterone appears likely to be safer than albumin, with a possible benefit on pregnancy rates[49].

Cryopreservation of all embryos

To avoid cycle cancellation, a proposal has been made to proceed with hCG administration and oocyte retrieval, but to cancel embryo transfer and to freeze the embryos that are of sufficient quality. This method is based on the assumption that late severe OHSS is observed exceptionally without pregnancy. Cancellation of embryo transfer is supposed to avoid enhancement of the syndrome by early secretion of hCG by the embryo. The frozen embryos may be transferred in subsequent cycles with an acceptable pregnancy rate[53]. The efficacy of this method remains controversial, because of several drawbacks[54]. First of all, for ethical reasons,

it is difficult to perform a controlled study. Second, early severe OHSS, resulting from exogenous hCG administration, is not avoided by the elective cryopreservation of all embryos. The third reason is that physicians encounter similar difficulties in determining the danger threshold when embryo transfer is postponed as for cycle cancellation: they therefore feel reluctant to propose it and patients find it difficult to accept, without evidence of low OHSS rates, as it is agreed that there is evidence of reduced pregnancy rates after frozen/thawed embryo transfers.

To optimize the efficacy of cryopreservation of all embryos in preventing early and late OHSS, some authors have proposed, after fresh-transfer cancellation, adding the continuation of GnRH-agonist administration after hCG injection (for 1 week); they have succeeded in preventing severe OHSS in high-risk patients (estradiol level > 5600 pg/ml, > 25 follicles of > 12 mm, > 20 collected oocytes)[55].

CONCLUSION

OHSS is a severe, life-threatening complication of ovarian stimulation in IVF and non-IVF treatment. Its prevention remains a priority objective for all physicians involved in the treatment of infertility, but they would be helped by better knowledge of the physiopathology of the syndrome. Thus, primary prevention, by screening patients and conducting the optimal treatment with consideration of risk factors, remains an essential point in the preventive strategy. The main difficulty for secondary prevention is the lack of a predictable relationship between the available data about ovarian response during the cycle and the risk of developing OHSS. When obvious indices of excessive ovarian response are present, all efforts should be made to avoid the occurrence of the severe form. Reducing hCG levels (exogenous and endogenous), enhancing luteolysis (withdrawal of follicular activity, coasting, follicular aspiration), and antagonizing the vascular effects (macromolecules), are the three levels of possible action for secondary prevention before the ultimate measure of cycle cancellation. All methods succeed in reducing the incidence and the severity of severe OHSS, but none of them, apart from cycle cancellation, is able to prevent it totally.

REFERENCES

1. Enskog A, Henriksson M, Unander M, *et al.* Prospective study of the clinical and laboratory parameters of patients in whom ovarian hyperstimulation syndrome developed during controlled ovarian hyperstimulation for *in vitro* fertilization. *Fertil Steril* 1999;71:808–14

2. Fauser BC, Van Heusden AM. Manipulation of human ovarian function: physiological concepts and clinical consequences. *Endocr Rev* 1997;18:71–106

3. Mathur RS, Jenkins JM. Severe OHSS: patients should be allowed to weigh the morbidity of OHSS against the benefits of parenthood. *Hum Reprod* 1999;14:2183–5

4. Knowler WC, Barrett-Connor E, Fowler SE, *et al.* Reduction in the incidence of type 2 diabetes with lifestyle intervention or metformin. *N Engl J Med* 2002;346:393–403

5. Amer SA, Gopalan V, Li TC, *et al.* Long term follow-up of patients with polycystic ovarian syndrome after laparoscopic ovarian drilling: clinical outcome. *Hum Reprod* 2002;17:2035–42

6. De Leo V, la Marca A, Ditto A, *et al.* Effects of metformin on gonadotropin-induced ovulation in women with polycystic ovary syndrome. *Fertil Steril* 1999;72:282–5

7. Morris RS, Karande VC, Dudkiewicz A, *et al.* Octreotide is not useful for clomiphene citrate resistance in patients with polycystic ovary syndrome but may reduce the likelihood of ovarian hyperstimulation syndrome. *Fertil Steril* 1999;71:452–6

8. Rimington MR, Walker SM, Shaw RW. The use of laparoscopic ovarian electrocautery in preventing cancellation of *in-vitro* fertilization treatment cycles due to risk of ovarian hyperstimulation syndrome in women with polycystic ovaries. *Hum Reprod* 1997;12:1443–7

9. Rongières-Bertrand C, Olivennes F, Righini C, *et al.* Revival of the natural cycles in *in-vitro* fertilization with the use of a new gonadotrophin-releasing hormone antagonist (Cetrorelix): a pilot study with minimal stimulation. *Hum Reprod* 1999;14:683–8

10. Tan SL, Child TJ. *In-vitro* maturation of oocytes from unstimulated polycystic ovaries. *Reprod Biomed Online* 2002;4:18–23

11. Hughes E, Collins J, Vandekerckhove P. Ovulation induction with urinary follicle stimulating hormone versus human menopausal gonadotropin for clomiphene-resistant polycystic ovary syndrome. *Cochrane Database Syst Rev* 2000;2:CD000087

12. Marci R, Senn A, Dessole S, *et al.* A low-dose stimulation protocol using highly purified follicle-stimulating hormone can lead to high pregnancy rates in *in vitro* fertilization patients with polycystic ovaries who are at risk of a high ovarian response to gonadotropins. *Fertil Steril* 2001;75:1131–5

13. El-Sheikh MM, Hussein M, Fouad S, *et al.* Limited ovarian stimulation (LOS), prevents the recurrence of severe forms of ovarian hyperstimulation syndrome in polycystic ovarian disease. *Eur J Obstet Gynecol Reprod Biol* 2001;94:245–9

14. Daya S. Updated meta-analysis of recombinant follicle-stimulating hormone (FSH) versus urinary FSH for ovarian stimulation in assisted reproduction. *Fertil Steril* 2002;77:711–14

15. The European and Middle East Orgalutran Study Group. Comparable clinical outcome using the GnRH antagonist ganirelix or a long protocol of the GnRH agonist triptorelin for the prevention of premature LH surges in women undergoing ovarian stimulation. *Hum Reprod* 2001;16:644–51

16. Al-Inany H, Aboulghar M. GnRH antagonist in assisted reproduction: a Cochrane review. *Hum Reprod* 2002;17:874–85

17. Lewit N, Kol S, Manor D, Itskovitz-Eldor J. Comparison of gonadotrophin-releasing hormone analogues and human chorionic gonadotrophin for the induction of ovulation and prevention of ovarian hyperstimulation syndrome: a case–control study. *Hum Reprod* 1996;11:1399–402

18. Fauser BC, de Jong D, Olivennes F, et al. Endocrine profiles after triggering of final oocyte maturation with GnRH agonist after cotreatment with the GnRH antagonist ganirelix during ovarian hyperstimulation for *in vitro* fertilization. *J Clin Endocrinol Metab* 2002;87:709–15

19. Olivennes F, Cunha-Filho JS, Fanchin R, et al. The use of GnRH antagonists in ovarian stimulation. *Hum Reprod Update* 2002;8:279–90

20. Thomas K, Searle T, Quinn A, et al. The value of routine estradiol monitoring in assisted conception cycles. *Acta Obstet Gynecol Scand* 2002;81:551–4

21. Anon. Human recombinant luteinizing hormone is as effective as, but safer than, urinary human chorionic gonadotropin in inducing final follicular maturation and ovulation in *in vitro* fertilization procedures: results of a multicenter double-blind study. *J Clin Endocrinol Metab* 2001;86:2607–18

22. Soliman S, Daya S, Collins J, et al. The role of luteal phase support in infertility treatment: a meta-analysis of randomized trials. *Fertil Steril* 1994;61:1068–76

23. Penzias AS. Luteal phase support. *Fertil Steril* 2002;77:318–23

24. Mathur RS, Akande AV, Keay SD, et al. Distinction between early and late ovarian hyperstimulation syndrome. *Fertil Steril* 2000; 73: 901–7

25. Christin-Maitre S, Rongieres-Bertrand C, Kottler ML, et al. A spontaneous and severe hyperstimulation of the ovaries revealing a gonadotroph adenoma. *J Clin Endocrinol Metab* 1998;83:3450–3

26. Balen AH, Braat DD, West C, et al. Cumulative conception and live birth rates after the treatment of anovulatory infertility: safety and efficacy of ovulation induction in 200 patients. *Hum Reprod* 1994;9:1563–70

27. Blankstein J, Shalev J, Saadon T, et al. Ovarian hyperstimulation syndrome: prediction by number and size of preovulatory ovarian follicles. *Fertil Steril* 1987;47:597–602

28. Delvigne A, Rozenberg S. Epidemiology and prevention of ovarian hyperstimulation syndrome (OHSS): a review. *Hum Reprod Update* 2002;8:559–77

29. Delvigne A, Rozenberg S. Preventive attitude of physicians to avoid OHSS in IVF patients. *Hum Reprod* 2001;16:2491–5

30. Delvigne A, Rozenberg S. A qualitative systematic review of coasting, a procedure to avoid ovarian hyperstimulation syndrome in IVF patients. *Hum Reprod Update* 2002;8: 291–6

31. D'Angelo A, Amso N. 'Coasting' (withholding gonadotrophins) for preventing ovarian hyperstimulation syndrome. *Cochrane Database Syst Rev* 2002;(3):CD002811

32. Egbase PE, Sharhan MA, Grudzinskas JG. Early unilateral follicular aspiration compared with coasting for the prevention of severe ovarian hyperstimulation syndrome: a prospective randomized study. *Hum Reprod* 1999;14:1421–5

33. Sher G, Zouves C, Feinman M, Maassarani G. 'Prolonged coasting': an effective method for preventing severe ovarian hyperstimulation syndrome in patients undergoing *in-vitro* fertilization. *Hum Reprod* 1995;10:3107–9

34. Benadiva CA, Davis O, Kligman I, et al. Withholding gonadotropin administration is an effective alternative for the prevention of ovarian hyperstimulation syndrome. Fertil Steril 1997;67:724–7

35. Tortoriello DV, McGovern PG, Colon JM, et al. 'Coasting' does not adversely affect cycle outcome in a subset of highly responsive in vitro fertilization patients. Fertil Steril 1998;69:454–60

36. Dhont M, Van der Straeten F, De Sutter P. Prevention of severe ovarian hyperstimulation by coasting. Fertil Steril 1998;70:847–50

37. Lee C, Tummon I, Martin J, et al. Does withholding gonadotrophin administration prevent severe ovarian hyperstimulation syndrome? Hum Reprod 1998;13:1157–8

38. Fluker MR, Hooper WM, Yuzpe AA. Withholding gonadotropins ('coasting') to minimize the risk of ovarian hyperstimulation during superovulation and in vitro fertilization–embryo transfer cycles. Fertil Steril 1999;71:294–301

39. Waldenström U, Kahn J, Marsk L, Nilsson S. High pregnancy rates and successful prevention of severe ovarian hyperstimulation syndrome by 'prolonged coasting' of very hyperstimulated patients: a multicentre study. Hum Reprod 1999;14:294–7

40. Dechaud H, Anahory T, Aligier N, et al. Coasting: a response to excessive ovarian stimulation. Gynecol Obstet Fertil 2000;28:115–19

41. Ohata Y, Harada T, Ito M, et al. Coasting may reduce the severity of the ovarian hyperstimulation syndrome in patients with polycystic ovary syndrome. Gynecol Obstet Invest 2000;50:186–8

42. Aboulghar MA, Mansour RT, Serour GI, et al. Reduction of human menopausal gonadotropin dose before coasting prevents severe ovarian hyperstimulation syndrome with minimal cycle cancellation. J Assist Reprod Genet 2000;17:298–301

43. Al-Shawaf T, Zosmer A, Hussain S, et al. Prevention of severe ovarian hyperstimulation syndrome in IVF with or without ICSI and embryo transfer: a modified 'coasting' strategy based on ultrasound for identification of high-risk patients. Hum Reprod 2001;16:24–30

44. Egbase PE, Al-Sharhan M, Grudzinskas JG. 'Early coasting' in patients with polycystic ovarian syndrome is consistent with good clinical outcome. Hum Reprod 2002;17:1212–16

45. Egbase PE, Makhseed M, Al Sharhan M, Grudzinskas JG. Timed unilateral ovarian follicular aspiration prior to administration of human chorionic gonadotrophin for the prevention of severe ovarian hyperstimulation syndrome in in-vitro fertilization: a prospective randomized study. Hum Reprod 1997;12:2603–6

46. Tay CC. Use of gonadotrophin-releasing hormone agonists to trigger ovulation. Hum Fertil (Camb) 2002;5:G35–7

47. Orvieto R, Ben-Rafael Z. The immune system in severe ovarian hyperstimulation syndrome. Isr J Med Sci 1996;32:1180–2

48. Tan SL, Balen A, el Hussein E, et al. The administration of glucocorticoids for the prevention of ovarian hyperstimulation syndrome in in vitro fertilization: a prospective randomized study. Fertil Steril 1992;58:378–83

49. Costabile L, Unfer V, Manna C, et al. Use of intramuscular progesterone versus intravenous albumin for the prevention of ovarian hyperstimulation syndrome. Gynecol Obstet Invest 2000;50:182–5

50. Graf MA, Fischer R, Naether OG, et al. Reduced incidence of ovarian hyperstimulation syndrome by prophylactic infusion of hydroxyaethyl starch solution in an in-vitro fertiliza-

tion programme. *Hum Reprod* 1997;12: 2599–602

51. Konig E, Bussen S, Sutterlin M, Steck T. Prophylactic intravenous hydroxyethyl starch solution prevents moderate–severe ovarian hyperstimulation in *in-vitro* fertilization patients: a prospective, randomized, double-blind and placebo-controlled study. *Hum Reprod* 1998;13:2421–4

52. Gökmen O, Ugur M, Ekin M, *et al.* Intravenous albumin versus hydroxyethyl starch for the prevention of ovarian hyperstimulation in an *in-vitro* fertilization programme: a prospective randomized placebo controlled study. *Eur J Obstet Gynecol Reprod Biol* 2001;96:187–92

53. Wada I, Matson PL, Troup SA, *et al.* Outcome of treatment subsequent to the elective cryopreservation of all embryos from women at risk of the ovarian hyperstimulation syndrome. *Hum Reprod* 1992;7:962–6

54. D'Angelo A, Amso NN. Embryo freezing for preventing ovarian hyperstimulation syndrome: a Cochrane review. *Hum Reprod* 2002;17: 2787–94

55. Endo T, Honnma H, Hayashi T, *et al.* Continuation of GnRH agonist administration for 1 week, after hCG injection, prevents ovarian hyperstimulation syndrome following elective cryopreservation of all pronucleate embryos. *Hum Reprod* 2002;17:2548–51

15

Health-economic considerations regarding single- versus double-embryo transfer

P. De Sutter and J. Gerris

INTRODUCTION

When discussing single-embryo transfer it is necessary not only to consider the medical and ethical advantages over double-embryo transfer[1], but also to analyze the cost-effectiveness of the single-embryo transfer approach. Is single-embryo transfer as cost-effective as double-embryo transfer, or will it only lead to an increase in the number of (costly) assisted reproductive technology (ART) procedures? If it were proved that single-embryo transfer was as cost-effective as double-embryo transfer, what about couples who actually wish to have two children, and for whom it would seem that having twins is an easy solution to their wish? For them, applying single-embryo transfer would mean more treatment cycles and this would therefore cost more.

The answer to the above questions should come from a health-economic analysis comparing single-with double-embryo transfer. Health-economic evaluations try to compare not only the effect of two treatments, but also their costs. There are different kinds of health-economic study[2]. Full economic evaluations, such as cost-effectiveness studies, analyze outcomes as discrete entities (pregnancy, birth, or death) and calculate the cost per outcome measure (for instance the cost per liveborn child). Cost-utility studies include morbidity and mortality in the outcome and, for example, measure quality-adjusted life years. Finally, cost–benefit analyses calculate costs as well as outcome measures in monetary units[3]. These studies are faced with the difficulty that it is not easy to convert outcome into monetary units. What is the price of a child? Of a prematurely born child? Or of a disabled child? How can one calculate or express the 'cost' of a deceased child? Besides full economic evaluations, there are costing studies and economic benefit studies that are easier to perform. Costing studies do not measure real costs, but estimate them. Economic benefit studies analyze the 'willingness to pay'. How much does a couple wish to pay to obtain a healthy child? It will not surprise anybody that 'willingness to pay' studies are subject to local social, political and ethical influences and that, in the field of infertility, there are few such studies that allow solid conclusions to be drawn[4].

Infertility is an important subject for health-economic evaluation, because of the high impact on society. A growing number of couples seek infertility treatment, and patients, insurance companies and governments wish to know how much a given treatment will cost. New and more successful drugs may be more expensive than older less successful drugs, therefore the decision for reimbursement should include an economic evaluation. The importance of health economics in assisted reproduction is illustrated by the studies comparing urinary and recombinant gonadotropins. Several meta-analyses have shown the superiority of recombinant gonadotropins over the older urinary products[5,6]. A few years later the same group of authors published a cost-effectiveness study showing that recombinant gonadotropins may be (much) more expensive in themselves, but, owing to their superiority, they are more cost-effective than the urinary products[7–9]. Some other nice examples of cost-effectiveness comparisons are described in a review paper by Garceau and co-workers[4]. For instance, they mention that natural-cycle *in vitro* fertilization (IVF) is more cost-effective than IVF in stimulated cycles[10] and that the transfer of two embryos is more cost-effective than the transfer of three embryos, owing to the increased neonatal care expenses of triplet pregnancies[11].

HEALTH-ECONOMIC COMPARISON OF SINGLE- AND DOUBLE-EMBRYO TRANSFER

In comparing single- with double-embryo transfer, we would ideally need a prospective randomized study including an economic evaluation. In the literature to date there are just two prospective randomized trials comparing single- with double-embryo transfer[12,13], and these do not offer data on costs of the procedures. These studies will not be discussed in detail here, since they will be described in more detail elsewhere in this book. Real-life health-economic evaluations are difficult to perform, and to date there is only one prospective non-randomized (but patient choice-based) study comparing single- with double-embryo transfer, which will be discussed below[14] (and manuscript in preparation). The problem of real-life studies, however, is that the number of patients to be included should be large enough to draw robust conclusions, which makes these studies time consuming and expensive. If the outcome is multiple pregnancy and its morbidity and mortality (as in a study comparing single- with double-embryo transfer), the number of patients to be included should be large enough to yield enough pregnancies complicated by premature birth to allow valuable economic evaluation. Also, costs will often have to be partially estimated and projected onto the whole group, a health-economic technique known as imputation, because cost data are not always available from all patients under study, which makes them costing studies, rather than full economic evaluations. Indeed, from every patient individual bills should be kept or be available from the health-care providers, and this proves to be a very difficult task.

THE WØLNER-HANSSEN AND RYDHSTROEM PAPER

Wølner-Hanssen and Rydhstroem[15] hypothesized in 1998 that the transfer of one embryo after IVF would lead to a lower rate of twin pregnancies at the cost of a lower take-home baby rate. At that time no data of randomized comparisons between single- and double-embryo transfer were available and these authors performed a comparison of actual results and costs of double-embryo transfer with hypothetical results and costs of single-embryo transfer. They considered the average implantation rate observed after double-embryo transfers to be the expected pregnancy rate after single-embryo transfer. It has been known since then that this is not completely correct, since the implantation rate after single-embryo transfer is higher than after double-embryo transfer. Indeed, of two embryos, both never have exactly the same implantation potential, and when performing single-embryo transfer it is always the one of the two which has the putative highest implantation potential that is chosen for transfer. However, in the paper several sensitivity analyses have been described, comparing single- with double-embryo transfer for varying pregnancy rates after single-embryo transfer. The Wølner-Hanssen and Rydhstroem paper was one of the first papers to emphasize that cost-effectiveness studies of IVF should not only be limited to the actual laboratory procedure costs, but also include costs for health care of the pregnant women and their offspring. The conclusion of their exercise was that, even when more treatments might be needed to achieve a similar take-home baby rate after transfer of one embryo when compared to two embryos, the lower twin pregnancy rate of the former approach caused it to be more cost-efficient than the latter.

MODELING

Put simply, a model allows conversion of input parameters such as effectiveness (e.g. pregnancy rate per cycle) and costs (e.g. of an IVF cycle) of procedures into outcome measures (e.g. children born) and their cost (e.g. cost per child born), based on a computer simulation. The model should be as complete as possible, including direct and indirect, short-term and long-term, measurable and unmeasurable costs. The mathematical simulation most often used is a decision-analytic model, called a Markov model[16], consisting of a tree structure in which each branch corresponds to a certain outcome occurring with a certain probability. Probabilities for each branch as well as costs of each particular outcome are obtained from meta-analyses, randomized trials, national registries, insurance data and expert opinions. A computer program allows a high number of virtual patients to enter the tree model and calculates the final outcomes and corresponding costs. Since the input parameters can be varied, the impact of each individual parameter on the output can be studied. This is called 'sensitivity analysis' but has the limitation that only one parameter can be varied at a time.

Incorporation of a distribution (including standard deviations or confidence limits) around all input parameters at once is achieved by the Monte Carlo method[17]. This probability sensitivity analysis method uses a random number generator that attributes values to each branch for a particular virtual patient and analyzes the corresponding outcome. The Monte Carlo simulation technique is superior to the classical sensitivity analysis approach, because it allows statistical testing, but confidence limits around input parameters are not always available.

DECISION-ANALYTICAL MODEL COMPARING SINGLE- WITH DOUBLE-EMBRYO TRANSFER

We have recently published a Markov model comparing single- with double-embryo transfer[18] created in Excel 97 (Microsoft Corporation, USA). Treatment efficiency estimates were obtained from published trials, costs from local hospital bills, and obstetric and neonatal outcome data of singleton and twin pregnancies from the Flemish register of perinatal activities[19]. We performed a sensitivity analysis using pregnancy rates for single- and double-embryo transfer from four different studies (two prospective randomized studies, one retrospective observational study and one retrospective case–control study) and found that the cost per child born was similar for single- and double-embryo transfer, irrespective of the pregnancy rates

used. For instance, using data from the study by Martikainen and colleagues[13], the cost per child born after single-embryo transfer was found to be 11 805 € whereas it was 10 966 € for double-embryo transfer. When 1000 couples had undergone three cycles of single-embryo transfer, they had obtained 634 children (versus 970 after three cycles of double-embryo transfer). However, the extra number of double-embryo transfer children (due to the twins in the double-embryo transfer group) was compensated for by the extra cost for neonatal care in the double-embryo transfer children, so that the cost per child born remained the same for the two groups.

Using data from the study of Gerris and co-workers[12], a single-embryo transfer child costs 9520 € compared to 9511 € for a double-embryo transfer child. Also, employing the pregnancy rates from two retrospective studies led to the same conclusion: single-embryo transfer 12 254 € versus double-embryo transfer 12 934 €[20], and single-embryo transfer 10 563 € versus double-embryo transfer 11 297 €[21]. Although the general conclusion of this mathematical exercise is that the cost per child born after single-embryo transfer is the same as after double-embryo transfer, it should not be forgotten that this model starts at the time of transfer and stops at hospital discharge. It is clear that the twins originating from double-embryo transfer increase the indirect and long-term costs, which were not included in the model. Twins have a perinatal mortality of 2.5% versus singletons' 0.6%[19], and it is well documented that the long-term morbidity is much higher with twins than with singletons[15]. There is more need for hospitalization, special education and training, owing to cerebral palsy and other handicaps following preterm birth. The message is clear: although double-embryo transfer leads to more children in fewer cycles, economically single-embryo transfer and double-embryo transfer are break-even; and in the long term single-embryo transfer definitely is more advantageous than double-embryo transfer.

SENSITIVITY ANALYSIS

Of course, the robustness of any model depends on the reliability of the data used for input. Pregnancy rates may vary widely between centers and therefore influence the analysis, yielding different results (although single- and double-embryo transfer costs remain similar in all instances, as discussed above). Also, the cost of the IVF procedure itself may vary widely, and finally the real costs of a premature twin birth are difficult to estimate. How does one calculate long-term costs of rehabilitation and special education for children with cerebral palsy?

In a situation where (only) IVF costs increase, the total cost would obviously increase as well, both for the single-embryo transfer and the double-embryo transfer strategy. The model predicts that the cost per child shows a linear correlation with the IVF cost, but that for single-embryo transfer this curve is steeper than for double-embryo transfer. Therefore, the cost per live-born child increases more rapidly for single-embryo transfer than for double-embryo transfer, indicating that in that scenario single-embryo transfer would become less cost-efficient than double-embryo transfer. However, if the model is run using increased IVF costs in conjunction with proportionally inflated costs for neonatal care, the total costs will again increase, but at all instances the cost per liveborn child remains the same for single-embryo transfer and for double-embryo transfer[22]. It can be expected that in some countries IVF costs as well as neonatal care expenses are higher than the figures used in the model, but sensitivity analysis shows that this does not affect the conclusion of the model.

REAL-LIFE ECONOMIC COMPARISON OF SINGLE- WITH DOUBLE-EMBRYO TRANSFER

As discussed above, the best approach for analyzing possible health-economic benefits of single- over double-embryo transfer is a real-life study. One such study has recently been performed in a two-center design[14] (manuscript in preparation). It was not randomized but based on patient choice. Patients younger than 38 years of age in their first IVF/ICSI cycle were offered the choice between the transfer of one embryo, if it was a high-quality embryo, or two embryos, irrespective of embryo quality. The clinical outcome results and the costs of single-embryo transfer were compared with those of double-embryo transfer, including the costs of the neonates up to the age of 3 months. The choice was

determined before the start of the cycle. In total, 408 women were included, of whom 367 (89.9%) had a transfer on day 3. Of these women 243 (66.2%) had chosen single-embryo transfer and 124 (33.8%) double-embryo transfer. It was agreed that single-embryo transfer would be performed only if a putative high-competence embryo were available; if not, the two best embryos were transferred. Therefore, in reality 206 patients received single-embryo transfer (56.1%) and 161 double-embryo transfer (43.9%). In the single-embryo transfer group the ongoing pregnancy rate was 40.3% without twins; in the double-embryo transfer group it was 40.4% with 27.7% ongoing twins. In the double-embryo transfer group, the mean duration of pregnancy was shorter (38.2 ± 2.1 vs. 39.1 ± 1.5 weeks; $p = 0.02$); there were more premature deliveries (21.3% versus 9.3%; $p = 0.09$); more low-birth-weight neonates (< 2500 g) (18.6% vs. 6.1%; $p = 0.066$); and neonatal hospitalizations were more frequent (18.6% vs. 4.1%; $p = 0.026$) and lasted longer (10.2 ± 9.6 vs. 6.1 ± 2.2 days; $p = 0.009$). All differences found were attributable to the twins after double-embryo transfer. The health-economic analysis showed higher total (mother plus children) costs after double-embryo transfer than after single-embryo transfer: $8790 \pm 10\,004$ € (double-embryo transfer) versus 4523 ± 3050 € (single-embryo transfer) ($p = 0.109$). This was entirely due to significantly higher neonatal costs after double-embryo transfer due to the twins: 3414 ± 8101 € (double-embryo transfer) versus 434 ± 954 € (single-embryo transfer) ($p < 0.001$) and not to differences in maternal costs: 5376 ± 4287 € (double-embryo transfer) versus 4089 ± 2661 € (single-embryo transfer) ($p = 0.152$) (Wilcoxon rank test used in all cases).

This study reconfirmed that judicious application of single-embryo transfer yields a high live birth rate similar to that of double-embryo transfer (approximately 40%). However, double-embryo transfer results in a twin gestation in about 25% of ongoing pregnancies, leading to the well-known risks of premature delivery, low birth weight and prolonged maternal and neonatal hospitalization. These result in a highly significant cost per child born after double-embryo transfer, which is entirely due to extremely elevated costs in some of the twins.

Of course in this study the costs of the IVF procedure were not included, which makes this real-life study different from the Markov model.

CONCLUSION

Health-economic evaluation of medical treatments is becoming increasingly important. There is no doubt that the avoidance of twins is mandatory from a purely medical and ethical point of view. However, also from an economic perspective, there are strong arguments in favor of single-embryo transfer. When comparing single- with double-embryo transfer using a Markov model, the cost-per-child-born is similar for single-embryo transfer and for double-embryo transfer, irrespective of the pregnancy rates used for both, and irrespective of the costs of procedures. Although more single-embryo transfer cycles are needed to yield the same amount of children as for double-embryo transfer, the extra cost for these extra cycles is more than compensated for by the increased neonatal care expenses due to the double-embryo transfer twins, as demonstrated in the real-life study. Since none of these studies have taken into account the long-term costs of children with cerebral palsy because of premature birth, it is clear that single-embryo transfer is to be preferred over double-embryo transfer, also from a purely economic perspective.

REFERENCES

1. ESHRE Campus Course Report. Prevention of twin pregnancies after IVF/ICSI by single embryo transfer. *Hum Reprod* 2001;16:790-800

2. Donaldson C. The state of the art of costing health care for economic evaluation. *Community Health Stud* 1990;14:341–56

3. McIntosh E, Donaldson C, Ryan M. Recent advances in the methods of cost–benefit analysis in healthcare. Matching the art to the science. *Pharmacoeconomics* 1999;15:357–67

4. Garceau L, Henderson J, Davis LJ, *et al.* Economic implications of assisted reproductive techniques: a systematic review. *Hum Reprod* 2002;17:3090–109

5. Out HJ, Mannaerts BMJL, Driessen SGAJ, *et al.* Recombinant follicle stimulating hormone (rFSH, Puregon) in assisted reproduction: more oocytes, more pregnancies. Results from five comparative studies. *Hum Reprod Update* 1996;2:162–71

6. Daya S, Gunby J. Recombinant versus urinary follicle stimulating hormone for ovarian stimulation in assisted reproduction. *Hum Reprod* 1999;14:2207–15

7. Daya S, Ledger W, Auray JP, *et al.* Cost-effectiveness modelling of recombinant FSH versus urinary FSH in assisted reproduction techniques in the UK. *Hum Reprod* 2001;16:2563–9

8. Sykes D, Out HJ, Palmer SJ, *et al.* The cost-effectiveness of IVF in the UK: a comparison of three gonadotrophin treatments. *Hum Reprod* 2001;16:2557–62

9. Silverberg K, Daya S, Auray JP, *et al.* Analysis of the cost effectiveness of recombinant versus urinary follicle-stimulating hormone in *in vitro* fertilization/intracytoplasmic sperm injection programs in the United States. *Fertil Steril* 2002;77:107–13

10. Nargund G, Waterstone J, Bland J, *et al.* Cumulative conception and live birth rates in natural (unstimulated) IVF cycles. *Hum Reprod* 2001;16:259–62

11. Liao XH, Decaestecker L, Gemmell J, *et al.* The neonatal consequences and neonatal cost of reducing the number of embryos transferred following IVF. *Scot Med J* 1997;42:76–8

12. Gerris J, De Neubourg D, Mangelschots K, *et al.* Prevention of twin pregnancy after *in-vitro* fertilization or intracytoplasmatic sperm injection based on strict criteria: a prospective

randomized clinical trial. *Hum Reprod* 1999;14:2581–7

13. Martikainen H, Tiitinen A, Tomas C, *et al.* One versus two embryo transfer after IVF and ICSI: a randomized study. *Hum Reprod* 2001;16:1900–3

14. De Neubourg D, Mangelschots K, Van Royen E, *et al.* Impact of patients' choice for single embryo transfer of a top quality embryo versus double embryo transfer in the first IVF/ICSI cycle. *Hum Reprod* 2002;17:2621–5

15. Wølner-Hanssen P, Rydhstroem H. Cost-effectiveness analysis of *in-vitro* fertilization estimated costs per successful pregnancy after transfer of one or two embryos. *Hum Reprod* 1998;13:88–94

16. Briggs A, Sculpher M. An introduction to Markov modelling for economic evaluation. *Pharmacoeconomics* 1998;13:397–409

17. Doubilet P, Begg CB, Weinstein MC, *et al.* Probabilistic sensitivity analysis using Monte Carlo simulation: a practical approach. *Med Decis Making* 1985;5:157–77

18. De Sutter P, Gerris J, Dhont M. A health-economic decision-analytic model comparing double with single embryo transfer in IVF/ICSI. *Hum Reprod* 2002;17:2891–6

19. SPE (Studiecentrum voor perinatale epidemiologie). *Perinatale activiteiten in Vlaanderen.* Brussels: SPE, 2000

20. Vilska S, Tiitinen A, Hydén-Granskog C, *et al.* Elective transfer of one embryo results in an acceptable pregnancy rate and eliminates the risk of multiple birth. *Hum Reprod* 1999;14:2392–5

21. De Sutter P, Van der Elst J, Coetsier T, Dhont M. Single embryo transfer and multiple pregnancy rate reduction after IVF/ICSI: a 5-year appraisal. *Reprod Biomed Online* 2003;6:464–9

22. De Sutter P, Gerris J, Dhont M. A health-economic decision-analytic model comparing double with single embryo transfer in IVF/ICSI: a sensitivity analysis [Letter]. *Hum Reprod* 2003;18:1361

16

Oncogenic risks related to assisted reproductive technologies

P. A. van Dop, H. Klip and C. Burger

ONCOGENEITY, SUBFERTILITY AND FERTILITY DRUGS

General considerations

An important issue in oncogenic risks related to assisted reproductive technologies (ART) is to assess the risk of cancer in subfertile versus fertile women before dealing with the risks of fertility drugs. Klip and associates[1] have summarized the data for several types of malignancy (Table 1)[2–10]. This question has been investigated in many case–control studies and in at least six cohort studies. According to these authors ovarian cancer risk among nulliparous or nulligravid women in most case–control studies was found to be weakly associated with unsuccessful attempts to conceive, with a history of physician-diagnosed subfertility, with expressed doubts about the ability to conceive or with the number of years of unprotected intercourse[1]. For gravid or parous women, subfertility has generally not been found to be associated with a significantly increased risk of ovarian cancer. The Collaborative Ovarian Cancer Group has published a well-conducted meta-analysis of case–control studies[11]. No significant differences in ovarian cancer risk were found according to marital status and gravidity, as indicators of subfertility. In addition, women who had tried to become pregnant for at least 2 years were at no greater risk than women who became pregnant within 1 year. However, after a total of ≥ 15 years of unprotected intercourse, nulligravid and gravid women experienced an increased risk of ovarian cancer (OR 1.6; 95% CI 1.2–2.2) compared to women with less

than 2 years of unprotected intercourse. Klip and colleagues stressed the importance of limitation of the use of the standardized incidence rates (SIR) in the above-mentioned studies, which are based on a comparison of cancer risk in subfertile women with that of the general population[1]. Since cohorts of subfertile women have lower parity rates than the general population and nulliparity is a strong risk factor for ovarian cancer, an increased SIR may be solely due to the confounding effect of nulliparity. Thus, results based only on the SIR are of little value when determining the relationship between subfertility (treatment) and ovarian cancer or other hormone-related cancers.

For that reason a comparison of cancer risk within a cohort of subfertile women is necessary for making a valid assessment of the independent effect of causes of subfertility. Only two such studies were large enough to analyze the effect of the cause of subfertility on cancer risk. The results are shown in Table 2[11,12]. The odds ratios for ovarian cancer were not significantly increased in women with subfertility: with tubal disease, idiopathic subfertility or ovulation disorders. One group found a 2.4 increased risk for ovarian cancer in patients with polycystic ovaries[12]. Based on the confidence interval this increase was on the edge of significance.

The cohort studies that have presented data on ovarian cancer risk in relation to different causes of subfertility are summarized in Table 3[2–4,7,8,10,13,14]. Two cohorts showed a significantly increased risk of ovarian cancer relative to the population rates for women with unexplained subfertility. Overall, however, the data presented in Table 3 do not favor

Table 1 Standardized incidence rates (SIR) for ovarian cancer, breast cancer, endometrial cancer and melanoma in cohorts of subfertile patients

Authors, year and country	Total	Mean follow-up (years)	Population	Ovarian cancer Obs	Exp	SIR	95% CI	Breast cancer Obs	Exp	SIR	95% CI	Endometrial cancer Obs	Exp	SIR	95% CI	Melanoma Obs	Exp	SIR	95% CI
Ron et al. 1987, Israel[2]	2575	12.3	diagnosed with subfertility	4	1.9	2.1	NS	15	14.1	1.1	NS	5	1.1	4.8	1.7–10.6	4	2.0	2.0	NS
Brinton et al. 1989, USA[3]	2335	19.4	evaluated for subfertility	11	8.6	1.3	NS	49	52.0	0.9	NS	11	12.8	0.9	NS	4	3.5	1.2	NS
Rossing et al. 1994, USA[4–6]	3837	6.9	evaluated for subfertility	11**	4.3	2.5	1.3–4.5	27	28.8	0.9	0.6–1.4					12	6.8	1.8	0.9–3.1
Venn et al. 1995, Australia[7]	5564	5.2*	evaluated for subfertility and exposed to IVF	3	1.8	1.7	0.6–5.3	16	17.9	0.9	0.6–1.5	2†	0.9	2.2	0.6–8.9	7	7.4	1.0	0.5–2.0
	4794	7.6*	evaluated for subfertility and unexposed to IVF	3	1.9	1.6	0.5–5.1	18	18.3	1.0	0.6–1.6	3†	0.9	3.5	1.1–10.8	9	7.6	1.2	0.6–2.3
Modan et al. 1998, Israel[8]	2469	21.4	diagnosed with subfertility	12	7.2	1.6	0.8–2.9	59	46.6	1.3	0.96–1.6	21	4.3	4.8	3.0–7.4	8	7.0	1.1	0.5–2.2
Potashnik et al. 1999, Israel[9]	780	18.0	infertile women exposed to FDs	1	1.5	0.7	0.0–3.8	16	9.6	1.7	0.9–2.7	2†	0.7	3.0	0.3–10.9				
	417	17.6	infertile women unexposed to FDs	1	0.7	1.4	0.0–7.5	4	5.0	0.8	0.2–2.0	0†	0.4	—	—				
Venn et al. 1999, Australia[10]	2065	7*	evaluated for subfertility and exposed to IVF	7	8	0.9	0.4–1.8	87	95.4	0.9	0.7–1.1	5†	4.6	1.1	0.5–2.6				
		10*	evaluated for subfertility and unexposed to IVF	6	5.2	1.2	0.5–2.6	56	59.2	0.95	0.7–1.2	7†	2.8	2.5	1.2–5.2				

NS, not significant; IVF, *in vitro* fertilization; FDs, fertility drugs

* Median years of follow-up; † body of the uterus; obs, observed cases; exp, expected cases; **invasive (*n* = 5) or borderline tumor (*n* = 4) and granulosa-cell tumors (*n* = 2)

Table 2 Cause of subfertility and ovarian cancer risk: case–control studies

Author, year and country	Total no. of cases	Total no. of controls	Type of control	Comparison	OR	95% CI	Adjustment				
							Family history	Age	Parity	FDs	Other variables*
Whittemore et al., 1992, USA[11]	2197	8893	H/P	ovulatory vs. no subfertility	2.1*	0.9–4.7	N	Y	N	N	sv
				tubal vs. no subfertility	1.3*	0.6–2.8	N	Y	N	N	sv
				unexplained/other vs. no subfertility	0.8*	0.6–1.1	N	Y	N	N	sv
Schildkraut et al., 1996, USA[12]	476	4081	P	diagnosed with PCOS vs. no PCOS	2.4	1.0–5.9	N	Y	Y†	N	ofe

H, hospital controls; P, population controls; N, no; Y, yes; s, study; v, age at diagnosis or interview; o, oral contraceptive use; f, subfertility; e, education
* Based on three case–control studies: The Cancer and Steroid Hormone study for the Centers of Disease Control and the National Institute of Child Health and Human Development
† Number of pregnancies with duration > 6 months

ASSISTED REPRODUCTIVE TECHNOLOGIES

Table 3 Cause of subfertility and ovarian cancer risk: cohort studies

Author, year and country	Mean follow-up	Total cohort size	Total no. of cases	Comparison	RR	95% CI	Adjustment Family history	Age	Parity	FDs	Other variables
Ron et al., 1987, Israel[2]	12.3	2575	4	unexplained vs. GP	6.1*	1.0–20.0	N	Y	N	N	vr
Brinton et al., 1989, USA[3]	19.4	2335	11	progesterone deficiency vs. GP	1.6*	NS	N	Y	N	N	v
				other causes vs. GP	1.1*	NS	N	Y	N	N	v
Rossing et al., 1994, USA[4]	6.9	3837**	11‡	ovulatory factors vs. GP	3.7*	1.4–8.1	N	Y	N	N	N
				ovulatory vs. non-ovulatory	2.2	0.6–8.2	N	Y	Y†††	N	wv
				anovulation vs. non-ovulatory	2.5	0.4–14.1	N	Y	Y†††	N	wv
				PCOS vs. non-ovulatory	2.4	0.2–22.5	N	Y	Y†††	N	wv
				oligomenorrhea vs. non-ovulatory	2.2	0.3–13.5	N	Y	Y†††	N	wv
Venn et al., 1995, Australia[7]	6.3§	10 358	6	unexplained vs. GP	7.0*	2.9–16.8	N	Y	N	N	N
				unexplained vs. known causes	19.2	2.2–165	N	Y	N	Y	N
Brinton et al., 1997, Sweden[13]	11.4	20 686	29	endometriosis†† vs. GP	1.9*	1.3–2.8	N	Y	N	N	N
Modan et al., 1998, Israel[8]	21.4	2496	12	progesterone deficiency vs. GP	0.8*	0.1–2.9	N	Y	N	N	vr
				mechanical/male vs. GP	2.7*	1.0–6.0	N	Y	N	N	vr
				unexplained vs. GP	1.9*	0.5–4.8	N	Y	N	N	vr

continued

Table 3 *continued*

Author, year and country	Mean follow-up	Total cohort size	Total no. of cases	Comparison	RR	95% CI	Adjustment				
							Family history	Age	Parity	FDs	Other variables
Rodriguez et al., 1998, USA[14]	12.0	198 247‡‡	797***	female subfertility vs. no subfertility	2.2	1.1–4.6	Y	Y	Y‡‡‡	N	reb mot
				male infertility vs. no subfertility	0.9	0.2–3.8	Y	Y	Y‡‡‡	N	hp reb
				unexplained vs. no subfertility	1.3	0.7–2.3	Y	Y	Y‡‡‡	N	mot hp reb mot hp
Venn et al., 1999, Australia[10]	7.8	29 666	13	tubal vs. GP	0.96*	0.4–2.1	N	Y	N	N	N
				male factor vs. GP	0.7*	0.2–2.7	N	Y	N	N	N
				endometriosis vs. GP	1.5*	0.5–4.6	N	Y	N	N	N
				unexplained vs. GP	2.6*	1.1–6.4	N	Y	N	N	N

GP, general population; N, no; Y, yes; PCOS, polycystic ovary syndrome; v, calendar year at diagnosis; r, ethnicity/race/country of origin; w, weight; e, education; b, body mass index; m, age at menarche; o, years of use of oral contraceptives; t, tubal ligation; h, years of estrogen replacement therapy use; p, menopausal status/age

*Standardized incidence rate; †median years of follow-up; ‡invasive ($n = 4$) or borderline tumor ($n = 5$) and granulosa-cell tumors ($n = 2$); **subcohort ($n = 135$) used in analysis; ††women hospitalized for endometriosis – fertility status unknown; ‡‡cohort of fertile and subfertile women; ***ovarian cancer deaths; †††parity at entry into cohort; ‡‡‡nulligravid women

a consistent risk increase or decrease associated with any of the specified subfertility disorders. Despite the size of the cohorts, owing to the overall low incidence of ovarian cancer the numbers in all of the above studies are small. Consequently, all studies have wide confidence intervals around the risk estimates. Therefore, conclusions of risk changes in subfertility alone must be made with caution.

Fertility drugs and ovarian cancer risk

In the USA, the number of women treated annually with fertility drugs nearly doubled between 1973 and 1991[1]. In The Netherlands, the sales of gonadotropins increased from 60 000 ampules per year in 1984 to almost 400 000 in 1990. Among others the paper of Whittemore and co-workers stirred anxiety on this subject[11].

The shortcomings of many studies on fertility drugs are retrospective study designs, mainly focused on ovarian cancers; small numbers of ovarian cancer cases; inconsistent reporting of fertility drug use; and inconsistent reporting of type of infertility.

Klip and co-workers published an extensive review of this subject, using identification of papers published between 1966 and 1999, examination of fertility drugs and specific causes of subfertility in relation to the risks of cancer (not only of the ovary, but also of the breast, endometrium and thyroid, and melanoma)[1]. They used SIRs to compare the observed versus the expected incidence of the studied malignancies. For the results of risks of ovarian cancer and subfertility in case–control studies we refer to Table 2, and for the details to the original paper[1]. The cohort studies with the same subject are shown in Table 3. Table 4 shows the results of fertility drugs and ovarian cancer risks in cohort studies. Rossing and colleagues studied the long-term use of clomiphene citrate[4]. A relative risk of 11 was found with significant confidence intervals. Adjustment for the presence of ovulatory abnormalities reduced the relative risk (RR) associated with the use of clomiphene citrate for ≥ 12 cycles to 7.7 (95% CI 1.0–60.1). The RR of ovarian cancer associated with long-term use (≥ 12 cycles) of clomiphene citrate was 9.1 (95% CI 1.0–86.5) among women without ovulatory abnormalities, and 7.4 (95% CI 1.0-53.1) among women with ovulatory abnormalities (compared with use of 0–11

cycles). Thus, among women both with and without ovulatory abnormalities, extended periods of subfertility treatment with clomiphene citrate were associated with an increased risk of ovarian malignancies. These authors[15] presented new analyses in response to criticism of the inclusion of granulosa cell tumors in the group of epithelial tumors. When women with granulosa cell tumors were eliminated from the analysis, exposure to 12 or more cycles of clomiphene citrate was still associated with an elevated risk for epithelial ovarian tumors (RR 6.7) but the 95% CIs were no longer significant (0.8–58.8).

Venn and associates published a large cohort study on this subject in IVF patients[7]. Because of the relatively short follow-up period in the first report, the number of ovarian cancer cases was rather small (n = 6). After adjustment for age and subfertility type, the RR for developing ovarian cancer after treatment with IVF was 1.5. A limitation of this study was that information on specific fertility drugs was not analyzed. In the second report of Venn and co-workers[10], seven cases of ovarian cancer in the exposed group were observed, and the SIR did not differ from that in the unexposed group (SIRs of 0.88 and 0.16, respectively). In this publication, the authors stratified the incidence of ovarian cancer according to the number of stimulated cycles and specific drugs that were used during IVF treatment. However, the numbers of ovarian cancers in the subgroups were too small to yield reliable risk estimates.

Fertility drugs and breast cancer risk

Breast cancer is the most common malignancy in women in developed countries and accounts for 30–35% of all malignancies in females. In the USA recent estimates of approximately 178 700 new cases and more than 43 500 breast cancer deaths per year have been published[1]. The role of subfertility in breast cancer must first be considered. Regarding this subject, only cohort studies are discussed. An overview including different types of hormonal disturbance is presented in Table 5[2,4,7–10]. In subfertility no statistically significant increase in risk for breast cancer has been demonstrated. The results of the oncogeneity of fertility drugs on breast cancer are shown in Table 6[2–4,7,9,10,16–18]. The two papers of Venn included 10 000 and nearly 30 000

Table 4   Use of fertility drugs (FDs) and ovarian cancer risk: cohort studies

Author, year and country	Mean follow-up (years)	Total cohort size	Total no. of cases	Comparison	RR	95% CI	Adjustment Family history	Age	Parity	Infertility*	Other variables
Ron et al., 1987, Israel[2]	12.3	2575	4	hMG vs. no FDs	no assoc	NS	n/a	n/a	n/a	n/a	n/a
				CC vs. no FDs	no assoc	NS	n/a	n/a	n/a	n/a	n/a
				other FDs vs. no FDs	no assoc	NS	n/a	n/a	n/a	n/a	n/a
Rossing et al., 1994, USA[4]	6.9	3837[††]	11[†]	CC vs. no CC	2.3	0.5–11.4	N	Y	Y[‡‡]	N	v
				1–11 cycles CC vs. no CC	0.8	0.1–5.7	N	Y	Y[‡‡]	N	v
				≥12 cycles CC vs. no CC	11.1	1.5–82.3	N	Y	Y[‡‡]	N	v
				hCG vs. no hCG	1.0	0.2–4.3	N	Y	Y[‡‡]	N	v
Venn et al., 1995, Australia[7]	6.3[‡]	10 358	6	IVF vs. no IVF	1.5	0.3–7.6	N	Y	N	Y	N
Modan et al., 1998, Israel[8]	21.4	2496	12	CC vs. GP	2.7**	0.97–5.8	N	Y	N	N	rd
Potashnik et al., 1999, Israel[9]	17.9	1197	2	1–2 cycles CC vs. GP	1.9**	0.0–10.5	N	Y	N	N	r
Venn et al., 1999, Australia[10]	7.8	29 666	13	CC vs. GP	2.5**	0.4–17.5	N	Y	N	N	N
				CC/hMG vs. GP	0.8**	0.2–3.1	N	Y	N	N	N
				hMG vs. GP	1.1**	0.2–8.1	N	Y	N	N	N
				hMG/GnRH-agonist vs. GP	0.5**	0.1–3.4	N	Y	N	N	N

hMG, human menopausal gonadotropin; CC, clomiphene citrate; hCG, human chorionic gonadotropin; IVF, in vitro fertilization; n/a, no information available; no assoc, no association; GP, general population; GnRH, gonadotropin releasing hormone; NS, not significant; N, no; Y, yes; d, calendar year at diagnosis; v, year of enrolment in study; r, country of origin

*Clinically assessed cause of subfertility, classified into subtypes; †invasive (n = 4) or borderline tumor (n = 5) and granulosa-cell tumors (n = 2);
‡median years of follow-up; **standardized incidence rate; ††subcohort (n = 135) used in analysis; ‡‡parity at entry into cohort

Table 5 Cause of subfertility and breast cancer risk: cohort studies

Author, year and country	Mean follow-up (years)	Total cohort size	Total no. of cases	Comparison	RR	95% CI	Adjustment Family history	Age	Parity	FDs	Other variables
Cowan et al., 1981, USA[16]	19.4	1083	17	progesterone deficiency vs. non-hormonal factors	1.8	0.6–5.1	N	N	N	N	N
Coulam et al., 1983, USA[17]	11.4	1270	12	chronic anovulation syndrome vs. GP	1.5*	0.8–2.6	N	Y	N	N	N
Ron et al., 1987, Israel[2]	12.3	2575	15	hormonal subfertility vs. GP	1.4*	NS	N	Y	N	N	dr
Brinton et al., 1989, USA[3]	19.4	2335	49	progesterone deficiency vs. GP	0.9*	NS	N	Y	N	N	d
				other causes vs. GP	1.0*	NS	N	Y	N	N	d
Rossing et al., 1994, USA[4]	6.9	3837†	27	ovulatory vs. non-ovulatory factors	1.0	0.4–2.5	N	Y	Y‡	N	d
Venn et al., 1995, Australia[7]	6.3	10 358	34	unexplained vs. known causes	0.8	0.2–3.1	N	Y	N	Y	N
				ovarian disorders vs. GP	1.8	0.4–5.6	N	Y	N	N	N
Garland et al., 1998, USA[18]	4.0	11 6678	251	ovulatory vs. non-ovulatory factors	0.4	0.2–0.9	Y	Y	Y	N	axmbgpo
Potashnik et al., 1999, Israel[9]	17.9	1197	20	FD users:							
				hormonal factor vs. GP	1.6*	0.6–3.2	N	Y	N	N	r
				mechanical factor vs. GP	1.5*	0.4–3.8	N	Y	N	N	r
				male factor vs. GP	1.8*	0.5–4.5	N	Y	N	N	r
				other factor vs. GP	3.9*	0.0–21.4	N	Y	N	N	r
				non-FD users:							
				hormonal factor vs. GP	1.8*	0.5–4.5	N	Y	N	N	r
Venn et al. 1999, Australia[10]	8.5	29 700	143	tubal vs. GP	0.6*	0.4–0.8	N	Y	N	N	N
				male factor vs. GP	1.3*	0.9–1.7	N	Y	N	N	N
				endometriosis vs. GP	1.0*	0.7–1.5	N	Y	N	N	N
				ovarian defects vs. GP	0.5*	0.2–1.6	N	Y	N	N	N
				unexplained vs. GP	1.3	0.9–1.8	N	Y	N	N	N

FD, fertility drugs; GP, general population; N, no; Y, yes; d, calendar year at entry; r, ethnicity, a, alcohol consumption; x, history of benign breast disease; m, age at menarche; b, body mass index; g, age at first full-term pregnancy; p, menopausal status; o, duration of use of oral contraceptives
*Standardized incidence rate; †subcohort ($n = 135$) used in analysis; ‡parity at entry into cohort

Table 6   Use of fertility drugs and breast cancer risk: cohort studies

Author, year and country	Mean follow-up (years)	Total cohort size	Total no. of cases	Comparison	RR	95% CI	Adjustment				Other variables
							Family history	Age	Parity	Infertility	
Ron et al., 1987, Israel[2]	12.3	2575	15	hMG vs. no FDs	no assoc	NS	n/a	n/a	n/a	n/a	n/a
				CC vs. no FDs	no assoc	NS	n/a	n/a	n/a	n/a	n/a
				other FDs vs. no FDs	no assoc	NS	n/a	n/a	n/a	n/a	n/a
Rossing et al., 1994, USA[4]	6.9	3837‡	27	CC vs. no CC	0.5	0.2–1.2	N	Y	Y††	N	wd
				1–5 cycles CC vs. no CC	0.4	0.2–1.4	N	Y	Y††	N	wd
				6–11 cycles CC vs. no CC	0.5	0.1–1.7	N	Y	Y††	N	wd
				≥ 12 cycles CC vs. no CC	0.6	0.2–2.4	N	Y	Y††	N	wd
				hCG vs. no hCG	0.5	0.2–1.8	N	Y	Y††	N	wd
Venn et al., 1995, Australia[7]	6.3**	10 358	34	IVF vs. no IVF	1.1	0.6–2.2	N	Y	N	Y	N
Modan et al., 1998, Israel[8]	21.4	2496	59	CC vs. GP	1.2†	0.7–1.9	N	Y	N	N	rv
				CC/hMG vs. GP	1.6†	0.7–3.4	N	Y	N	N	rv
Potashnik et al., 1999, Israel[9]	17.9	1197	20	1–2 cycles CC vs. GP	2.6†	1.2–5.0	N	Y	N	N	r
				3–5 cycles CC vs. GP	1.3†	0.4–3.4	N	Y	N	N	r
				≥ 6 cycles CC vs. GP	0.9†	0.2–2.7	N	Y	N	N	r
				≥ 1000 mg CC vs. GP	2.5†	1.2–4.6	N	Y	N	N	r
				1001–2000 mg CC vs. GP	1.2†	0.2–3.5	N	Y	N	N	r
				≥ 3000 mg CC vs. GP	2.1†	0.3–4.2	N	Y	N	N	r
Venn et al., 1999, Australia[10]	8.5	29 700	143	CC vs. GP	0.9†	0.3–2.3	N	Y	N	N	N
				CC/hMG vs. GP	1.2†	0.9–1.6	N	Y	N	N	N
				hMG vs. GP	0.99†	0.6–1.8	N	Y	N	N	N
				hMG/GnRH-agonist vs. GP	0.8†	0.6–1.4	N	Y	N	N	N

hMG, human menopausal gonadotropin; FDs, fertility drugs; CC, clomiphene citrate; hCG, human chorionic gonadotropin; IVF, in vitro fertilization; GP, general population; GnRH, gonadotropin releasing hormone; n/a, no information available; NS, not significant; no assoc, no association; N, no; Y, yes; v, calendar year at diagnosis; r, ethnicity/country of origin; w, weight; d, year of enrolment in study
*Clinically assessed cause of subfertility, classified into subtypes; †standardized incidence rate; ‡subcohort (n = 135) used in analysis; **median years of follow-up; ††parity at entry into cohort

persons, respectively[7,10]. It can be concluded that the use of fertility drugs did not increase the risk for breast cancer in either of these two large study groups, or in the other studies.

Fertility drugs and endometrial cancer risk

In most industrialized countries, cancer of the corpus uteri is about as frequent as ovarian cancer, accounting for 6% of all new cancers. Recent estimates from the USA show that, yearly, 36 100 women are diagnosed with cancer of the corpus uteri. Owing to the relatively good prognosis, fewer than 6% (6300) will die from this disease[1].

The SIRs from different cohort studies are summarized in Table 1, showing a significant positive association in four studies[2,7,8,17]; and no association in one study[3]. At present there is general agreement that subfertility is a risk factor for endometrial cancer, particularly in the case of hormonal disorders.

Use of fertility drugs in relation to the risk of endometrial cancer has been studied in only two papers. Ron and colleagues[2], showed after 12 years of follow-up, found no significant increase in risk. A SIR of 6.8 after 21 years of follow-up was demonstrated. In the SIR of 6.8 was included the subgroup with subfertility, but, without fertility drugs, the SIR would be 3.3. According to one author the different causes of subfertility in the two groups largely explained the difference in risk estimates between the treated and untreated groups[8]. In one study by Venn and co-workers, cancer of the uterus was not associated with IVF treatment or any of the specific fertility drugs examined, but the risk estimate was based on very small numbers ($n = 5$)[10].

Fertility drugs and melanoma risk

Increased risk of cutaneous melanoma in women has been associated with delayed childbearing and low parity[19]. However, these associations have not been observed consistently[20]. Risk data are summarized in Table 1. A biological mechanism for an effect of fertility drugs on the development of cutaneous melanoma is unclear. Some epidemiological studies[2] have suggested a possible increase in melanoma risk in relation to hormonal subfertility and/or its treatment. Owing to the small number of melanoma cases that occurred in the studies, the observed associations may have been chance findings[2,6,8]. The largest study to date showed no increase in melanoma risk due to subfertility[10].

Fertility drugs and thyroid cancer risk

Since incidence rates of thyroid cancer are much higher in females than in males, a role of hormonal factors has long been suspected[21]. In summary, studies published to date have not shown convincing evidence of an association between thyroid cancer risk and subfertility, or its treatment.

General conclusions on fertility drugs and cancer risk

The shortcomings of the present data on cancer risk and the use of fertility drugs are retrospective study designs, small numbers of (ovarian) cancer cases, inconsistent reporting of fertility drug use and inconsistent reporting of type of infertility. For these reasons no convincing relationship has been found between fertility drugs and risks for ovarian, breast, endometrial and thyroid cancer. Also, the risk for cutaneous melanoma is not amplified by fertility drugs. However, fertility specialists must become aware that consistent observations of increased risk of endometrial cancer for women with infertility, particularly due to hormonal disorders, have been published.

ONCOGENEITY OF *IN VITRO* FERTILIZATION TREATMENT

General considerations

Klip and colleagues have carried out a well-designed, detailed and large study (the OMEGA study) on this subject (unpublished data). The methodology is based on cancer risk in a nationwide historical cohort of 25 152 women treated for subfertility in The Netherlands between 1980 and 1995. In total, 19 136 women received one or more cycles of IVF, whereas 6016 patients did not undergo IVF. In 13 216 patients, detailed medical data (cause of subfertility, gynecological surgery, details of fertility treatment) were collected from the medical records of the 12 participating IVF clinics. Cancer incidence until 1997 was ascertained through linkage with the population-based Netherlands Cancer Registry. Causes of death were obtained through the women's general practitioners. Women were asked to complete a mailed questionnaire that inquired about reproductive variables and the occurrence and age at onset of specific medical conditions. The observed numbers of hormone-related cancers were compared with the numbers expected on the basis of age and calendar period-specific cancer incidence rates in the Dutch population. SIRs and the Cox proportional hazards model were used to compare cancer risk directly between IVF-exposed and -unexposed women.

Another large cohort study is that of Venn and associates, who also reported on IVF and the risk of cancer[7]. A total of seven ovarian cancer cases in the exposed group were observed, and the SIR did not differ from that in the unexposed group (SIRs of 0.88 and 0.16, respectively). The small numbers of ovarian cancers precluded subgroup analysis. The Venn study did not include a confirmation of the data of the questionnaire with the medical records, as was included in the OMEGA study by Klip and colleagues.

Other studies on cancer risk and IVF cannot be compared with the paper of Klip and colleagues or that by Venn and colleagues for reason of sample size only, so the conclusions have less weight.

It can be concluded that, in the first 6 years following IVF treatment, significantly increased risks of tumors of the ovary, endometrium, breast and melanoma can be excluded, based on the present data. Even in large studies, the internal comparisons are still limited by small numbers of cases.

Oncogenic effects in offspring after *in vitro* fertilization

Over the past decade attention has increasingly been focused on the long-term health effects of ART such as IVF in both women and their offspring. From the same dataset for the analysis of cancer risks in women who underwent IVF, Klip and associates analyzed the cancer risks in offspring after IVF treatment[22].

A large population-based historical cohort was studied that was initially designed to examine the risk of gynecological disorders in women who underwent IVF. Children were included in the exposed group, if they were conceived by IVF or by other related fertility techniques ($n = 9484$). The unexposed group consisted of 7532 children whose mothers were diagnosed with subfertility disorders, but who were conceived naturally. All cohort members were asked to complete a mailed questionnaire that inquired about reproductive variables and cancer in the offspring (response rate 66.9%). During an average follow-up period of 6.0 years, 16 cancers were observed in the combined exposed and unexposed group, whereas 15.5 were expected (SIR 1.0; 95% CI 0.6–1.7). Direct comparison between children conceived after ART and naturally conceived children revealed no increased risk for childhood malignancies (risk ratio 0.8; 95% CI 0.3–2.3).

Despite the small numbers of observed cancer cases, these findings demonstrated that children conceived by ART had no greatly increased risk of cancer during childhood compared to the general population and the internal reference group.

In another paper on this subject, with a large sample size, a record-linkage cohort design was used to investigate the incidence of cancer in children born after IVF[23]. All conceptions using assisted reproductive technologies between 1979 and 1995 at two clinics in Victoria, Australia that resulted in a live birth were included. Data on births were linked with a population-based cancer registry to determine the number of cases of cancer that occurred. The SIR was calculated by comparing the observed number of cases to the expected number of cases. The final cohort included 5249 births. The median length of follow-up was 3 years, 9 months (range 0–15 years). In all, 4.33 cases of cancer were expected and six were observed, giving a SIR of 1.39 (95% CI 0.62–3.09).

From this study it can be concluded that children conceived using IVF and related procedures did not have a significantly increased incidence of cancer in comparison to the general population.

There is also a small Israeli study on his subject[24]. A cohort of 332 children from 1254 women who underwent IVF treatment was compared with the expected age-adjusted rates of the general population during the respective time period. No cancer case was found in the study group, whereas 1.7 cases were expected.

It can be concluded that the available data do not show an increased cancer risk in the offspring of mothers who underwent IVF.

General conclusions about oncogenic risks and fertility treatment

Fertility drugs

No convincing relationship exists between fertility drugs and cancer risks. A consistent observation is the increased risk of endometrial cancer for women with infertility due to hormonal disorders[1]. An association between ovulation induction and ovarian cancer does not necessarily indicate a causal effect. Infertility alone is an independent risk factor for the development of ovarian cancer. Nulliparous women with refractory infertility may harbor a particularly high risk of ovarian cancer, irrespective of their use of fertility drugs.

In vitro fertilization

From the data of the present literature it can be concluded that fertility drugs and IVF do not increase the risk of breast and ovarian cancer. There is, however, concern about the risk of endometrial cancer. The small increased risk of endometrial cancer is apparently not correlated with hormone use but rather with the polycystic ovary syndrome.

Cancer risks in offspring

The three largest studies have shown no increase in cancer in offspring after IVF. The studied populations were large and the incidence of cancer was low. Huge populations are needed to reach power.

REFERENCES

1. Klip H, Burger CW, Kenemans P, et al. Cancer risk associated with subfertility and ovulation induction: a review. *Cancer Causes Control* 2000;11:319–44

2. Ron E, Lunenfeld B, Menczer J, et al. Cancer incidence in a cohort of infertile women. *Am J Epidemiol* 1987;125:780–90

3. Brinton LA, Melton LJ, Malkasian GD Jr, et al. Cancer risk after evaluation for infertility. *Am J Epidemiol* 1989;129:712–22

4. Rossing MA, Daling JR, Weiss NS, et al. Ovarian tumors in a cohort of infertile women. *N Engl J Med* 1994;331:771–6

5. Rossing MA, Daling JR, Weiss NS, Moore DE, Self SG. Risk of breast cancer in a cohort in infertile women. *Gynecol Oncol* 1996;60:3–7

6. Rossing MA, Daling JR, Weiss NS, et al. Risk of cutaneous melanoma in a cohort of infertile women. *Melanoma Res* 1995;5:123–7

7. Venn A, Watson L, Lumley J, et al. Breast and ovarian cancer incidence after infertility and *in vitro* fertilisation. *Lancet* 1995;346:995–1000

8. Modan B, Ron El R, Lerner-Geva L, et al. Cancer incidence in a cohort of infertile women. *Am J Epidemiol* 1998;147:1038–42

9. Potashnik G, Lerner-Geva L, Genkin L, et al. Fertility drugs and the risk of breast and ovarian cancers: results of a long-term follow-up study. *Fertil Steril* 1999;71:853–9

10. Venn A, Watson L, Bruisma F, et al. Risk of cancer after use of fertility drugs with *in-vitro* fertilisation. *Lancet* 1999;354:1586–90

11. Whittemore AS, Harris R, Intyre J. Characteristics relating to ovarian cancer risk: collaborative analysis of 12 US case–control studies. II. Invasive epithelial ovarian cancers in white women. Collaborative Ovarian Cancer Group. *Am J Epidemiol* 1992;136:1184–203

12. Schildkraut JM, Schwingl PJ, Bastos E, Evanoff A, Hughes C. Epithelial ovarian cancer risk among women with polycystic ovary syndrome. *Obstet Gynecol* 1996;88:554–9

13. Brinton LA, Gridley G, Persson I, Baron J, Bergqvist A. Cancer risk after a hospital

discharge diagnosis of endometriosis. *Am J Obstet Gynecol* 1997;176:572–9

14. Rodriguez Tatham LM, Calle EE, Thun MJ, Jacobs EJ, Heath CW Jr. Infertility and risk of fatal ovarian cancer in a prospective cohort of US women. *Cancer Causes Control* 1998;9:645–51

15. Rossing MA, Daling JR, Weiss NS. Risk of ovarian cancer after treatment for infertility. *N Engl J Med* 1995;332:1302

16. Cowan LD, Gordis L, Tonascia JA, Jones GS. Breast cancer incidence in women with a history of progesterone deficiency. *Am J Epidemiol* 1981;114:209–17

17. Coulam CB, Annegers JF, Kranz JS. Chronic anovulation syndrome and associated neoplasia. *Obstet Gynecol* 1983;61:403–7

18. Garland M, Hunter DJ, Colditz GA, *et al.* Menstrual cycle characteristics and history of ovulatory infertility in relation to breast cancer risk in a large cohort of US women. *Am J Epidemiol* 1998;147:636–43

19. Gallagher RP, Elwood JM, Hill GB, *et al.* Reproductive factors, oral contraceptives and risk of malignant melanoma: Western Canada Melanoma Study. *Br J Cancer* 1985;52:901–7

20. Holman CD, Armstrong BK, Heenan PJ. Cutaneous malignant melanoma in women: exogenous sex hormones and reproductive factors. *Br J Cancer* 1984;50:673–80

21. McTiernan AM, Weiss NS, Daling JR. Incidence of thyroid cancer in women in relation to reproductive and hormonal factors. *Am J Epidemiol* 1984;120:423–35

22. Klip H, Burger CW, de Kraker J, *et al.* Risk of cancer in the offspring of women who underwent ovarian hyperstimulation for *in-vitro* fertilization. *Hum Reprod* 2001;16:2451–8

23. Bruinsma F, Venn A, Lancaster P, *et al.* Incidence of cancer in children born after *in-vitro* fertilization. *Hum Reprod* 2000;15:604–7

24. Lerner-Geva L, Toren A, Chetrit A, *et al.* The risk for cancer among children of women who underwent *in vitro* fertilization. *Cancer* 2000; 88:2845–7

17

Genetic considerations regarding azoospermic and severely oligozoospermic men

S. Repping, J. de Vries and F. van der Veen

INTRODUCTION

Subfertility, defined as 1 year of unprotected intercourse without conception, affects 10–15% of couples. According to the World Health Organization (WHO), in 47% of subfertile couples semen parameters are impaired[1]. However, as subfertility can be caused by a combination of various female and male factors, the WHO criteria for semen analysis are of limited diagnostic value for establishing the contribution of impaired spermatogenesis to subfertility. Therefore, the exact prevalence of subfertility exclusively based on impaired spermatogenesis is not known. Nevertheless, both azoospermia and severe oligozoospermia are generally considered to be significant causes of subfertility.

There are hardly any means to treat impaired spermatogenesis directly, the only examples being treatment with a dopamine agonist in case of hyperprolactinemia and treatment with gonadotropins in case of hypogonadotropic hypogonadism. To circumvent the absence of treatment of impaired spermatogenesis in the vast majority of cases, intracytoplasmic sperm injection (ICSI) was invented, allowing fertilization and thereby pregnancy with only minute amounts of spermatozoa[2]. However, there is still some concern regarding the health of ICSI-conceived offspring. Although major birth defects do not seem to be increased in children born after ICSI, the fertility status of these children is not known, as the oldest children are yet to enter

puberty[3]. If the impaired spermatogenesis phenotype is genetic in origin, transmission of the phenotype to offspring via ICSI seems likely. This potential transmission requires investigation of the genetic causes of impaired spermatogenesis to ensure proper counseling of affected couples.

At first, a hereditary cause of impaired spermatogenesis may seem an oxymoron. As stated before, fertility is a combination of both male and female factors, and spontaneous pregnancies can occur with nearly azoospermic males. Epidemiological studies have shown that impaired spermatogenesis can be familial and hereditary, indeed suggesting an underlying genetic cause[4,5]. These epidemiological studies have not been able to identify the precise genetic mechanism underlying impaired spermatogenesis but have indicated that it is most likely to be a complex disease, in which several different factors play a role.

At this time, we know of only a few genetic causes that explain some cases of impaired spermatogenesis. These genetic causes and their clinical implications are discussed in this chapter.

STRUCTURAL AND NUMERICAL CHROMOSOME ABNORMALITIES

The first group of genetic causes are structural or numerical chromosome abnormalities. Structural chromosomal abnormalities, such as translocations and inversions, are found in approximately 2% of infertile males. In approximately 4% of men with azoo- or oligozoospermia numerical chromosomal abnormalities are found by cytogenetic studies[6]. The most common numerical chromosomal abnormalities in azoospermic men are abnormalities involving the sex chromosomes. Klinefelter's syndrome, in which patients show a 47,XXY karyotype, is the most frequent form. Owing to these chromosomal abnormalities, proper chromosome pairing during meiosis is impaired, giving rise to spermatogenic disruption and the impaired spermatogenesis phenotype. Other abnormalities of a similar nature, e.g. mosaics such as 47,XXY/46,XY have been described, which also show impaired spermatogenesis.

Y-CHROMOSOME DELETIONS

Most research on the genetic causes of male infertility has focused on genetic aberrations of the Y chromosome. This specialized chromosome contains many genes that are involved in spermatogenesis, and deletions involving these genes are relatively frequent in infertile males[7]. The frequency of deletions on the Y chromosome in men with impaired spermatogenesis varies between 6 and 13%, depending on the phenotypic criteria of the population of infertile men studied.

Suspicion of involvement of the Y chromosome in male infertility originally arose from cytogenetic evidence reported over 25 years ago. This study showed terminal Y-chromosome deletions detectable by light microscopy in a very small percentage (five out of 1170; 0.5%) of azoospermic men[8]. It was postulated that the Y chromosome contained a so-called azoospermia factor (AZF). Since then an intense search has ensued for these AZF genes, i.e. genes that control spermatogenesis and which may be defective in infertile but otherwise normal males. During the past 10 years, we have come to understand that at least five deletions on the long arm of the Y chromosome exist: AZFa, P5/proximal-P1 (formerly known as AZFb), P5/distal-P1, AZFc and gr/gr deletions (Figure 1)[9–11].

Our knowledge of the human Y chromosome has recently increased tremendously with the completion of the annotated sequence of the male-specific region of the human Y chromosome (MSY)[7]. The MSY is the part of the chromosome that does not recombine with the X chromosome during meiosis. Flanking the MSY there are two segments that still undergo meiotic recombination with the X chromosome: pseudo autosomal region 1 and 2 (PAR 1 and 2; Figure 1). One of the most striking features of the MSY is the high prevalence of repetitive sequences. These sequences are arranged in direct and inverted repeats, including eight major palindromes – inverted repeats without any intervening sequence. As will be discussed further in this chapter, these repeats are responsible for maintaining MSY sequence integrity throughout evolution, but also form the substrates through which deletions arise on the MSY.

In contrast to previous thinking, we now know that the MSY contains at least 78 genes, of which 60 are expressed exclusively or predominantly in the testes[7]. It appears that the Y chromosome has evolved to become an essential chromosome for male reproduction, making deletions on this chromosome potential threats for male fertility.

AZFa deletions

AZFa deletions are very uncommon and only a few patients have been described. The AZFa region spans approximately 800 kilobases (kb) and contains two functional single-copy genes: USP9Y and DBY[12]. All patients affected by AZFa deletions described to date are azoospermic and have no germ cells in their testes (Sertoli cell only syndrome)[8]. Interestingly, one patient with a de novo point mutation in USP9Y has been described who has maturation arrest with a few pachytene spermatocytes developing into mature sperm in some seminiferous tubules[13]. Thus, the phenotype of men with complete AZFa deletions appears to be the result of the removal of both genes.

P5/proximal-P1 deletions

Originally it was thought that there were three non-overlapping deletion intervals on the Y chromosome[9]. The absence of a detailed map of the Y chromosome at that time, however, precluded the detection of the deletion boundaries of these intervals. With the use of the MSY sequence, it was found that deletions encompassing AZFb in fact extend from palindrome P5 into the proximal arm of the P1 palindrome and remove 1.5 Mb of the

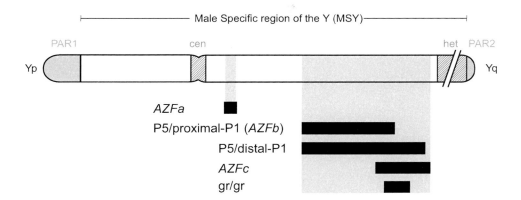

Figure 1 Schematic diagram of deletions on the Y chromosome found in men with impaired spermatogenesis. The part of the Y chromosome that does not recombine with the X chromosome during meiosis is called the male specific region of the Y (MSY). Flanking the MSY there are two regions that still recombine with the X chromosome called pseudo autosomal regions 1 and 2 (PAR1 and PAR2, darker shading). The short and long arms are separated by the centromere (cen) and the long arm contains a large block of heterochromatin (het) that varies in length between different individuals. The location and size of the five regions frequently deleted in men with impaired spermatogenesis are shown as black bars

AZFc region[10]. Thus, these regions overlap and do not represent separate deletion intervals, as was originally thought. The P5/proximal-P1 deletion (formerly known as *AZFb*) removes a total of 33 genes or transcripts and has a total length of 6.2 Mb, nearly a quarter of the entire euchromatic MSY (Figure 1). P5/proximal-P1 deletions are slightly more common than deletions of the *AZFa* region, but remain rare, being found in only approximately 1% of men with impaired spermatogenesis. The phenotype of men affected by P5/proximal-P1 deletions is azoospermia with testicular maturation arrest. Because the deletions involve many genes and no deletions have yet been described that affect only one gene or gene family, the contribution of the individual genes in the P5/P1 region to the azoospermic phenotype is unknown.

P5/distal-P1 deletions

The proximal breakpoint of P5/distal-P1 deletions is similar to that of P5/proximal-P1 deletions. In contrast, the distal breakpoint lies – as the name implies – in the distal arm of the P1 palindrome. The deletion overlaps with nearly all of *AZFc*, sparing only the last approximately 500 kb. The

deletion is in fact the largest (7.6 Mb) deletion in the human genome for which deletion boundaries and complete nucleotide sequences are known. The P5/distal-P1 deletion affects 44 genes or transcripts and is found in similar frequencies to those of P5/proximal-P1 deletions. Also, the phenotype of men affected by this deletion is similar: azoospermia with testicular maturation arrest[10].

AZFc deletions

Deletions of the *AZFc* region are found in approximately 12% of azoospermic men and in 6% of severely oligozoospermic men, and represent the most common known genetic cause of impaired spermatogenesis[14]. The region is constructed of massive areas of absolute sequence identity called amplicons, which are arranged in direct repeats, inverted repeats or palindromes. The *AZFc* region spans 3.5 Mb and contains eight distinct gene families with a total of 21 transcription units that are all expressed exclusively or predominantly in the testes[14].

The *deleted in azoospermia* (*DAZ*) gene family, which is one of the eight gene families located within *AZFc*, was one of the first spermatogenesis genes identified on the human Y chromosome[15]. The human *DAZ* genes were shown to be transcribed specifically in spermatogonia and in early primary spermatocytes[16]. *DAZ* is present in four near-identical copies (99.9%) arranged in two clusters with two genes each[17].

The *DAZ* genes have an autosomal homolog called *DAZL*, which is located on chromosome 3. During evolution, some time after the split of Old and New World monkeys approximately 30 million years ago, the *DAZL* gene was transposed to the Y chromosome[18]. Once *DAZL* was transposed to the Y, it was amplified and pruned until it became the modern-day *DAZ* gene family. It was shown recently that in fact there is yet another *DAZ* family homolog in humans, termed *BOULE*[19]. The exact interaction and possible functional overlap between *DAZ*, *DAZL* and *BOULE* remain to be determined.

Although all *AZFc* deletions seem to be identical on a genomic scale, men with these deletions show a high phenotypic diversity in contrast to men with either *AZFa* or P5/P1 deletions[20]. Some men with an *AZFc* deletion are azoospermic while others are only oligozoospermic. The specific histological defect in the testes, whether maturation arrest or Sertoli cell only, is also quite variable. It is therefore likely that other stochastic factors, genetic or environmental in origin, contribute to the specific phenotype.

Most *AZFc* deletions occur *de novo*, but they may occasionally be present in the 'fertile' father of the infertile male, as illustrated by reports showing natural transmission of *AZFc* deletions from apparently fertile men[21]. However, in these cases, the father may very well have been oligozoospermic, as ~5% of even severely oligozoospermic men can have children without any fertility treatment.

gr/gr Deletions

The recently described gr/gr deletion occurs in about 3% of men with impaired spermatogenesis. The deletion removes 1.6 Mb of the *AZFc* region and nine genes with testes specific expression (Figure 1). It does not completely eliminate any of the *AZFc* gene families but instead reduces the copy number of eight such families. For instance, only two of the four *DAZ* genes are affected by this deletion. The existence of deletions that affect only part of *AZFc* had been noted before, but the precise

nature and size of these deletions as well as their effect on spermatogenesis was unclear[22,23]. In contrast to other Y-chromosome deletions, the gr/gr deletion is often transmitted from father to son indicating that the deletion is incompletely penetrant[11].

Deletion mechanism

Most Y-chromosome deletions seem to be caused by ectopic (non-allelic) homologous recombination between highly similar or identical sequences which, as said before, are found on the MSY in great abundance. The *AZFa* region is bounded on each side by two sequence stretches of approximately 10 kb which are 94% identical to each other. Homologous recombination between these two sequence stretches results in dropout of the intervening *AZFa* region. Interestingly, these two sequence stretches belong to the HERV15 class of endogenous retroviruses, suggesting that viral sequences, which are ubiquitous in the human genome, can form potential targets for deletions. Although all *AZFa* deletions fall within these two 10-kb regions, the precise breakpoints can differ slightly between patients[12].

Both P5/proximal-P1 and P5/distal-P1 deletions are caused by homologous recombination between homologous sequences in the P5 palindrome and the P1 palindrome. The 100-kb region in the center of P5 is nearly identical to the two mini-palindromes in P1 : P1.1 and P1.2. Interestingly, some deletion junctions show no sign of homologous recombination, although the deletion breakpoints still cluster around the center of P5 and the mini-palindromes in P1. Apparently, these sites form deletion hotspots[10].

The sequence of *AZFc* reveals the same mechanism as for *AZFa* and P5/P1 deletions, but on a larger scale[14]. In this case the substrates for homologous recombination are two repeats that are over 99.9% identical and are 229 kb in length. Precise breakpoint determination for *AZFc* deletions is virtually impossible, because of the extremely high similarity between the two flanking repeats. Interestingly, the frequency with which these deletions occur seems to correspond to the length of the stretch of homology. Deletions of *AZFc*, caused by homologous recombination between 229-kb repeats, are far more common than deletions of P5/P1 bounded by 100-kb homologous sequences and even more common than *AZFa* deletions, which are caused by repeats of only 10 kb in length.

Homologous recombination between repeats located within the *AZFc* region cause gr/gr deletions. In fact, deletion nomenclature is based on the targets for homologous recombination: the amplicons g1-r1-r2 and g2-r3-r4, abbreviated as gr/gr. In this case the targets for homologous recombination are 610 kb in length[11].

Besides causing deletions on the MSY and thereby negatively affecting fertility, these repeats also have a positive effect. In the absence of a partner during meiosis, which is essential to allow repair of mutations that may have arisen, the MSY can use these repeats to maintain DNA integrity. This process is known as Y–Y gene conversion and involves unidirectional exchange of DNA sequences between repeats. It is thought that through this mechanism the MSY has been able to keep intact the structure of its many genes throughout evolution, thereby preventing the decay of the chromosome[7,24].

OTHER GENETIC CAUSES

The only other established genetic cause of impaired spermatogenesis is mutations in the *CFTR* gene. Such mutations, which are present in 1–2% of infertile males, are found only in men with congenital bilateral absence of the vasa deferentia (CBAVD)[25]. Some of these patients present with CBAVD and have no respiratory component of cystic fibrosis while having one of the common mutations in the *CFTR* gene.

Other reported genetic causes of impaired spermatogenesis are still heavily disputed, in contrast to the above-mentioned structural or numerical chromosome abnormalities, the deletions of the Y chromosome and *CFTR* mutations. For instance, mutations or an expansion of CAG repeat lengths in the androgen receptor (*AR*) gene have been described in subfertile men, but strong arguments for an association are still lacking.

Apart from the described genetic causes, the vast majority of cases of impaired spermatogenesis are classified as idiopathic, as no etiology is known. Nevertheless, it is believed that many of these idiopathic cases will in due time be proven to be genetic in origin. Indeed, several animal studies have provided good candidate genes, but their involvement in human impaired spermatogenesis awaits further research.

SCREENING FOR GENETIC CAUSES – COUNSELING REGARDING OFFSPRING

Although the combined frequency of genetic abnormalities found is only approximately 15%, screening for these abnormalities in men with impaired spermatogenesis prior to starting assisted reproduction is essential. Karyotyping and Y-chromosome deletion analysis should be performed in all men with impaired spermatogenesis undergoing ICSI treatment. Screening for *CFTR* mutations should be performed in men with CBAVD. The outcome of these tests will determine how the couples should be counseled before starting treatment with regard to potential effects on their offspring.

The chance of transmitting a structural chromosome abnormality depends on the aberration found. Several reports have indicated that in men with Klinefelter's syndrome the chance for numerical chromosome abnormalities occurring in their offspring is rather low. This is so because the majority of spermatozoa from men with Klinefelter's syndrome appear to have a normal haploid gene content[26].

In contrast, all male offspring from men with Y-chromosome deletions will have the same deletion as their infertile father without any expansion. With the use of fluorescence *in-situ* hybridization (FISH) techniques, it has been shown that all spermatozoa from *AZFc*-deleted men carry the same deletion that was originally detected in their somatic cells[27]. Thus it seems that, if a patient carries a deletion on the Y chromosome as determined by analysis of his blood, all of his spermatozoa will have the same deletion, as will all of his sons when these spermatozoa are used for ICSI.

As no patients are described that are mosaic for cells with and cells without a Y-chromosome deletion, it can be assumed that most Y-chromosome deletions arise in the testes of the fertile father, and not during embryogenesis. The deletions which arise in the testes of the fertile father are apparently caused by an accidental homologous recombination between repeats on the MSY. The exact frequency of the occurrence of these deletions in the testes is unknown, although it is estimated that approximately 1 in 4000 newborn boys carries a Y-chromosome deletion[14]. Whether these deletions might occur more frequently in the deficient testes of a patient with impaired spermatogenesis is a subject for further investigation. The result of deletions on the Y chromosome is impaired spermatogenesis and not necessarily a failure to father offspring naturally. The degree of impairment (mild oligozoospermia, severe oligozoospermia or azoospermia) differs between different deletions and between different patients with the same deletion. Whether these men are able to induce pregnancies naturally depends on the fertility of their sexual partners. The fact that even men with *AZFc* deletions can, in some instances, father children without the use of ICSI, illustrates the ability of some partners of men with minute amounts of spermatozoa to conceive naturally. As some deletions, such as gr/gr deletions, potentially have a less dramatic impact on spermatogenesis, these could very well be transmitted naturally more often. The use of ICSI could contribute considerably to the spreading of these deletions and, as a consequence, reduced overall fertility within the human population.

Finally, the risk of transmission in patients with *CFTR* mutations will depend largely on the genotype of the female partner. Therefore, partners of men with *CFTR* mutations will need to be tested as well.

CONCLUSIONS

The use of ICSI has increased tremendously over the past decade and currently allows even men with only minute amounts of spermatozoa in their testes to father children. In the majority of cases, there is no obvious explanation for the impaired spermatogenesis phenotype. If the cause of the deficient sperm production is genetic in origin, chances are that male offspring from ICSI will inherit the aberration and thus be infertile as well. Studies on the role of Y-chromosome deletions in male infertility have given new insights into this transmission of male infertility via ICSI. Through evolution, the Y chromosome acquired a specialized role in spermatogenesis, making it highly useful in studying the genetic causes of male infertility. Aberrations on the Y chromosome are currently found in approxi-

mately 10% of infertile males. Most, although not all, of these males still possess some degree of spermatogenesis resulting in enough spermatozoa to perform ICSI. The presence of Y-chromosome deletions does not decrease the fertilization or pregnancy rate thereby enabling these men to father children with the same efficiency as non-Y-deleted men undergoing ICSI. However, the Y-chromosome deletion is transmitted to all male offspring, as all Y-bearing spermatozoa carry the deletion as well.

Research into the many other testes-specific genes on the Y chromosome and on other chromosomes will be necessary to help elucidate the complex process of spermatogenesis and eventually enable screening for aberrations in these genes in men with impaired spermatogenesis. Of special interest are genes located on the X chromosome, as the X chromosome seems to have acquired several spermatogenesis genes as well during the course of evolution[28]. However, as infertility affects the ability to transmit genes to the next generation, the mode of inheritance of genetic aberrations causing infertility is difficult to investigate. The only straightforward method of investigating the genetic basis of infertility therefore seems to be large-scale association studies comparing infertile men with idiopathic spermatogenic failure to normospermic controls.

In our view, genetic counseling should be provided to all infertile males, whether or not an abnormality is detected prior to starting treatment. The frequencies with which genetic aberrations are found in men with impaired spermatogenesis are about 15%. However, if no abnormalities are found in a man with impaired spermatogenesis, this does not obviate the likelihood of there being a genetic cause for his azoospermia or severe oligozoospermia.

It is apparent that there is likely to be frequent transmission of male infertility from the ICSI father to his male offspring regardless of current testing. Every couple must decide for themselves whether they wish to consider this risk. Future studies of genes involved in spermatogenesis, not only on the human Y chromosome but also on other chromosomes as well as in other species, will hopefully lead to a better understanding of the genetic causes of male infertility and enable proper counseling of couples undergoing assisted reproductive technologies such as ICSI.

REFERENCES

1. World Health Organization. Towards more objectivity in diagnosis and management of male infertility. *Int J Androl* 1987;7:1–53

2. Palermo G, Joris H, Devroey P, Van Steirteghem AC. Pregnancies after intracytoplasmic injection of single spermatozoon into an oocyte. *Lancet* 1992;340:17–18

3. Van Steirteghem A, Bonduelle, M, Devroey P, Liebaers I. Follow-up of children born after ICSI. *Hum Reprod Update* 2002;8:111–16

4. Lilford R, Jones AM, Bishop DT, Thornton J, Mueller R. Case-control study of whether subfertility in men is familial. *Br Med J* 1994;309:570–3

5. Gianotten J, Westerveld GH, Leschot NJ, *et al.* Familial clustering of impaired spermatogenesis; no evidence for a common genetic inheritance pattern. *Hum Reprod* 2003;in press

6. Tuerlings JH, de France HF, Hamers A, *et al.* Chromosome studies in 1792 males prior to intra-cytoplasmic sperm injection: the Dutch experience. *Eur J Hum Genet* 1998;6:194–200

7. Skaletsky H, Kuroda-Kawaguchi T, Minx PJ, *et al.* The male-specific region of the human Y chromosome is a mosaic of discrete sequence classes. *Nature* 2003;423:825–37

8. Tiepolo L, Zuffardi O. Localization of factors controlling spermatogenesis in the nonfluorescent portion of the human Y chromosome long arm. *Hum Genet* 1976;34:119–24

9. Vogt PH, Edelmann A, Kirsch S, *et al.* Human Y chromosome azoospermia factors (AZF) mapped to different subregions in Yq11. *Hum Mol Genet* 1996;5:933–43

10. Repping S, Skaletsky H, Lange J, *et al.* Recombination between palindromes P5 and P1 on the human Y chromosome causes massive deletions and spermatogenic failure. *Am J Hum Genet* 2002;71:906–22

11. Repping S, Skaletsky H, Brown LG, *et al.* Polymorphism for a 1.6-Mb deletion of the human Y chromosome persits through balance between recurrent mutation and haploid selection. *Nat Genet* 2003;in press

12. Sun C, Skaletsky H, Rozen S, *et al.* Deletion of azoospermia factor a (AZFa) region of human Y chromosome caused by recombination between HERV15 proviruses. *Hum Mol Genet* 2000;9:2291–6

13. Sun C, Skaletsky H, Birren B, *et al.* An azoospermic man with a *de novo* point mutation in the Y-chromosomal gene USP9Y. *Nat Genet* 1999;23:429–32

14. Kuroda-Kawaguchi T, Skaletsky H, Brown LG, *et al.* The AZFc region of the Y chromosome features massive palindromes and uniform recurrent deletions in infertile men. *Nat Genet* 2001;29:279–86

15. Reijo R, Lee TY, Salo P, *et al.* Diverse spermatogenic defects in humans caused by Y chromosome deletions encompassing a novel RNA-binding protein gene. *Nat Genet* 1995;10:383–93

16. Menke DB, Mutter GL, Page DC. Expression of DAZ, an azoospermia factor candidate, in human spermatogonia. *Am J Hum Genet* 1997;60:237–41

17. Saxena R, de Vries JWA, Repping S, *et al.* Four DAZ genes in two clusters found in the AZFc region on the human Y chromosome. *Genomics* 2000;67:256–67

18. Saxena R, Brown LG, Hawkins T, *et al.* The DAZ gene cluster on the human Y chromosome arose from an autosomal gene that was transposed, repeatedly amplified and pruned. *Nat Genet* 1996;14:292–9

19. Xu EY, Moore FL, Pera RA. A gene family required for human germ cell development evolved from an ancient meiotic gene conserved in metazoans. *Proc Natl Acad Sci USA* 2001;98:7414–19

20. Oates RD, Silber S, Brown LG, Page DC. Clinical characterization of 42 oligospermic or azoospermic men with microdeletion of the AZFc region of the Y chromosome, and of 18 children conceived via ICSI. *Hum Reprod* 2002;17:2813–24

21. Saut N, Terriou P, Navarro A, Levy N, Mitchell MJ. The human Y chromosome genes BPY2, CDY1 and DAZ are not essential for sustained fertility. *Mol Hum Reprod* 2000;6:789–93

22. de Vries JW, Hoffer MJV, Repping S, Hoovers JMN, Leschot NJ, van der Veen F. Reduced copy number of the DAZ genes in sub- and infertile men. *Fertil Steril* 2002;77:68–75

23. Fernandes S, Huellen K, Goncalves J, *et al.* High frequency of DAZ1/DAZ2 gene deletions in patients with severe oligozoospermia. *Mol Hum Reprod* 2002;8:286–98

24. Rozen S, Skaletsky H, Marszalek JD, *et al.* Abundant gene conversion between arms of palindromes in human and ape Y chromosomes. *Nature* 2003;423:873–6

25. Chillon M, Casals T, Mercier B, *et al.* Mutations in the cystic fibrosis gene in patients with congenital absence of the vas deferens. *N Engl J Med* 1995;332:1475–80

26. Shi Q, Martin RH. Aneuploidy in human spermatozoa: FISH analysis in men with constitutional chromosomal abnormalities, and in infertile men. *Reproduction* 2001;121:655–66

27. de Vries JW, Repping S, Oates R, Carson R, Leschot NJ, van der Veen F. Absence of deleted in azoospermia (DAZ) genes in spermatozoa of infertile men with somatic DAZ deletions. *Fertil Steril* 2001;75:476–9

28. Wang PJ, McCarrey JR, Yang F, Page DC. An abundance of X-linked genes expressed in spermatogonia. *Nat Genet* 2001;27:422–6

18

Preimplantation genetic diagnosis: risks and complications

I. Liebaers, K. Sermon and E. Van Assche

INTRODUCTION

Preimplantation genetic diagnosis (PGD) is a medical procedure involving *in vitro* fertilization (IVF), oocyte or embryo biopsy and genetic analysis of the polar bodies and/or blastomeres before transfer of an embryo to the uterus. As an alternative to prenatal diagnosis, this procedure allows couples at risk of transmitting a hereditary disease to have unaffected children. The first PGDs, involving sex determination with transfer of XX embryos because of sex-linked disease in the family, were reported in 1990 by Handyside and associates[1].

Today, after 10 years, a few thousand of IVF/PGD cycles for high genetic risk conditions have been performed, indicating that it is not yet a widely available routine procedure. This is related to the complexity of the procedure both at the clinical level and at the laboratory level. To establish a genetic diagnosis at the single-cell level, two currently used types of genetic test can be applied. They are based on the polymerase chain reaction (PCR) to detect gene defects or on fluorescent *in situ* hybridization (FISH) to detect chromosomal aberrations. In this chapter, the conditions for which PGD can be offered will be discussed as part of the genetic counseling procedure. The clinical procedure will briefly be mentioned, emphasizing the differences from regular IVF. Particularities about single-cell PCR and single-cell FISH will be stressed. Practical clinical applications, outcomes as well as risks and complications, will also be discussed.

PGD for aneuploidy screening (PGD-AS) will not be discussed, because its main aim is not to avoid transmission of a known genetic disease but to improve the outcome of IVF, thereby lowering the risk of age-related trisomies in older women[2]. This type of PGD will be discussed in Chapter 19.

HEREDITARY DISEASES AND GENETIC COUNSELING

Hereditary diseases can be classified into a few categories, the main ones being chromosomal aberrations, monogenic diseases, multifactorial diseases and mitochondrial diseases[3]. Diagnosis of these conditions is based on personal and familial history, clinical signs, complementary tests such as specific genetic tests, e.g. karyotyping, DNA tests or targeted biochemical tests looking for deficient gene products[3]. In a continuously growing number of conditions such a specific diagnosis can be established either because a new causal gene has been described or because novel technology has emerged[4–6]. Nevertheless, in a number of conditions the genetic defect has not yet been found and the diagnosis is based on clinical signs only or on indirect biological evidence. In any case, based on the available information, affected families will be counseled concerning the prognosis of the condition, its recurrence risk and the possible options to avoid the transmission of the condition to the next generation[7]. PGD can be one of these options, and although PGD can be considered as a very early form of prenatal diagnosis it cannot replace prenatal diagnosis in all cases. This means that, before this option is given to a couple at risk, one has to make sure that the cause of the disease can be seen at the chromosomal or gene level and that an adequate single-cell FISH or PCR assay is available or can be developed. Therefore, to date only in case of a chromosomal aberration or in case of a monogenic condition with a proven mutation or assigned to a specific locus, may PGD be an option[8–11].

OVARIAN STIMULATION, FERTILIZATION AND EMBRYO TRANSFER

For PGD, the IVF treatment of the patients is comparable to a regular IVF treatment. However, it is important to realize that, while avoiding hyperstimulation, as many embryos and therefore as many oocytes as possible should be collected, to limit the risk of not having even one embryo to transfer[12]. In case of autosomal recessive (AR) diseases, only one out of four embryos will be discarded because they are affected; in case of autosomal dominant (AD) diseases, one out of two embryos will have to be discarded. In case of X-linked recessive diseases, the situation is comparable to AR conditions if the diagnosis is based on mutation detection followed by the elimination of affected male embryos only, while it will be comparable to AD conditions if carrier female embryos are also discarded or if the diagnosis is based on embryo sexing with transfer of only XX embryos[13]. In any case, because of genetic testing, fewer embryos will be available for transfer than in regular IVF. This is even more so in cases of structural chromosomal aberrations and more in particular in cases of reciprocal translocations, because apparently as many as 80% of the embryos will have to be discarded because of imbalances for the tested chromosomes[8,14,15]. Another particularity of PGD is the mandatory use of intracytoplasmic sperm injection (ICSI) when a PCR-based diagnostic procedure is used, even in the presence of normal sperm parameters. This is to avoid an erroneous diagnosis due to contamination of the PCR by sperm DNA from sperm lodged in the zona pellucida after regular IVF[10,16,17]. For the same reason the oocytes have to be perfectly devoid of possibly contaminating granulosa cells before ICSI and embryo biopsy[17]. In case of a FISH-based diagnostic procedure and adequate sperm quality, IVF can be used to fertilize the oocytes[14]. Embryo transfer and further follow-up is not different from routine IVF/ICSI.

OOCYTE AND EMBRYO BIOPSY

In most centers, PGD is performed on day-3 embryos when 6–10 blastomeres are counted (Figure 1). Usually in the morning, a hole is made in

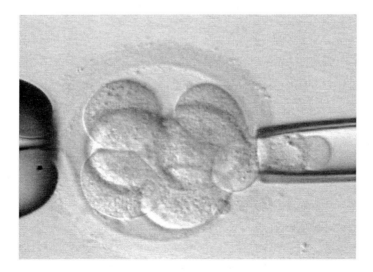

Figure 1   Embryo biopsy. A cleavage-stage eight-cell embryo 3 days after fertilization. On the left, a holding pipette immobilizes the embryo by gentle suction. On the right, a hole was made in the zona pellucida with a laser. With a biopsy pipette with an outer diameter of 35 μm and an inner diameter of 30 μm, one nucleated blastomere is being aspirated

the zona pellucida of all embryos, either mechanically by making a slit with a sharp needle[18,19] or by using as little as possible of acidic Tyrode's solution[20] or by laser drilling[8,21,22].

No prospective comparative study is available to indicate which of these procedures is better than the other. A retrospective study demonstrated that acidic Tyrode's drilling and laser drilling were equivalent, but that the laser biopsy procedure was faster[23]. After zona drilling, at least one blastomere will be removed from the embryo, usually by aspiration[20,22]. A second blastomere may be taken either when the first cell is anucleate or lysed, or to improve the accuracy of the diagnosis[22]. In the latter situation, the diagnosis is accepted only if the result of the second blastomere confirms the result of the first. Of course, this approach may lead to the loss of unaffected embryos, but it will limit the number of misdiagnoses. Only one major PGD center systematically biopsies two blastomeres; others do it more selectively and according to the disease and the diagnostic approach used[8,14,24]. The matter of debate here is that taking a biopsy of two cells may be detrimental to the embryo when compared to taking a biopsy of one cell. Although a retrospective comparative study has not shown a difference, a prospective study is needed to clarify the matter and help set guidelines for good clinical PGD practice[25].

Polar body biopsy as a means of preconceptual genetic diagnosis rather than PGD was first reported in 1992 by Verlinsky and colleagues[18]. The biopsy of the first polar body is a particularly elegant method aimed at diagnosing the genotype of an oocyte before fertilization and thus before creating an embryo. A drawback is that it can be used only if the woman carries a dominant gene defect or a chromosomal aberration, and possibly for couples at risk for an autosomal recessive disease. It cannot be used if the male partner is the carrier of a dominant trait, or for sexing of the embryo if the woman is a carrier of an X-linked disease. Moreover, crossing over or recombination may lead to a heterozygous first polar body, leading to inconclusive results. If, in such a heterozygous polar body, allele drop out (ADO) occurs, this may even lead to a misdiagnosis. The solution to this is also to analyze the second polar body, but of course this is only possible after fertilization[26]. Nevertheless,

the pioneering center is still using this approach to a great extent, even combining it with biopsy of one blastomere of the embryo if indicated[27].

Blastocyst biopsy has been carried out, but only to a limited extent to date[28].

DIAGNOSIS OF SINGLE-GENE DEFECTS BY THE POLYMERASE CHAIN REACTION

A PCR-based diagnosis allows the direct or indirect detection of a known gene mutation. PCR is the first step in the detection procedure, aiming at the amplification of the DNA sequence of interest, present in two copies in the biopsied cell, by using adequately chosen upstream and downstream primers[10,17]. Once amplified the DNA fragments can be further treated and analyzed in order to differentiate affected from unaffected embryos. Whereas initially mainly simplex non-fluorescent PCR assays visualizing the mutations were used to establish the diagnosis of an embryo, today diagnoses are increasingly based on duplex or multiplex PCR assays, identifying the mutations along with a linked DNA sequence or identifying the presence or absence of a series of well-chosen intragenic and extragenic linked markers[10,17] (Figures 2–4). The main advantage of using linked markers is to avoid misdiagnosis by more readily identifying endogeneous or exogenous DNA contamination or ADO, two pitfalls complicating single-cell diagnosis that will be discussed later.

Another advantage is that for certain more or less common diseases caused by mostly private mutations – i.e. mutations limited to one family – the use of linked markers spread over the entire gene will in the end allow PGD to be offered to most families without much delay. The way this will be achieved is by first identifying interesting, i.e. informative, intragenic and extragenic markers for a given gene. Often these markers are microsatellites. Second, in a given family, the informative potential of two such markers, preferably intragenic and upstream and downstream of the mutation, is tested. Third, if informative (i.e. if the difference between healthy alleles and mutated alleles can be determined) the single-cell assays for the particular markers are developed. The efficiency and accuracy of these assays are evaluated by analyzing up to 50 single cells (lymphocytes, lymphoblasts, fibroblasts,

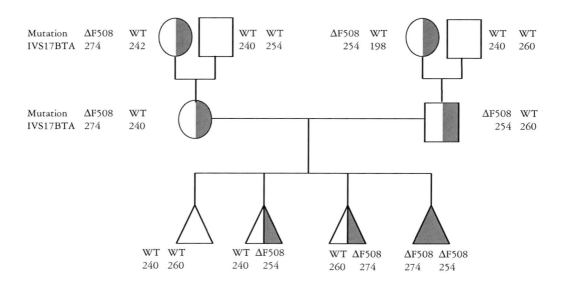

Figure 2 Segregation of the linked marker IVS17BTA in a couple asking for preimplantation genetic diagnosis (PGD) because both partners are healthy carriers of the most common ΔF508 mutation in the *CFTR* gene for cystic fibrosis. They are informative for the linked marker IVS17BTA. By examining DNA from the parents of both partners, we learn that, in the female, the ΔF508 mutation segregates with IVS17BTA 274 (shaded) and the wild type (WT) sequence with IVS17BTA 240. In the male, the segregation is ΔF508/IVS17BTA 254 (shaded) and WT/IVS17BTA 260. Embryos inheriting both WT alleles + IVS17BTA 240/260 are homozygous normal and therefore healthy. Embryos inheriting WT/IVS17BTA240 + ΔF508/IVS17BTA254 or WT/IVS17BTA260 + ΔF508/IVS17BTA274 are healthy carriers. Embryos inheriting ΔF508/ΔF508 and IVS17BTA274/240 are affected and should not be transferred

amniocytes, etc) carrying the mutation of interest or heterozygous for the markers. The aim is to obtain at least 90% amplification efficiency and less than 5% ADO and contamination. For a second family with the same disease but due to a different mutation, the informative linked markers may be different and therefore other single-cell assays may have to be developed. In the end, a panel of single-cell assays for markers spread over the entire gene will be available. At that point, in case of a new request, the panel of markers can be tested in the family, usually the couple and an affected child or parent, and the single-cell assays will be available for immediate clinical application[29].

DIAGNOSIS OF GENDER OR CHROMOSOMAL ABERRATIONS BY FLUORESCENT *IN SITU* HYBRIDIZATION

A FISH-based diagnosis allows the enumeration and identification of sex and other chromosomes as well as the detection of chromosomal microdeletions and of imbalances in case of other structural chromosomal aberrations such as translocations. Here, the correct fluorescent DNA probes have to be chosen. Most of the time, commercially available probes are used. For the identification of sex chromosomes, highly repetitive fluorescence-labeled probes, usually green for the X chromosome and red for the Y chromosome, are used[30]. Currently often chro-

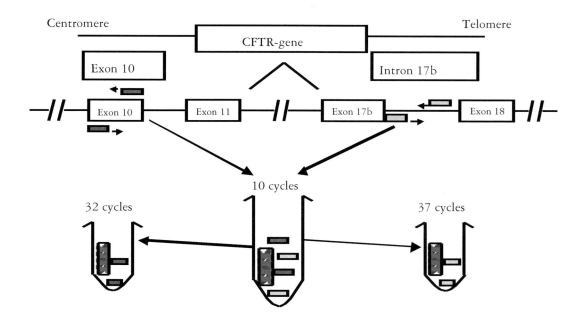

Figure 3   Analysis of the ΔF508 mutation and the linked IVS17BTA marker in the CFTR gene. The CFTR gene is shown in a box on the long arm of chromosome 7 between the centromere and the telomere. Within the CFTR gene, exons 10, 11, 17b and 18 are shown in boxes. The ΔF508 mutation is in exon 10, which is amplified with the shaded primers. The linked marker IVS17BTA is in intron 17b between exon 17b and exon 18 and is amplified with the hatched primers. With a duplex polymerase chain reaction (PCR) of 10 cycles, using the two specific primer sets (shaded), two DNA fragments are amplified. The mixture of the two PCR products is then used as a template in two separate PCR reactions. In the left hand tube, the shaded primer set is added to further amplify the ΔF508/WT sequences in 32 cycles, and in the right hand tube, the hatched primer set is added to further amplify the IVS17BTA marker sequence in 37 cycles. Thereafter, the DNA fragments will be analyzed on an automated DNA sequencer

mosomes 13, 18 and 21, identified by differently labeled probes, are counted as well[2].

For microdeletions such as the 22q11 deletion occurring in the velocardiofacial syndrome locus, specific probes combined with a differently labeled control probe on the same arm of the same chromosome are used[31].

For translocations, specific probe mixtures have to be designed. For Robertsonian translocations most of the time two telomeric and/or region-specific probes, labeled with different fluorochromes (one for each chromosome involved) are applied. Usually for the most common Robertsonian translocation der(13;14)(q10;q10) the region-specific probe 13q14 labeled green and the 14q telomeric

probe labeled orange are used (Figure 5). For reciprocal translocations the probe mixture used will depend on the specific breakpoints of the chromosomes involved in the translocation. Usually a mixture of three probes is used – two centromeric probes labeled with different fluorochromes for the chromosomes involved and one labeled with still another fluorochrome on the telomeric side of one of the breakpoints. In this way, balanced embryos (normal or with a balanced translocation) can be differentiated from unbalanced embryos (partial monosomies or partial trisomies)[11,32,33]. For the reciprocal translocation t(3;8)(p25;q12) (Figure 5) the centromeric probes for chromosomes 3 and 8 (labeled red and yellow, respectively) and the p-

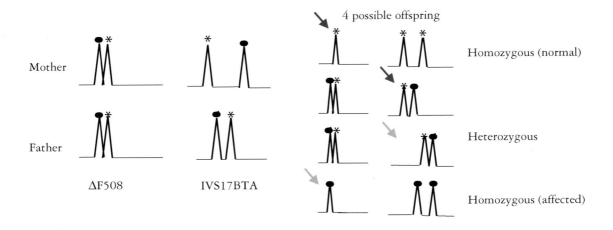

Figure 4   Schematic results of an electrophoresis and fragment analysis after duplex polymerase chain reaction (PCR) for ΔF508 and IVS17bTA. The left electrophoretic result shows that both partners carry the ΔF508 mutation: the mutated allele is marked with a circle, while the normal allele is marked with an asterisk. The middle electrophoretic result shows the IVS17bTA for both parents: the mother has a 240 and a 274 (segregating with ΔF508; circle) allele, while the father carries a 254 (segregating with the ΔF508) and a 260 allele (asterisk). The right electrophoresis shows the four possible offspring, each time with the alleles marked with an asterisk (healthy) or circle (affected). If patterns indicated with a black arrow and marked with a circle are seen together, allele drop out (ADO) of the ΔF508 mutation is suspected. If patterns with the shaded arrow are seen together, ADO of the wild-type allele is suspected. When a combination with the arrows is seen (homozygous normal/abnormal for ΔF508 and heterozygous for IVS17bTA), ADO of one of the ΔF508 alleles can be assumed

telomeric probe for chromosome 3 (labeled green), were used. To develop a family-specific FISH PGD assay, preclinical development is carried out on lymphocytes of both partners. The aim is to obtain 90% hybridization efficiency without cross-hybridization. Sometimes a new probe mixture is also tested on blastomeres of spare research embryos before a PGD is clinically applied[33].

APPLICATION OF PREIMPLANTATION GENETIC DIAGNOSIS IN THE CLINIC

Over the past 10 years, a few thousand PGDs have been performed worldwide, most of them in a few larger centers in the US and Europe[9,15]. However, more and more centers offering PGD are emerging,

either carrying out diagnoses themselves or collaborating with the larger centers by performing the biopsy and sending the blastomeres or polar bodies to the main center for diagnosis. The result of the PGD is then forwarded as soon as possible to the satellite center, which can take care of the transfer and further look after the patients.

PGD has so far been requested and offered to three groups of couples. In all of these couples a pre-existing genetic condition was the reason for proposing PGD. However, some of these couples suffered from concurrent infertility, either because of their genetic condition or for another unrelated reason. These patients needed IVF if they wanted children of their own. A second group of couples are those who are normally fertile and can achieve pregnancy spontaneously. Some of these have indeed

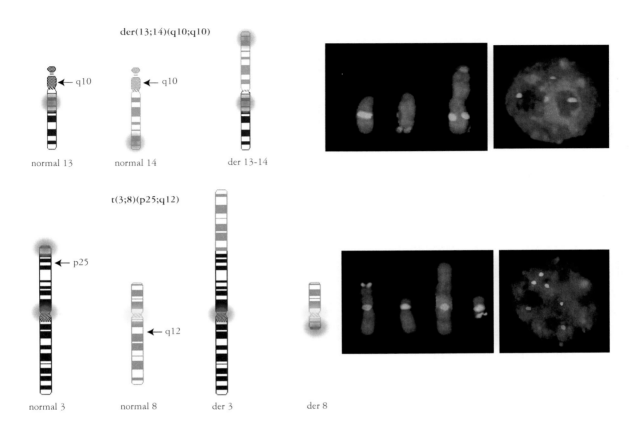

Figure 5   Fluorescent *in situ* hybridization results on the translocation chromosomes and blastomeres from a carrier of the Robertsonian translocation der(13;14)(q10;10) and a carrier of the reciprocal translocation t(3;8)(p25;q12), respectively. The probe mixtures that were used are mentioned in detail in the text

experienced pregnancy before, but underwent the trauma of prenatal diagnosis followed by termination of pregnancy once or more than once, and found the burden too great.

Others, and so far the largest group of couples, refuse prenatal diagnosis because of their objection to termination of pregnancy for moral, religious or psychological reasons but find PGD acceptable[9,16].

In cases of monogenic diseases, the purpose of the PGD is usually to avoid the transmission of the disease to the offspring. In a few instances, however, PGD is combined with an IVF treatment that is needed to enable the couple to have offspring and, in particular unaffected offspring. This, for example, is the case for men with cystic fibrosis (CF) or men with congenital bilateral absence of the vas deferens (CBAVD) who have a partner who is a heterozygous carrier of a CF mutation. By combin-

ing IVF with ICSI and PGD, their 1/4 or even 1/2 risk of conceiving a child affected with CF can be reduced to almost zero[34,35]. A similar situation may occur in male patients with myotonic dystrophy whose sperm quality may become so impaired that natural conception is no longer an option for them. Again, IVF with ICSI and PGD will help them to overcome their infertility as well as their 1/2 risk of having affected children[36].

The list of monogenic conditions for which PGD can now be offered is continuously growing and can be divided into three categories. Some of them are quite frequent and are caused by only one mutation, as is the case in myotonic dystrophy, Huntington's disease (Figure 6) and fragile X syndrome[24,36,37]. Once such a condition can be detected at the single-cell level, most couples requesting PGD can be helped almost immediately. However, whereas this

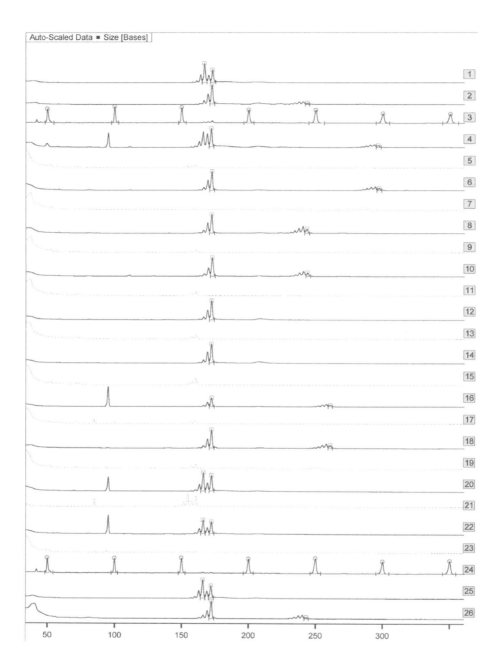

Figure 6 Example of preimplantation genetic diagnosis for Huntington's disease. Electrophoresis of polymerase chain reaction products of the CTG triplet repeat stretches on control DNA from the couple at risk and their embryos: lane 1, unaffected mother with two healthy alleles with 20 and 22 repeats; lane 2, carrier father with one 'healthy' allele with 20 repeats and one expanded allele with 44 repeats; lane 3, molecular weight standard (50–350 bp); lanes 4 and 6, two blastomeres from embryo 1 (affected); lanes 8 and 10, two blastomeres from embryo 2 (affected); lanes 12 and 14, two blastomeres from embryo 3: an unaffected homozygous (20/20 repeats) embryo; lanes 16 and 18, two blastomeres from embryo 4 (affected); lanes 20 and 22, two blastomeres from embryo 5: a heterozygous (18/20 repeats) healthy embryo. Embryos 3 and 5 can therefore be transferred

is true for myotonic dystrophy and Huntington's disease, it is only partially true for the fragile X syndrome[37]. Next are the recurrent conditions caused by many different mutations such as CF, Duchenne's muscular dystrophy, Marfan's disease and neurofibromatosis type I. Here the multiplex linked marker approach will in the end probably allow acceptance of most of the couples for treatment within a reasonable time lapse, but this is not yet the case. These couples often have to wait several months before their PGD is ready for clinical application. Finally, there are the rare conditions caused by different mutations such as most of the metabolic diseases. Here, custom-made PCR assays have to be developed which is time and therefore money consuming. In this case even more than elsewhere, collaborative efforts should be made.

In case of chromosomal aberrations, especially translocations, the situation is different in that often these conditions lead to recurrent miscarriages or infertility due to oligoasthenoteratospermia. Here not only will PGD avoid the birth of an affected child due to chromosomal imbalance but ICSI combined with PGD will also circumvent the miscarriages and the infertility. Especially in case of reciprocal translocations, the available data indicate that PGD is a valuable approach to these couples because the pregnancy rate is reasonable as long as one or two balanced embryos can be selected for transfer out of a majority of unbalanced embryos[8,14,15].

OUTCOME AND FOLLOW-UP

It is difficult to tell how many IVF/PGD cycles have been performed to date. It is also difficult to provide an exact take-home-baby rate or to give extended information on the health of the children born. Based on the information in the literature and on our own results, the overall estimated ongoing pregnancy rate is around 20% per oocyte retrieval. This rate increases to around 25% per transfer of at least one embryo, because, in a number of cycles, no embryos are available for transfer (e.g. in case of reciprocal translocations). The age range of these patients is broad (between 20 and 40 years). The success rate of the treatment will therefore differ according to the age of the patients. If one looks at the success rate in a different way, around 40% of

the patients will achieve pregnancy after a mean of two treatment cycles, meaning that some are pregnant after the first IVF/PGD cycle but others need seven cycles, and some never become pregnant[16]. When pregnant, up to 25% of these pregnancies will spontaneously miscarry. Therefore, the take-home-baby rate is probably closer to 20% per transfer.

Reporting 1000–2000 children born after PGD is again no more than a rough estimate. From about 400–500 of these children follow-up data are available. These show that they seem to be at least as healthy as other IVF/ICSI children, indicating that the biopsy of the embryo causes no harm if the embryo survives the biopsy[9,15,38].

RISKS AND COMPLICATIONS

The risks and complications of PGD seem to be limited. Some of the risks are related to the IVF/ICSI treatment in itself, and therefore not directly related to PGD. These risks are mainly the risk of hyperstimulation as well as the risk of multiple pregnancies. Careful monitoring and transfer of no more than two but preferably one embryo will decrease this risk. The risk of monozygotic twinning has still to be evaluated. Removing two blastomeres as compared to one blastomere from an embryo may be detrimental to further embryo development and thus lower the chance of implantation or ongoing pregnancies. The risk of misdiagnosis exists beyond doubt. Almost every large center has reported it at least once. This risk is inherent to the single-cell PCR and the single-cell FISH and to the mosaicism existing, if not in every, at least in many, cleavage-stage embryos. In case of a PCR-based single-cell assay, a misdiagnosis can occur due to contamination by carry-over of PCR product or DNA from cellular debris from maternal or paternal origin or from the operator. Also, ADO, the non-amplification of one allele, can cause a misdiagnosis[9,17]. Finally, mosaicism may in certain conditions lead to an incorrect diagnosis[8,14]. One can take care of most of these problems by careful preclinical work-up of each diagnostic assay and by only accepting diagnoses based on two cells or by doing multiplex PCR assays on one cell[10,17]. Even then, however, a low risk of misdiagnosis will remain. Therefore, a control prenatal diagnosis should be offered to the couple[16]. They can then decide which risk they want to take: either a misdiagnosis risk estimated to be around 3–4% or the risk of miscarriage due to chorionic villus biopsy or to amniocentesis of around 0.5–1%[9,15].

For PGD assays based on single-cell FISH, a misdiagnosis can occur due to a missing signal, to cross-over hybridization or to overlapping signals. Again, analyzing two cells may lower the risk of misdiagnosis[8,14]. Here too, prenatal diagnosis after PGD is recommended.

As mentioned before, the babies born seem as healthy as IVF and ICSI babies, but larger numbers and a longer follow-up period are needed to confirm this[9,15,38].

A major drawback of PGD is its cost, mainly due to the labor-intensive single-cell analyses to be performed. Perhaps in the future innovative technology may reduce the cost, but this will not occur in the near future.

When PGD was first reported, ethical discussions occurred because of embryo selection, but the procedure has now been accepted by many in most countries. Germany and Ireland are exceptions. The ethical debate has now focused on certain applications of PGD such as social sexing, accepted by some in any circumstances or within the frame of family balancing, but totally unacceptable for others[9,39–44]. Another application of the procedure, which by some is considered a step too far, is PGD with HLA typing of the embryos to create a child within a family having to care for a sick child in need of a transplantation of HLA-matched hematopoietic stem cells[27,39,45].

PERSPECTIVES

Technology is evolving, also in the field of PGD. Continuous efforts are being made to improve the efficiency and the quality of the genetic tests at the single-cell level. The use of comparative genomic hybridization to analyze not only one or a few chromosome imbalances, but the whole chromosome complement in each embryo, has recently made the transition from the research laboratory to the clinic[5,46–49]. Real-time PCR and minisequencing are new techniques being used at the single-cell level for diagnosis of gene defects[6,50].

Microarray technology in PGD can be used both for the detection of chromosome imbalances and for

gene mutations or for single nucleotide polymorphisms[6]. Cryopreservation of biopsied embryos followed by thawing and replacement in the uterus has recently been improved and has led to pregnancies[51]. The final aim in the field of PGD is to make the procedure available to all couples confronted with a high recurrence risk for a genetic condition with a reasonable success rate and at a reasonable cost.

CONCLUSIONS

PGD is now an established procedure that can be proposed as an option to couples at high risk of transmitting an inherited disease. Couples who, besides their genetic risk, are also infertile and need IVF may more readily benefit from PGD. Nevertheless, an increasing number of fertile couples make use of this novel procedure in order to avoid termination of pregnancy after prenatal diagnosis. However, it is important to realize that, today, PGD cannot replace prenatal diagnosis in all cases. This has to be carefully evaluated before offering PGD. Moreover, patients should be informed in detail about the procedure, preferably by a written informed consent form, explaining at least the ovarian stimulation procedure with the risk of hyperstimulation, the relatively low take-home-baby rate of around 20% per cycle or even per transfer, the risk of misdiagnosis of probably 3–4%, for which a control prenatal diagnosis is recommended, and finally the still relatively small number of young children born (very few after cryopreservation) who in general seem to be in good health but for whom follow-up studies are required.

REFERENCES

1. Handyside A, Kontogianni E, Hardy K, Winston R. Pregnancies from biopsied human preimplantation embryos sexed by Y-specific DNA amplification. *Nature (London)* 1990; 344:768–70

2. Wilton L. Preimplantation genetic diagnosis for aneuploidy screening in early human embryos: a review. *Prenat Diagn* 2002;22: 312–18

3. Rimoin DL, Connor M, Pyeritz R, Korf B, eds. *Emery and Rimoin's Principles and Practice of Medical Genetics*, 4th edn. London: Churchill Livingstone, 2002;36:961–81

4. www.ncbi.nlm.nih.gov/omim/searchomin. html

5. Wells D, Levy B. Cytogenetics in reproductive medicine: the contribution of comparative genomic hybridization (CGH). *BioEssays* 2003;25:289–300

6. Syvänen A-C. From gels to chips: 'minisequencing' primer extension for analysis of point mutations and single nucleotide polymorphisms. *Hum Mut* 1999;13:1–10

7. Harper P. *Practical Genetic Counselling*, 5th edn. London: Arnold, 2001

8. Braude P, Pickering S, Flinter F, Ogilvie CM. Preimplantation genetic diagnosis. *Nature Rev Genet* 2002;3:941–53

9. ESHRE PGD Consortium Steering Committee. ESHRE Preimplantation Genetic Diagnosis Consortium: data collection III (May 2001). *Hum Reprod* 2002;17:233–46

10. Thornhill AR, Snow K. Molecular diagnostics in preimplantation genetic diagnosis. *J Mol Diagn* 2002;4:11–29

11. Munne S. Preimplantation genetic diagnosis of numerical and structural chromosomal abnormalities. *Reprod Biomed Online* 2002;4:183–96

12. Vandervorst M, Liebaers I, Sermon K, et al. Successful preimplantation genetic diagnosis is related to the number of available cumulus–oocyte complexes. *Hum Reprod* 1998;13:3169–76

13. Vandervorst M, Staessen C, Sermon K, et al. The Brussels' experience of more than 5 years of clinical preimplantation genetic diagnosis. *Hum Reprod Update* 2000;4:364–73

14. Pickering S, Polidoropoulos N, Caller J, et al. Strategies and outcomes of the first 100 cycles of preimplantation genetic diagnosis at the Guy's and St. Thomas' Center. *Fertil Steril* 2003;79:81–90

15. Report of the 11th Annual Meeting of International Working Group on Preimplantation Genetics. Preimplantation genetic diagnosis: experience of 3000 clinical cycles. *Reprod BioMed Online* 2001;3:49–53

16. Liebaers I, Sermon K, Staessen C, et al. Clinical experience with preimplantation genetic diagnosis and intracytoplasmic sperm injection. *Hum Reprod* 1998;13(Suppl 1):186–95

17. Sermon K. Current concepts in preimplantation genetic diagnosis (PGD): a molecular biologist's view. *Hum Reprod Update* 2002;8:1–10

18. Verlinsky Y, Rechitsky S, Evsikov S, et al. Preconception and preimplantation diagnosis for cystic fibrosis. *Prenat Diagn* 1992;12:103–10

19. Cieslak J, Ivakhnenko V, Wolf G, et al. Three-dimensional partial zona dissection for preimplantation genetic diagnosis and assisted hatching. *Fertil Steril* 1999;71:308–13

20. Ao A, Ray P, Harper J, et al. Clinical experience with preimplantation genetic diagnosis of cystic fibrosis (ΔF508). *Prenat Diagn* 1996;16:137–42

21. Boada M, Carrera M, De La Iglesia C, et al. Successful use of a laser for human embryo biopsy in preimplantation genetic diagnosis: report of two cases. *J Assist Reprod Genet* 1998;15:302–6

22. De Vos A, Van Steirteghem A. Aspects of biopsy procedures prior to preimplantation genetic diagnosis. *Prenat Diagn* 2001;21:767–80

23. Joris H, De Vos A, Janssens R, *et al*. Comparison of the results of human embryo biopsy and outcome of PGD after zona drilling using acid Tyrode medium or a laser. *Hum Reprod* 2003;16:1896–1902

24. Sermon K, Goossens V, Seneca S, *et al*. Preimplantation diagnosis for Huntington's disease (HD): clinical application and analysis of the HD expansion in affected embryos. *Prenat Diagn* 1998;18:1427–36

25. Van de Velde H, De Vos A, Sermon K, *et al*. Embryo implantation after biopsy of one or two cells from cleavage-stage embryos with a view to preimplantation genetic diagnosis. *Prenat Diagn* 2000;20:1030–7

26. Verlinsky Y, Cieslak J, Freidine M, *et al*. Polar body diagnosis of common aneuploidies by FISH. *J Assist Reprod Genet* 1996;13:157–62

27. Strom C, Ginsberg N, Rechitsky S, *et al*. Three births after preimplantation genetic diagnosis for cystic fibrosis with sequential first and second polar body analysis. *Am J Obstet Gynecol* 1997;178:1298–306

28. Veiga A, Sandalinas M, Benkhalifa M, *et al*. Laser blastocyst biopsy for preimplantation diagnosis in the human. *Zygote* 1997;5:351–4

29. Eftedal I, Schwartz M, Bendtsen H, *et al*. Single intragenic microsatellite preimplantation genetic diagnosis for cystic fibrosis provides positive allele identification of all CFTR genotypes for informative couples. *Mol Hum Reprod* 2001;7:307–12

30. Staessen C, Van Assche E, Joris H, *et al*. Clinical experience of sex determination by fluorescent *in situ* hybridisation for preimplantation genetic diagnosis. *Mol Hum Reprod* 1999;5:392–9

31. Iwarsson E, Ährlund-Richter L, Inzunza J, *et al*. Preimplantation genetic diagnosis of DiGeorge syndrome. *Mol Hum Reprod* 1998;4:871–5

32. Scriven P, Handyside A, Mackie Ogilie C. Chromosome translocations: segregation modes and strategies for preimplantation genetic diagnosis. *Prenat Diagn* 1998;18:1437–49

33. Van Assche E, Staessen C, Vegetti W, *et al*. Preimplantation genetic diagnosis and sperm analysis by fluorescence *in situ* hybridisation for the most common reciprocal translocation t(11;22). *Mol Hum Reprod* 1999;5:682–90

34. Liu J, Lissens W, Silber S, *et al*. Birth after preimplantation diagnosis of the cystic fibrosis ΔF508 mutation by polymerase chain reaction in human embryos resulting from intracytoplasmic sperm injection with epididymal sperm. *J Am Med Assoc* 1994;272:1858–60

35. Goossens V, Sermon K, Lissens W, *et al*. Improving clinical preimplantation genetic diagnosis for cystic fibrosis by duplex-PCR using two polymorphic markers or one polymorphic marker in combination with the detection of the ΔF508 mutation. *Mol Hum Reprod* 2003;9:559–67

36. Sermon K, De Vos A, Van de Velde H, *et al*. Fluorescent PCR and automated fragment analysis for the clinical application of preimplantation genetic diagnosis of myotonic dystrophy (Steinert's disease). *Mol Hum Reprod* 1998;4:791–6

37. Platteau P, Sermon K, Seneca S, *et al*. Preimplantation genetic diagnosis for fragile Xa syndrome: difficult but not impossible. *Hum Reprod* 2002;17:2807–12

38. Strom C, Levin R, Strom S, *et al*. Neonatal outcome of preimplantation genetic diagnosis by polar body removal: the first 109 infants. *Pediatrics* 2000;106:650–3

39. Shenfield F, Pennings G, Devroey P, *et al*. The ESHRE Ethics Task Force. Taskforce 5: preimplantation genetic diagnosis. *Hum Reprod* 2003;18:649–51

40. Robertson J. Extending preimplantation genetic diagnosis: the ethical debate. Ethical issues in new uses of preimplantation genetic diagnosis. *Hum Reprod* 2003;18:465–71

41. de Wert G. Ethics of assisted reproduction. In Fauser B, Bouchard P, Hsueh A, *et al.*, eds. *Reproductive Medicine. Molecular, Cellular and Genetic Fundamentals.* London: Parthenon Publishing, 2003;645–65

42. Malpani A. The use of preimplantation genetic diagnosis in sex selection for family balancing in India. *Reprod BioMed* 2002;4:16–20

43. Pennings G. Personal desires of patients and social obligations of geneticists: applying preimplantation genetic diagnosis for non-medical sex selection. *Prenat Diagn* 2002;22:1123–9

44. Ray P, Munnich A, Nisand I, *et al.* Sex selection by preimplantation genetic diagnosis: should it be carried out for social purposes? Is preimplantation genetic diagnosis for 'social sexing' desirable in today's and tomorrow's society? *Hum Reprod* 2003;18:463–4

45. Pennings G, Schots R, Liebaers I. Ethical considerations on preimplantation genetic diagnosis for HLA typing to match a future child as a donor of haematopoietic stem cells to a sibling. *Hum Reprod* 2002;17:534–8

46. Voullaire L, Slater H, Williamson R, Wilton L. Chromosome analysis of blastomeres from human embryos by using CGH. *Hum Genet* 2000;105:210–17

47. Wells D, Delhanty J. Comprehensive chromosomal analysis of human preimplantation embryos using whole genome amplification and single cell comparative gnomic hybridisation. *Mol Hum Reprod* 2000; 6:1055–62

48. Wilton L, Williamson R, McBain J, *et al.* Birth of a healthy infant after preimplantation confirmation of euploidy by comparative genomic hybridisation. *N Engl J Med* 2001; 345:1537–41

49. Wells D, Escudero T, Levy B, *et al.* First clinical application of comparative genomic hybridisation and polar body testing for preimplantation genetic diagnosis of aneuploidy. *Fertil Steril* 2002;78:543–9

50. Fiorentino F, Magli MC, Podini D, *et al.* The minisequencing method: an alternative strategy for preimplantation genetic diagnosis of single gene disorders. *Mol Hum Reprod* 2003;9:399–410

51. Jericho H, Wilton L, Gook D, Edgar D. A modified cryopreservation method increases the survival of human biopsied cleavage stage embryos. *Hum Reprod* 2003;18:568–71

19

Preimplantation aneuploidy screening: myths and facts

J. Van der Elst

WHY ANEUPLOIDY SCREENING MAY HELP EMBRYO SELECTION *IN VITRO*

Numerical chromosome anomalies are found in up to 21% of spontaneous abortions[1]. Of these, trisomies for sex chromosomes and autosomal chromosomes 13, 16, 18 and 21 account for 50% of chromosomally abnormal abortions. The only identifiable risk factor is increasing maternal age with the incidence of trisomies rising from 0.6% to 2.2% from age 35 to age 40 onwards. Prenatal genetic diagnosis is now being offered to all women of > 35 years of age. Fetal cells for karyotyping are obtained either by chorionic villus sampling or by amniocentesis. In both cases, however, the finding of chromosomal abnormalities will place the patient before the heartbreaking choice of termination of pregnancy.

When pregnancy is attempted through *in vitro* fertilization (IVF), embryos are developing in a laboratory environment and embryo selection has to be carried out before transfer into the uterus. Selection of the embryo that will implant and lead to a living healthy child is a daily challenge for embryologists. Generally selection is roughly based on external embryo morphology. The available tool is an inverted microscope with a magnification potential of at least × 300. The embryo is carefully inspected and scored for number of blastomeres, percentage of fragmentation and multinucleation[2]. For many years, worldwide IVF experience has taught that this type of selection is necessary but not sufficient for invariable detection of the vital and genetically normal embryos. It is tempting to obtain information from the inside of the embryo

and to unravel genetic clues that the outside cover cannot show. Aneuploidy screening to identify those embryos with the characteristic euploid set of human chromosomes could be the first step on this genetic path. Fluorescent *in situ* hybridization (FISH) to screen the number of chromosomes in embryos before implantation was introduced by Munné and colleagues to increase the pregnancy rate and reduce the risk of delivering trisomic offspring in older patients undergoing IVF[3]. Chromosomal analysis of *in vitro* cleavage-stage embryos for chromosomes X, Y, 13, 18 and 21 revealed that aneuploidy was the most common abnormality in morphologically normal embryos and that aneuploidy increased significantly with increasing maternal age[4–6]. From these results it is clear that the decline in ongoing embryo implantation with advancing maternal age is related to an increase of chromosomal aneuploidy in cleavage-stage embryos.

From a theoretical point of view, it would seem that aneuploidy screening could help to transfer only normal embryos and that this policy could increase pregnancy and implantation rates, in particular in older patients. Can current aneuploidy screening technology really make this promise come true? Are we selecting the right embryo for implantation by FISH? The real question is not whether we will find aneuploidies — because we most certainly will — but rather whether the results that we obtain with current screening panels give an accurate picture of the whole embryo. We must first answer the question of whether there is a solid basis for introducing aneuploidy screening in assisted reproductive technologies (ART) and, if there is, make the promise into a fact.

IS FLUORESCENT *IN SITU* HYBRIDIZATION FOR ANEUPLOIDY SCREENING OF BLASTOMERES A MIRACLE TOOL?

The basic technique

The basic strategy for aneuploidy screening is embryo biopsy at the eight-cell stage on day 3 of development. One or two blastomeres are taken as being representative of the whole embryo. Aneuploidy screening is performed by means of FISH for a panel of 5–9 chromosomes[6–8]. The test kit includes fluorescent probes for the five chromosomes X, Y, 13, 18 and 21, extendable with probes for chromosomes 16, 22, 14 and 15. The genetic test is run during a time frame compatible with IVF, so that results are available by day 4 or 5 of embryo development. When aneuploidy screening of these blastomeres for the specific chromosome panel shows normality, the counterpart embryo can be transferred.

It is evident from blastomere aneuploidy screening that the above expectation is too simplistic. There are several pitfalls that may compromise the outcome of aneuploidy screening. Some of these are related to the technical aspects of the procedure, whereas others are related to mosaicism of the embryo.

Technical errors of fluorescent *in situ* hybridization

FISH technology is based on the hybridization of fluorescent color-labeled probes on complementary DNA sequences specific for every chromosome. Each chromosome can be labeled but only a restricted number can be visualized simultaneously, because of the limitation in fluorochromes available and the risk of obtaining overlapping signals. Signals for the five chromosomes X, Y, 13, 18 and 21 are generally visualized in a first hybridization round followed by a second round with two to four additional chromosomes (14, 15, 16, 22). The rationale for correct diagnosis is that each signal represents a true chromosome constitution. False positives originate mainly from signal splitting due to DNA stretching during fixation or due to occurrence of non-synchronous S-phase, causing replicating chromosomes or chromosome domains to show two signals instead of one. False negatives can be due to overlapping signals or loss of DNA during fixation.

Mosaicism

Embryo mosaicism is the coexistence of several chromosomally different cell lines in the embryo. This specific phenomenon can obviously interfere with correct diagnosis in preimplantation diagnosis, where it is expected that the biopsied blastomeres are a mirror image of the counterpart embryo.

Thirty per cent of IVF embryos are mosaics[6]. Mosaics of three different types have been found: chaotic mosaics, where few normal diploid blastomeres exist, together with on average 84% of abnormal cells that show random chromosome distribution; diploid/polyploid mosaics with on average 43% of the cells being abnormal; and mosaics arising from mitotic non-disjunction or anaphase lagging in cleaving embryos, which show on average 65% of abnormal cells.

Preimplantation genetic misdiagnosis

Technical FISH errors as well as the rather frequent occurrence of embryo mosaicism illustrate the fact that the risk of classifying an abnormal embryo as normal and vice versa is a worrying cause of misdiagnosis in preimplantation genetic diagnosis (PGD). This risk is estimated to be 7.2%, with 5.6% due to mosaicism[6].

For the sake of completeness, PGD by polar body analysis has to be mentioned. Verlinsky and Kuliev developed this technique to screen the genetic status of the oocyte before conception[9]. This method does not take into account post-mitotic errors but is ethically more acceptable and does not take away biological material involved in embryo development. Since most PGD laboratories offer blastomere screening, polar body analysis will not be discussed here. More in-depth information about PGD by polar body analysis can be obtained from recent reviews[6,9].

OUTCOME OF ANEUPLOIDY SCREENING IN CLEAVAGE-STAGE EMBRYOS

The link between increased maternal age and the increased incidence of both abortion and aneuploidy makes it easy to understand that the outcome of IVF treatment with PGD is a subject of study in women of advanced maternal age. In addition to this group, two other distinct groups of patients with poor prognosis have been focused on: those with recurrent miscarriage and those with repeated implantation failure after IVF. In these two situations, chromosome abnormalities may be suspected as an underlying cause of the infertility. Recurrent miscarriage is defined here as three or more consecutive spontaneous abortions before 20 weeks of gestation with the parents having normal karyotypes. Repeated implantation failure is defined as at least three successive failed IVF cycles.

Gianaroli and co-workers analyzed embryos with the classic five-chromosome panel X, Y, 13, 18 and 21 in patients older than 38 years and in couples with at least three unsuccessful previous IVF attempts[10]. More than half of the embryos were abnormal. Transfer of only normal embryos resulted in a 28% implantation rate that was significantly higher than the 12% implantation rate in a control group with zona assisted hatching without blastomere biopsy.

Later, a more extensive chromosome screen panel for five to nine chromosomes (X, Y, 13, 14, 15, 16, 18, 21 and 22) was introduced by Munné and colleagues[11]. The rationale for this was that chromosomes 15, 16 and 22 are most frequently involved in cleavage-stage embryo aneuploidy and chromosomes 14, 15, 16 and 22 are common in spontaneous abortions whereas trisomies for X, Y, 13, 18 and 21 are compatible with fetuses reaching term delivery[6]. The nine-chromosome screening panel may thus have a higher impact on implantation than the first five-chromosome screening panel that was chiefly designed to prevent trisomic offspring. First reports with the nine-chromosome screening panel showed rather high ongoing pregnancy rates of 50% and 33%, albeit in non-controlled trials[6].

Controlled trials have to be carried out before the true benefit for patients can be estimated. Gianaroli and associates reported a study in patients ≥ 36 years of age or with at least three previous failed IVF cycles[7]. Randomization between PGD or embryo culture without PGD but with assisted hatching was performed on the basis of patients' voluntary decision. It was shown in this controlled trial that the use of a six-to-nine chromosome screening panel resulted in a significant increase in both implantation and ongoing pregnancy rates in the PGD group versus the control group with assisted hatching (22.5% vs. 10.2%; 37% vs. 27%, respectively). The advantage was particularly clear for women aged 38 years or older.

A large multicenter IVF study by Munné and co-workers in patients ≥ 35 years of age retrospectively compared pregnancy outcome in a PGD group undergoing aneuploidy screening for five to six chromosomes versus a matched control group without PGD[12]. Whereas the fetal heart rate per transferred embryo was similar, long-term outcome showed a higher rate of ongoing pregnancies and deliveries in the PGD group due to a decrease in spontaneous abortions. This retrospective matched control study was further refined, and the authors concluded that, in women of an average age of 40 years, a significant improvement in implantation rate can be obtained by PGD for aneuploidy screening versus matched controls (18% vs. 11%)[13]. These promising results, however, are limited to patients who have at least eight normally fertilized zygotes and no more than one previous failed IVF cycle.

An ongoing prospective randomized study in patients of advanced maternal age has been reported on an intermediate basis by Staessen and associates[14]. Patients of ≥ 37 years of age were randomized either to have PGD for a seven-chromosome screen panel on day 3 followed by culture and transfer on day 5 or not to have PGD but immediate blastocyst culture and transfer on day 5. Pregnancy rates were similar in both PGD and control groups and, although more embryos were transferred in the control group, PGD seemed to have a positive impact on implantation rates (23.1% vs. 11.8% in the control group).

Conclusions from PGD studies for recurrent miscarriage and repeated implantation failure are further weakened by the rather small sample sizes. PGD in patients with recurrent miscarriage showed a high number of chromosomal errors, but the pregnancy rate was not increased by means of PGD[15]. Gianaroli and co-workers did not find an increased pregnancy outcome by PGD for patients with at least three previously failed IVF cycles[7]. Kahraman and associates found that pregnancy rates for advanced maternal age and repeated implantation failure were similar, but this was a selected group of patients with severe male factor and the mean age of the patients with repeated implantation failure was significantly lower (30.3 years) than in the group with advanced maternal age (37.1 years)[16].

WHICH COUPLES CAN BENEFIT FROM ANEUPLOIDY SCREENING AFTER IVF/ICSI?

Studies on PGD should lead to a reliable strategy for improving patient treatment. What can we learn from the current studies on aneuploidy screening? Do the results allow us to alter current treatment strategies, and can we predict an improved outcome in the patient groups for whom they were designed?

Advanced maternal age: decreased pregnancy loss and reduction of trisomic offspring

Patients with advanced maternal age seem to be a primary target group. This seems logical, since it is known that aneuploidy is the main cause of reproductive failure in women of advanced age. Progress can be made by extending the chromosome screening panel and by refining the age categories and the optimal embryo cohort for performing PGD in a cost-effective manner. Besides the increase in implantation rates, another important benefit of PGD in older patients is the reduction or prevention of trisomic pregnancies that might develop to term. A large number of deliveries after PGD will be needed before it can be concluded that PGD will effectively reduce the number of trisomic conceptuses. Nevertheless, in 241 fetuses the rate of trisomies after PGD for aneuploidy was lower (0.4%) than that expected in a population of the same age range (6.66%)[6].

Recurrent miscarriage and repeated implantation failure: the tough cases

PGD series are still rather small for these two groups with a poor prognosis, but the picture that seems to emerge is one in which PGD only marginally improves the outcome in recurrent miscarriage and does not seem to affect the outcome in patients with repeated implantation failure. From the European Society of Human Reproduction and Embryology PGD consortium data collection for 2001[17], the pregnancy rate per embryo transfer was 36% after PGD for advanced maternal age, 32% in case of recurrent miscarriage but only 11% in patients with recurrent implantation failure with embryo transfer performed in only 63% of cycles, mostly because all biopsied embryos were abnormal. Information on repetitive abnormality of the whole embryo cohort may, however, be useful in cycle closure.

CAN ANEUPLOIDY SCREENING HELP IN THE REDUCTION OF MULTIPLE GESTATIONS?

The only workable strategy to prevent multiple pregnancies is to replace only one embryo[18–20]. Because elective single-embryo transfer is mostly restricted to patients with a good prognosis, it seems paradoxical to combine single-embryo transfer with PGD. Moreover, the good results obtained by elective single-embryo transfer may be compromised by unnecessary invasion of the embryo.

The role of PGD in the prevention of multiple pregnancies is mainly to discourage the transfer of all available embryos in women of advanced maternal age, with a risk not only of multiple pregnancy but also of trisomic pregnancies.

CURRENT MESSAGES ON MYTHS AND FACTS REGARDING ANEUPLOIDY SCREENING

The mission is to select the right embryo. The tools are plain non-invasive embryo morphology and invasive aneuploidy screening by FISH. For young patients with a good prognosis, one may rely on embryo morphology. However, increasing female age brings increased gamete instability and entails increased chromosomal abnormalities in oocytes and *in vitro* embryos. The problem is that embryo morphology does not necessarily reflect the chromosomal composition. Therefore, advanced maternal age is considered an indication for aneuploidy screening. Also, recurrent miscarriage and repeated implantation failure after IVF are considered indications for aneuploidy screening, since chromosomal abnormalities can play a role.

At this time it appears that aneuploidy screening may be beneficial only by increasing implantation rates in patients where the sole indication is advanced maternal age. Can we hope for more? With the most common chromosome screening panel (X, Y, 13, 18 and 21) we have detected chromosomes involved in trisomies in embryos that can develop for several weeks into a clinically recognizable pregnancy or even go to term. Selecting against these chromosomes does not necessarily prevent embryo implantation. If we wish to increase implantation by aneuploidy screening, then the chromosomes we are screening for should be those involved in implantation failure, or we should be able to screen the full karyotype as may be possible in the future by comparative genomic hybridization[21,22]. If not, we cannot expect miracle gains on that level. Even then, owing to the occurrence of mosaicism, PGD can never be fully predictive.

Aneuploidy screening can be a remedy only if aneuploidy is the core of the problem. For increased maternal age it is a fact that the risk of oocyte and embryonic chromosomal abnormalities increases. However, in other conditions the oocyte or the embryo can carry a defective default setting, causing repeated chromosomal instabilities and perhaps by other mechanisms than advanced maternal age. In these cases, aneuploidy may be diagnosed by aneuploidy screening, but unfortunately this will not improve the outcome.

The myth is that current aneuploidy screening is a cure for chromosomal diseases. The fact is that aneuploidy screening seems to be an effective tool for specific target populations (advanced maternal age) and that the more chromosomes we analyze the closer we will be to tackling the core of the problem. For those target populations where this is not effective, it can help in defining further patient management options: donor gametes, embryo donation or adoption.

Further data collection will determine whether aneuploidy screening is another fashion in IVF/ICSI or has a future in routine ART. PGD cannot turn an abnormal embryo into a normal embryo. Aneuploidy screening detects, but nature selects.

REFERENCES

1. Hassold TJ, Chen N, Funkhouser T, et al. A cytogenetic study of 1000 spontaneous abortions. *Ann Hum Genet* 1980;44:151–78

2. Van Royen E, Mangelschots K, De Neubourg D, et al. Characterization of a top quality embryo, a step towards single embryo transfer. *Hum Reprod* 1999;14:2345–9

3. Munné S, Lee A, Rosenwaks Z, et al. Diagnosis of major chromosome aneuploidies in human preimplantation embryos. *Hum Reprod* 1993;8:2185–91

4. Munné S, Alikani M, Tomkin G, et al. Embryo morphology, developmental rates and maternal age are correlated with chromosome abnormalities. *Fertil Steril* 1995;64:382–91

5. Munné S, Magli C, Cohen J, et al. Positive outcome after preimplantation diagnosis of aneuploidy in human embryos. *Hum Reprod* 1999;14:2191–9

6. Munné S. Preimplantation genetic diagnosis of numerical and structural chromosome abnormalities. *Reprod Biomed Online* 2002;4: 183–96

7. Gianaroli L, Magli C, Ferraretti AP, et al. Preimplantation diagnosis for aneuploidies in patients undergoing *in vitro* fertilization with a poor prognosis: identification of the categories for which it should be proposed. *Fertil Steril* 1999;72:837–44

8. Bahçe M, Escudero T, Sandalinas M, et al. Improvements of preimplantation diagnosis of aneuploidy by using microwave-hybridization, cell recycling and monocolor labeling of probes. *Mol Hum Reprod* 2000;9:849–54

9. Verlinsky Y, Kuliev A. Polar body biopsy. In Gardner DK, Weissman A, Howles CM, Shoam Z, eds. *Textbook of Assisted Reproductive Techniques*. London: Martin Dunitz, 2001:333–40

10. Gianaroli L, Magli MC, Ferraretti AP, *et al.* Preimplantation genetic diagnosis increases the implantation rate in human *in vitro* fertilization by avoiding the transfer of chromosomally abnormal embryos. *Fertil Steril* 1997;68:1128–31

11. Munné S, Magli C, Bahçe M, *et al.* Preimplantation diagnosis of the aneuploidies most commonly found in spontaneous abortions and live births: XY, 13, 14, 15, 16, 18, 21, 22. *Prenat Diagn* 1998;18:1459–66

12. Munné S, Magli C, Cohen J, *et al.* Positive outcome after preimplantation diagnosis of aneuploidy in human embryos. *Hum Reprod* 1999;14:2191–9

13. Munné S, Sandalinas M, Escudero T, *et al.* Improved implantation after preimplantation genetic diagnosis of aneuploidy. *Reprod BioMed Online* 2003;7:91–7

14. Staessen C, Van Assche E, Platteau P, *et al.* The impact of blastocyst transfer with or without preimplantation genetic diagnosis for aneuploidy screening in couples with advanced maternal age. *Hum Reprod* 2001;16 (Abstract Book 1):23

15. Pellicer A, Rubio C, Vidal F, *et al. In vitro* fertilization plus preimplantation genetic diagnosis in patients with recurrent miscarriage: an analysis of chromosome abnormalities in human preimplantation embryos. *Fertil Steril* 1999;71:1033–9

16. Kahraman S, Bahçe M, Samli H, *et al.* Healthy births and ongoing pregnancies obtained by preimplantation genetic diagnosis in patients with advanced maternal age and recurrent implantation failure. *Hum Reprod* 2000;15:2003–7

17. ESHRE PGD Consortium Steering Committee. ESHRE Preimplantation Genetic Diagnosis Consortium: data collection III (May 2001). *Hum Reprod* 2002;17:233–46

18. Dhont M. Single embryo transfer. *Semin Reprod Med* 2001;19:251–8

19. Gerris J, De Neubourg D, Mangelschots K, *et al.* Elective single day 3 embryo transfer halves the twinning rate without decrease in the ongoing pregnancy rate of an IVF/ICSI programme. *Hum Reprod* 2002;17:2626–31

20. De Sutter P, Van der Elst J, Coetsier T, Dhont M. Single embryo transfer and multiple pregnancy rate reduction in IVF/ICSI: a 5 year appraisal. *Reprod Biomed Online* 2003;6:464–9

21. Wells D, Delhanty JDA. Comprehensive chromosomal analysis of human preimplantation embryos using whole genome amplification and single cell comparative genomic hybridization. *Mol Hum Reprod* 2000;6:1055–62

22. Wilton L. Preimplantation genetic diagnosis for aneuploidy screening in early human embryos: a review. *Prenat Diagn* 2002;22:521–8

20

Congenital anomalies after *in vitro* fertilization/ intracytoplasmic sperm injection

M. Bonduelle

INTRODUCTION

Congenital anomalies and *in vitro* fertilization

Since the birth of Louise Brown in 1978, *in vitro* fertilization (IVF) has become a widely used treatment for infertile couples and has spread gradually throughout the Western world. Even though great concern was voiced at the introduction of IVF, a formal and systematic evaluation of the outcome of this high-tech procedure was not carried out and relatively few studies on the children were undertaken. Gradually, IVF became accepted as a safe technique, mostly on the basis of the information in registries with retrospectively collected data[1–3]. One early study mentioned a statistically relevant increase in two types of birth defect in IVF as compared to the general population: neural tube defects and transposition of the great vessels[4]. This report was not confirmed by other studies in the 1980s. However, in one later Swedish retrospective cohort study on 5856 IVF babies[5], the risk of neural tube defects (hydrocephaly risk ratio 5.7, anencephaly risk ratio 12.9) and of esophageal atresia (risk ratio 3.9) was significantly higher in the IVF group than in the control group. In another Swedish study, all 9111 children born in Sweden after IVF (1982–97) were compared to a population-based control group[6]. An excess of congenital malformations was found, which disappeared when confounders such as year of birth, maternal age,

parity and period of unwarranted childlessness were taken into account. A three-fold risk was observed in the incidence of some specific conditions: neural tube defect, alimentary atresia and omphalocele. In one recent study on 837 IVF children (and 301 children born after intracytoplasmic sperm injection; ICSI) the odds ratio for a major birth defect in IVF singletons at the age of 1 year was 2.0 (95% confidence interval 1.5–2.9) after adjustment for maternal age, parity, sex of the infant and correlation between siblings[7]. This study led to a new debate on the risk of congenital anomalies after IVF.

Congenital anomalies and intracytoplasmic sperm injection

When ICSI was introduced by the Belgian group of Van Steirteghem it was considered from the start as a risky procedure[8]. ICSI is indeed a more invasive procedure than classic IVF, since one spermatozoon is injected through the oocyte membrane and fertilization can ensue from sperm that could never have been used previously in fertility treatment[9]. Two types of risks were mentioned by several authors: ICSI procedure-dependent and ICSI procedure-independent risk factors. In the latter case, the risk relates to the cause of infertility (which can be an inheritable condition) leading to the need to perform ICSI and to the adverse consequences of the use of spermatozoa that in many cases would otherwise not have been fit or mature enough to achieve fertilization.

Since its introduction, ICSI has spread over the world and different initiatives to collect data on the children have been undertaken. The first reports were published by the Belgian group on a gradually growing cohort of ICSI children. In a prospective study on a cohort of 1987 ICSI children, Bonduelle and colleagues failed to find any increased risk of major congenital malformations as compared to the general population based on registries, but found an increased risk of chromosomal aberrations, mostly sex-chromosomal aneuploidies[10]. A group in Western Australia reinterpreted the data on one of the publications on a still limited group of 423 children, and came to the conclusion that the Belgian children had a higher incidence of congenital malformations compared to those in the Australian Birth Register[11,12]. However, reclassification was performed without knowledge of the entire clinical background, and comparisons were made between Belgian and Australian populations (which contain children from different ethnic origin with a possibly higher malformation rate and a different socioeconomic background not taken into account in the analysis), as countered in the discussion[12]. Other fertility centers have collected their own data. The European Society of Human Reproduction and Embryology (ESHRE) Task Force collected data from different centers in Europe performing ICSI, but information on malformations in the children was incomplete[13]. In a Danish cohort of 730 ICSI children, no increase in major malformation data was found as compared to the general population[14]. In a Swedish study on 1139 children born after ICSI compared to a control group of all births in Sweden (using data compiled in the Swedish Medical Birth Registry), a slight increase in congenital (major or minor) malformations was found, mainly as a result of the high rate of multiple births. One particular malformation, hypospadias, was found more frequently in the ICSI children, and the authors deduced that this may be related to paternal subfertility[15,16]. This was also confirmed in the Swedish study on all infants born after assisted reproductive technologies (ART) in Sweden between 1982 and 97: 9111 children were compared to a population-based control group[7]. In a subgroup of this cohort, a group of 1639 children born after ICSI, the risk of hypospadias was greater (relative risk (RR) 2.9, 95% CI 1.4–5.4). In the recent study by Hansen and co-workers on 837 IVF children and 301 ICSI children, the odds ratio for a major birth defect in ICSI as compared to natural conception in singletons at the age of 1 year was 2.0 (95% CI 1.5–2.9) in both ICSI and in IVF after adjustment for maternal age, parity, sex of the infant and correlation between siblings[7]. A German prospective cohort study compared the major malformation rate in 3372 ICSI children compared to those in a prospective birth register (Mainzer Modell)[17]. Major malformation rate was calculated from the data of all liveborn and stillborn children, as well as from all spontaneous and induced abortions, beginning at the 16th week of gestation. In the ICSI cohort, 8.6% of the infants and in the control cohort, 6.9% of the infants had a major malformation. This resulted in a crude RR of 1.25 (95% CI 1.11–1.40). Adjustment for different demographic variables, genetic background or other medical variables possibly leading to a modification of the RR was not carried out in this study.

THEORETICAL REASONS FOR CONCERN IN *IN VITRO* FERTILIZATION AND INTRACYTOPLASMIC SPERM INJECTION

In vitro fertilization procedure

In retrospect, it is astonishing that no more controlled studies on the outcome of the children were initiated at the introduction of IVF in 1978. A number of concerns were raised and animal data suggested a possible risk due to *in vitro* culture techniques. General concerns included: an altered hormonal environment, the loss of a selective mechanism against morphologically abnormal sperm *in vivo* and point mutations due to various chemical exposures in the *in vitro* procedure. Since 1993 it was known that adult phenotypes could be affected by epigenetic events in early mouse embryos and in 1998 an unusually large offspring syndrome in sheep was observed and related to imprinted genes. In 1991 it was further shown that this fetal overgrowth in sheep after sheep embryo culture was related to epigenetic changes in the *IGF2R* gene[18]. It was thus clear from animal research that culture of preimplantation embryos affected fetal development and expression of imprinted genes. Only recently this mechanism has also been documented in humans, since the first reports on imprinting syndromes in ICSI and IVF children have been published.

Intracytoplasmic sperm injection procedure

At the introduction of the ICSI technique much more attention was given to the possible adverse effects for the children, and controlled studies on the outcome of the children were prospectively initiated[17,19]. Two types of risk were mentioned by several authors: procedure-dependent and procedure-independent risk factors.

Intracytoplasmic sperm injection-independent risk

Concerning this risk factor there is no doubt that spermatozoa used for ICSI have higher levels of defects which are in turn likely to have an adverse effect on embryo development, e.g. increased levels of aneuploidy in the spermatozoa and higher risks of transmitting an already existing genetic disease or transmitting gene defects related to the fertility problem, such as congenital bilateral absence of the vas deferens (CBAVD)/cystic fibrosis (CF), Yq11 mutations or higher levels of DNA damage[20].

A major concern was also the bypassing of the natural selection process. ICSI indeed circumvents several steps necessary in the natural fertilization process such as spermatozoa–zona pellucida binding and penetration, and fusion of the spermatozoon–oocyte membrane. The zona pellucida–spermatozoa binding selects for human spermatozoa with progressive motility, normal morphology and functional competence. It was shown that a lower percentage of chromosomally abnormal sperm (compared to the percentage of abnormal spermatozoa in the semen sample) bind to the zona pellucida, leading to the conclusion that the zona pellucida selects against spermatozoa with chromosomal aberrations and in particular against aneuploidy[21]. It is still unclear what the underlying mechanism of this selection is. However, other researchers argue that, even in spontaneous conceptions, there is no natural selection of spermatozoa[22].

Microinjection of sperm carrying a chromosomal anomaly such as an aneuploidy or a structural defect of the chromosomes is probably the major cause of the higher rate of chromosomal anomalies found in the ICSI fetuses that we observed. Both factors (bypassing the natural selection process and using sperm bearing a chromosomal anomaly) might lead to a higher percentage of chromosomally abnormal embryos after ICSI. In practice, this would lead to a higher number of aneuploid ICSI embryos as well as to higher percentages of early embryo loss or later pregnancy loss.

Intracytoplasmic sperm injection-dependent risk

The risk related to the procedure itself, which involves the penetration of the zona pellucida and oocyte cytoplasm, may result in a number of problems such as possible damage to the internal structure of the oocyte leading to aneuploidy and an increased risk of chromosomal anomalies due to the ICSI procedure itself. As chromosomal anomalies are one of the causes of congenital anomalies they should also be taken into account in evaluating the risk of an ART procedure.

Other risk factors include the injection of biochemical contaminants, e.g. polyvinylpyrrolidone, used to slow down spermatozoal motility, which possibly damages cell organelles or interferes with normal embryo development.

The injection of foreign, sperm-associated exogenous DNA (e.g. viral or bacterial DNA) or paternal mitochondrial DNA possibly leading to infectious or other diseases, presenting a possible risk of disease in children[23]. To date, no reports of diseases due to this contamination have been reported in the literature.

The transmission of mitochondrial DNA (mt-DNA) is strictly regulated and specific to each species. In many mammalian systems, paternal mt-DNA is eliminated very early during embryonic development. However, it is possible that the paternal mitochondria could be extruded into those cells destined to become trophoblasts and may act as a regulator of the fate of embryonic cell. In ICSI manipulation of the oocyte can result in the introduction of paternal mt-DNA, which can result in mixed mt-DNA populations being transmitted to the offspring, thus contravening the strict maternal inheritance of mt-DNA to the offspring[24]. Interestingly, in the few studies that have looked at the transmission of mt-DNA in embryonic as well as in extra-embryonic tissues, human offspring have not harbored paternal mt-DNA[24].

As in IVF, a higher risk of imprinting disorders was also suspected in ICSI, owing to two mechanisms. The ICSI embryo is exposed to *in vitro* culture; it is known from research that the mammalian genome undergoes widespread reprogramming and is susceptible to external factors. On the other hand, it was suspected that imprinting might be less complete at the time of fertilization if testicular sperm were used. Particularly the use of spermatids instead of the use of mature spermatozoa has been considered as involving a higher risk of imprinting disorders.

CAUSES OF MALFORMATION SYNDROMES

Congenital malformations arise from three major known mechanisms: genetic (responsible for 15–25%), environmental (causing approximately 10%, including maternal infections, uteroplacental problems and maternal exposition to drugs and other toxins) and multifactorial diseases (combined effect of genetic and environmental factors, responsible for 20–25%). A small percentage (0.5–1%) is attributed to the process of twinning. Within the genetic diseases, the majority are related to chromosome anomalies (10–15%), whereas a minority are related to single-gene defects (2–10%). Other mechanisms such as imprinting problems leading to multiple congenital anomaly syndromes such as Beckwith–Wiedemann syndrome or to a higher incidence of childhood cancer fall beyond this classification, but could be related to changes in the early embryonic environment. If a syndrome is visible at birth, it is reported as a congenital anomaly.

DIFFERENT PITFALLS TO CONSIDER WHEN ASSESSING CONGENITAL ANOMALIES AFTER ASSISTED REPRODUCTIVE TECHNOLOGIES

From the introduction of ART it has appeared that observing major congenital anomalies is not a straightforward task. Variable malformation rates have been reported and different conclusions have been drawn. ART children have been compared to children born after natural conception, for whom data were recorded in a registry. These data have led to reassuring attitudes towards the ART procedures with regard to major malformations. For a number of reasons, however, it is not possible to compare these data sets[25]. In the following sections we give an overview of the possible problems encountered when interpreting different studies.

Overview of the risk factors

If children born after ART are compared to children in the general population or to a selected control group out of the general population, we must be aware that different types of risk factor can be present in the two populations.

Demographic variables

In several studies on ART children it has been shown that there is an influence of factors such as maternal age, number of years of unwanted childlessness, parity, exposure to environmental agents, smoking and drinking habits, social class, and singleton or multiple pregnancies. If findings are not corrected for these variables, which are often different in ART children compared to the general population, a bias will be induced.

General health

General health expressed in number of fertility patients with chronic conditions such as diabetes and hypertension can be compromised and should be recorded. On the other hand, social class may be lower and exposure to toxins, nutritional and general health problems may be worse in the general population group.

Genetic background

Genetic background is also different in both populations and can be expressed as the number of miscarriages, pregnancy losses, number of malformed fetuses or children, pregnancy complications and premature delivery, leading to a higher number of neonatal complications, such as low birth weight and prematurity. Genetic diseases in the parents or their relatives can also be different. It is known that a number of underlying diseases (such as myotonic dystrophy) are at the origin or contribute to the fertility problem in the male and influence the outcome of the pregnancy course in the female. Chromosomal anomalies in the parents such as Turner mosaics can influence the pregnancy outcome. Malformation rates in the parents of ICSI children are slightly higher and are another risk factor for the outcome of ART children[26]. This genetic background could place the ART children in a higher risk situation, independent of the risk factors directly related to the treatment.

Assisted reproductive technology treatment in itself

ART treatment in itself can influence pregnancy outcome. In ART, both for IVF and for ICSI, hormonal ovarian stimulation can lead to changes in the endometrium and an altered embryological and early hormonal environment. This has been shown by a few studies on the outcome of cryopreserved IVF embryos, where perinatal results were better, indicating that hyperstimulation or changes in the endometrium might have a negative effect on the pregnancy outcome. Controlled ovarian stimulation in itself (without other fertility treatment) has been claimed to be responsible for a higher malformation rate[4], but this was not confirmed by other studies[27]. It will remain difficult to separate the effects of the hormonal therapy from the effects of the embryo culture, transfer or further manipulation, unless ART is more frequently carried out without controlled ovarian stimulation, in a natural cycle.

Exposure of the embryo to culture conditions and manipulation can be a source of risk factors for further normal development. For ICSI children in particular, more risk factors were enumerated in relation to procedure-dependent or procedure-independent problems.

Registration of congenital anomalies

Observation bias

The incidence of birth defects is often determined from birth registries, which record major anomalies in all or selected hospitals. When ART children stay in neonatal units, neonatologists tend to examine these children in a more exhaustive way. Ultrasound investigations and eye examinations leading to detection of non-symptomatic anomalies are often carried out in these units. In this way overestimation of the rate of anomalies can occur. Some anomalies such as undescended testes, hydronephrosis

and polycystic kidney disease are not necessarily reported in general neonatal surveys. In the study by Wennerholm and co-workers on congenital malformations in ICSI children, a substantial number of conditions had to be omitted as congenital malformations in order to avoid observation bias, since they were recorded only for the ICSI children, but not for the children in the general population in the medical birth registry of Sweden[16]. An opposite observation bias might exist if an increased anomaly rate in ART children is not detected. This is certainly the case when information is obtained only from written questionnaires obtained from the parents and even from the pediatricians and gynecologists, who do not always take the time to fill in all the extra questionnaires of a study. In the survey by Palermo and associates, only 20% of the children were examined in the center and for the remaining 80% reports from pediatricians and gynecologists were requested[28]. This explains the fact that the malformation rate in this study was only 1.55%, which is less than the 2–3% observed in the general population.

Definition and classification system

Several definitions are used to classify a malformation as of a major or a minor type (or as not a malformation). If these definitions are not exactly the same, the percentages of observed major malformations will differ. Definitions used are sometimes broader ('a major anomaly is one with adverse effect on either the function or social acceptability of the individual') or more restricted ('a major malformation is one resulting in death or causing serious handicap, requiring surgical correction or medical therapy').

Even if standardized coding systems are used such as the International Classification of Diseases (ICD)[29], where malformations are named and defined individually, additional guidelines or definitions are necessary to classify the malformations listed into major and minor conditions. Moreover, every classification system has guidelines on how to classify borderline cases and rules about certain conditions not to be reported.

One chapter in the ICD-10 is devoted to malformations (Chapter 17), but a number of congenital anomalies are not retained in this chapter and can be found in several other chapters. In the study by

Wennerholm and colleagues, the malformations described were limited to those described in Chapter 17 of the ICD-10, counting all the malformations listed in the Q codes and applying internal guidelines (set up by the authors for this purpose) to classify malformations into major and minor malformations[16]. In the study by Loft and colleagues, unspecified diagnoses were added for those conditions which did not have a specific ICD-10 diagnosis, such as facial paralysis, pilonidal cyst and amniotic band syndrome[14]. In the study by Ludwig and Katalinic, major malformations were defined as structural defects of the body/organs that affect viability and quality of life and require medical intervention[17]. This classification system is also based on the British Paediatric Association Classification of Diseases (which is a five-digit code extension of ICD-9). The term 'congenital malformation' in the EUROCAT system refers to structural defects (congenital malformations, disruptions and dysplasias), chromosomal abnormalities, inborn errors of metabolism and hereditary diseases[30]. No formal definition of a major anomaly is applied. For EUROCAT, all conditions, both major and minor, are to be reported, except for a standard list of minor anomalies, not to be reported.

Minor malformations can be defined as those malformations that are not major. They are relatively frequent structural alterations that pose no significant health or social burden. They are nonetheless important, since their presence increases the risk of a major malformation. The presence of two or more minor anomalies is an indication that a major defect may be present as well[31]. If a minor malformation occurs in 4% or more of the normal population from the same ethnic background it is called a normal variation. Minor malformations may be a normal variant in the newborn, but if they do not disappear later in childhood the same condition can become a minor malformation. If minor conditions are reported in the literature, the percentages vary greatly, depending on the experience and the interest of the examiner. Even in the literature on specific searches for minor malformations, the figures vary between 7.3%[32] and 40.7%[31]. The only way to limit the interobserver differences for the examination of minor anomalies is therefore to work with a standardized checklist on which the conditions to be reported are listed and

described. Even so there can be interobserver differences; ideally the same investigator should examine both case and control groups.

Bonduelle and co-workers used a pragmatic definition in order to avoid classification differences for major and minor malformations[19]. Major malformations were defined as those malformations that generally cause functional impairment or require surgical correction. For borderline situations where it was not clear from follow-up data up to 1 year whether a malformation should be considered major, identical guidelines for both ICSI and IVF files were followed. The remaining malformations were considered minor. Minor malformations were considered synonymous with structural abnormality and were recorded using a checklist (containing a list of 237 items) constructed on the basis of the textbook on minor malformations by Aase[33].

Inclusion of prenatal anomalies

Birth defect registries do or do not record the malformations in stillborn infants or in pregnancies terminated for a fetal anomaly. Moreover, cut-off points from when to include a stillborn or a termination are often defined differently (from 16 to 28 weeks). Prenatal detection of anomalies may be higher in ART pregnancies than in the general population, as a result of closer surveillance in much-wanted pregnancies after infertility treatment and as a result of social class differences and differences in the decision-making process on termination being influenced by the history preceding the conception. One also needs to know the total number of fetal losses at > 20 weeks of pregnancy with or without malformations, and the number of stillborns in the general population, in order to calculate the figure of the total malformation rate ((affected livebirths + affected fetal deaths + induced abortions for malformations) divided by (livebirths + stillbirths)). This figure gives the best estimate of congenital malformations from early pregnancy onwards. However, all these data are often unknown for the general population. Ideally one should also take embryonic losses into account, but then other factors than congenital malformations such as hormonal environment in early pregnancy might influence the figures.

If results from ART were compared to those in the general population, it would be better to separate the prenatally detected anomalies from malformations detected at birth, since in registration of prenatal anomalies even more detection bias may be present. Indeed, if the fetus is not terminated, a number of non-detected fetal anomalies may lead to spontaneous miscarriage and be lost to registration as a congenital anomaly.

On the other hand, if only congenital malformations at birth are taken into account, a great variation in the figures is to be expected. From one population to another the detection rate and termination policy can be different, and this interferes with the natural course of pregnancies and congenital malformations at birth.

Only if a study applies exactly the same prenatal screening battery in the study group as in the controls, can prenatal data registration be considered similar. This methodology can be applied only in prospective studies and is the best method for evaluating the rate. In the study of Bonduelle and colleagues[19] as well as those of Ludwig and Katalinic[17] and Hansen and colleagues[7], prenatal malformations were also taken into account.

Duration of follow-up period

A more or less protracted time interval can lead to another surveillance bias. The time period during which the malformations are observed is of the utmost importance. We know from the EUROCAT Registry that we can expect that approximately 30% of the congenital anomalies registered from the prenatal period up to 1 year of age will be observed between 1 month and 1 year (40% of the congenital anomalies are observed between birth and 1 month and 30% prenatally).

Timing of the observation is variable in the literature, sometimes restricted to the neonatal period or until 30 months, sometimes only vaguely described. For this reason, too, results from the different studies cannot be adequately compared.

Temporal changes

The time period during which study and control groups are examined should be simultaneous in order to limit a number of minor changes due to time-related variables. These could for instance be the experience of the examiner, changes in laboratory procedures, patient selection or environmental variables.

Sample size

Sample size has to be adequate to allow for meaningful conclusions to be drawn. If the sample size is inadequate, no adequate power can be obtained. In order to detect an increase of 2% in malformation rate (e.g. from 3 to 5%), with a power of 80% (alpha = 5%), 3000 children are needed. If only 244 children are available, only a three-fold increase in the malformation rate (from 3 to 9%) can be detected.

Lost to follow-up rate

If only a small proportion of children are lost to follow-up, the remaining subjects may be assumed to be representative. However, if a higher percentage of children are lost to follow-up, this can lead to a skewing of the observed anomaly rate. This has been documented by Aylward and co-workers, who reported that the profile of the children who withdrew at any time from a study (a multicenter clinical trial) was different from that of those who remained. Medical and biological variables, environmental quality, ethnic background and center were factors determining the timing of the dropout[34]. These data show that a high follow-up rate minimizes the bias that can occur from sampling a slightly better/different subpopulation due to losses in follow-up.

Control groups and study protocol

In order to check for differences in congenital anomaly rates, control groups must ideally be selected for similar characteristics of a number of maternal demographic and health characteristics, known to influence the pregnancy outcome. If this is not possible then these variables should be recorded in the control population, which should allow adjustment for these variables to be made if the patient population is large enough. Identical follow up of pregnancy and birth is needed in order to record all the important variables influencing the number of congenital anomalies.

EVALUATION OF MALFORMATIONS IN ASSISTED REPRODUCTIVE TECHNOLOGIES

The ideal study design

The ideal study design for detecting congenital anomalies is prospective, using a patient population and a control group born after natural conception. Prospective evaluation should begin as soon as pregnancy is recognized (by ultrasound), around 7 weeks of gestation[25]. Pre-existing chronic conditions, diseases during pregnancy and drug intake should be recorded. A number of influencing factors such as maternal age, maternal education and occupation, number and type of previous conceptions, number of years of childlessness, exposures to toxins and drugs, alcohol and cigarette smoking and social and ethnic background should be recorded. Special attention should also be given to the genetic background in terms of genetic diseases or malformations in the parents and to the infertility background. Towards the end of the teratogenic period, at around 12 weeks of pregnancy, early pregnancy events should be recorded, including infections, toxic agents or medication. Details on the findings of scheduled ultrasound evaluations (12 weeks, 22 weeks) should be recorded in both the study and the control group. Abortions and pregnancy terminations should be recorded, including timing and findings at pathological examination. These findings allow calculation of a more precise total malformation rate. Neonatal assessment should be performed in a standardized way with a systematic search for major and minor malformations. Definitions of major malformations should be standardized and minor anomalies limited to a list of items to record. If a major malformation is defined as a malformation causing functional impairment (and death) or requiring surgery, these outcomes are (usually) measurable. A minor cardiac malformation, such as a foramen ovale or atrial septal defect type II that will close spontaneously, will be classified as minor, whereas an atrial septal defect type I that is always pathological and will probably need surgery will be classified as major. All data should be recorded on files designed for the purpose and questions should be asked in a standardized way. Asking for pre-existing medical conditions or asking explicitly whether hypertension or diabetes is present leads to different types of answer.

Usually examiners are pediatricians or neonatologists. Additional expertise in genetics can help in describing and recognizing some anomalies and in classifying a number of anomalies in syndromes. However, if geneticists examine the children, as was the case in our study, the number of anomalies detected will be higher than in a standardized pediatric examination. Ideally, both pediatric and genetic assessment should be carried out. Internal anomalies (found by screening) should also be separated from external anomalies. If a neonate undergoes routine ultrasound examination of the brain and agenesis of the corpus callosum is found, which has no clinical symptoms at that age, this anomaly is an incidental finding (at that age), which should not be included in the neonatal malformations. However, if a cardiac anomaly is found by screening for hypotonia and poor sucking, this anomaly is symptomatic and should therefore be included. Finally, anomaly detection should be restricted to a specific time interval after birth.

Using this approach, the main drawbacks are recruitment bias and dropout. Recruitment bias can be limited by early inclusion in the study, whereas dropout can be reduced by giving extensive information and receiving informed consent at the start, and further intensive interacting by the research team and the patients during the study.

Comparison of registry data

If no specific control group is available, comparison of the congenital malformation rate in ART (or in any specific group at risk) can be done on the basis of a General Population Registry. The study group of children can be identified in the registry and the number of prenatal and neonatal congenital anomalies recorded for the study group over a specific time period can be compared to the children of the general population during the same time period. Often only a limited number of maternal and paternal variables are recorded in such registries, which limits the possibility of adjustment for influencing factors. When comparing malformation rates between the general population and the ART population it is important to realize that closer surveillance and more detailed reporting in the group at risk is still a source of observation bias, as documented in the Swedish study by Wennerholm and colleagues[16].

EVALUATION OF THE MAJOR PUBLISHED STUDIES

In vitro fertilization compared to the general population in evaluation of major studies

Different large studies based on register data analysis gave contradictory results. A Danish study by Westergaard and co-workers comparing 2140 IVF children with the general population did not observe differences in major malformation rate (Table 1)[35]. In contrast, Ericson and Källèn found an increased rate (OR 1.47) of major malformations in a very large dataset of 7523 Swedish IVF children[6]. Anthony and colleagues found an increased rate (OR 1.20) in 4224 Dutch IVF children[36]. Hansen and associates found an increased rate in 837 Australian IVF children[7]. After confounders were taken into account the difference disappeared in the Swedish and the Dutch studies, but remained in the Australian study even after adjusting for maternal age, parity, sex and sibling correlation (OR 2.0; 95% CI 1.5–2.9). However, this study did not control for a number of variables (as explained in the next paragraph), which are likely to have been different in the two populations and could have led to different results.

Intracytoplasmic sperm injection compared to the general population of major risks

Retrospective studies comparing intracytoplasmic sperm injection children to registers

Two Swedish studies based on register-based data analysis have shown an increase in major malformations in ICSI and in ICSI plus IVF (Table 2)[6,15,16]. However, after adjustment for maternal age, year of birth and multiple births[14,16], as well as time of unwanted childlessness[6], the difference disappeared.

The Australian study conducted by Hansen and colleagues[7] observed congenital malformations at the age of 1 year in a limited group of 301 ICSI children, 837 IVF children and a group of 4000 children born after natural conception. All ART children were retrospectively identified from the Reproductive Technology Register, and control children were identified in a Midwives Notification System. Congenital malformations in ICSI regis-

tered in a Birth Defects Registry were found in 8.6% (95% CI 5.7–12.4) (26/301) compared to 4.2% (95% CI 3.6–4.9) in the population born after natural conception ($p < 0.001$). After adjustment for maternal age, parity, sex and sibling correlation, the odds ratio for malformations in ICSI compared to the general population was 2.0 (95% CI 1.3–3.2). After exclusion of conditions detected because of closer surveillance, the odds ratio (OR) for malformations in ICSI was 1.8 (95% CI 1.1–2.9). When only singletons or term singletons were considered, the OR remained significant. Although the authors adjusted for different variables, they could not adjust for number of years of infertility or other sociodemographic factors such as ethnic background, which could have been different in the two populations. Observation bias due to the fact that the observers were not blinded could also have been present. Although the group of ICSI children was small in this study, being compared to a large control group led to statistical significance. However, it cannot be excluded that the higher rate of congenital malformations in the ICSI /IVF group occurred by chance.

Prospective studies comparing intracytoplasmic sperm injection children to control groups

Only one study on ICSI children was designed prospectively to compare a group of ICSI children ($n = 3372$) with a selected control group from the general population ($n = 30\,940$)[17]. This German prospective cohort study compared the major malformation rate in ICSI children in 59 different ICSI centers all over Germany with the malformation rates in a prospective birth register (Mainzer Modell) where children were examined according to exactly the same criteria as the ICSI cohort up to the age of 8 weeks of life. Major malformation rate was calculated on the data of all liveborn and stillborn children, as well as on all spontaneous and induced abortions, beginning with the 16th week of gestation. In the ICSI cohort 8.6% of the infants (291/3372) and in the control cohort 6.9% of infants (2140/30 940) had a major malformation. This resulted in a crude relative risk (RR) of 1.25 (95% CI 1.11–1.40). Adjustment for different demographic variables, genetic background or other medical variables possibly leading to a modification of the RR was not performed in this study. More

Table 1 Malformations after *in vitro* fertilization (IVF) in the literature

Authors	Number of children	Major malformations	Method	Number of control children	Major malformations	Malformation per organ system
Westergaard et al.*, 1999[35]	2245 (2140 IVF, 105 ICSI)	4.8% major in IVF + ICSI (ns) 1.7% major in ICSI	ICD-10 IVF register linked to MBR and to four registers, through identification number; follow-up to 7 days	2245 MBR; matched for maternal age, parity, multiplicity, year of birth	4.6% major (NS)	not considered
Ericson and Källén[†] 2001[6]	9175 (7523 IVF, 1652 ICSI, estimated numbers)	5.3% major in IVF 7.1% major in ICSI 5.6% major in IVF + ICSI OR 1.47 (95% CI 1.34–1.61) OR 0.89 (95% CI 0.74–1.06) adjusted	ICD-8-9-10 identification of all children born after IVF/ICSI through MBR, divided into major and mild/variable; follow-up to 7 days (up to 1 year for cytogenetics and cardiology; incomplete up to 2 years); adjustment for period of unwanted childlessness, year of birth, maternal age, singleton/twins	1 690 577		3-fold increase of neural tube defects, omphalocele, alimentary tract atresia; RR 2.9 (95% CI 1.4–5.4) hypospadias in ICSI
Hansen et al.[‡], 2002[7]	837 IVF	9.0% major in IVF OR 2.0 (95% CI 1.5–2.9) adjusted	ICD-9/British Paediatric Association/ major and minor classification; pre- and postnatal follow-up up to 1 year; adjustment for maternal age, parity, sex, sibling correlation	4000 naturally conceived	4.2% major ($p < 0.001$)	increase in musculoskeletal chromosomal cardiovascular urogenital anomalies
Anthony et al.**, 2002[36]	4224, undefined small proportion of ICSI	OR 1.20 (95% CI 1.01–1.43) OR 1.03 (95% CI 0.86–1.23) adjusted	national perinatal database classification (NPD) system, questionnaire to IVF parents, tracing of IVF children in NPD; pre- and postnatal follow-up to 8–28 days; adjustment for maternal age, parity, ethnicity	314 605 controlled for confounding maternal factors		increase in crude OR of cardiovascular and minor malformations; could be ascertainment bias

ICSI, intracytoplasmic sperm injection; MBR, Medical Birth Registry; RCM, Registry for Congenital Malformations
*In liveborn and stillborn children born after 28 weeks and in induced abortions; †in births, birth is defined as all liveborn or stillborn babies born after 28 weeks of gestation; ‡in births, records on pregnancies of at least 16 weeks of gestation; **in liveborn and stillborn children and terminations; ‡in liveborn and stillborn children born after 28 weeks of gestation

Table 2 Malformations after intracytoplasmic sperm injection (ICSI) in the literature

Authors	Number of children	Major malformations	Method	Number of control children	Major malformations	Malformation per organ system
Palermo et al.*, 1996[28]	578	1.55% major	definition of major malformation 20% examined and 80% reports from pediatricians and gynecologists	no		not considered
Loft et al.†, 1999[14]	730	2.7% major	ICD-10 divided into major and minor; Q codes; follow-up period 1–30 months; questionnaire to the parents (response rate 94%) and validation through discharge charts	no		not considered
Wennerholm et al.‡, 2000[16]	1139	5.0% major OR 1.75 (95% CI 1.19–2.58) OR 1.19 (95% CI 0.79–1.81) adjusted	ICD-9-10 divided into major and minor; identification of all children born after ICSI through MBR and RCM; follow-up of newborns; stratification for delivery hospital, year of birth, maternal age, singleton/twins	Medical Birth Registry (MBR); exclusion of conditions reported in ICSI not reported in the MBR		RR 3.0 (95% CI 1.09–6.5) for hypospadias
Bonduelle et al.**, 2002[19]	2840	3.4% major** 4.2% major (total) R.R. 0.94 (95% CI 0.66–1.07)	definition of major malformation; information from different sources; pre- and postnatal; follow-up of newborns up to 2 months	2955 (IVF)	3.8% major** 4.7% major (total)†† NS	not increased compared to IVF
Hansen et al.‡‡, 2002[7]	301	8.6% major in ICSI OR 2.0 (95% CI 1.3–3.2) adjusted	ICD-9 / British Paediatric Association/ major and minor classification; pre- and postnatal; follow-up to 1 year; adjustment for maternal age, parity, sex, sibling correlation of risk of birth defects	4000 naturally conceived	4.2% major (p < 0.001)	increase of musculoskeletal chromosomal anomalies
Ludwig et al.***, 2002[17]	3372	8.6% major RR 1.25 (95% CI 1.11–1.40)	definition of major malformation (EUROCAT Report 7); pre- and postnatal; follow-up of newborns up to 8 weeks	30 940 prospective birth registry		increase of cardiovascular and internal urogenital malformations
Ludwig 2003, personal communication†††		RR 1.13 (95% CI 0.98–1.30) adjusted	adjustment for parental malformations, previous malformed child, diabetes, maternal age, environment			

IVF, in vitro fertilization; RCM, Registry for Congenital Malformations
*In neonates; †in liveborns ≥ 24 weeks of gestation, terminations excluded; ‡in births, birth is defined as all liveborn or stillborn babies born after 28 weeks of gestation, terminations excluded; ‡‡in births, birth is defined as all liveborn and stillborn children ≥ 20 weeks of gestation; **in liveborns ≥ 20 weeks of gestation; ††in liveborn and stillborn children ≥ 20 weeks and in induced abortions at ≥ 12 weeks of gestation; ‡‡in liveborn and stillborn children and terminations; ***in liveborn and stillborn children and in spontaneous or induced abortions at > 15 weeks of gestation; †††oral communication Serono Symposia Brussels 10 years of ICSI

specifically, a higher risk for cardiovascular malformations and for internal urogenital malformations was found. For the latter, parental genetic factors might be involved.

Although this study design has tried to avoid major pitfalls, some criticism can be formulated. Pregnancies conceived after ICSI were assessed from throughout Germany, whereas naturally conceived pregnancies came from one limited geographical area. Only 44% of the ICSI pregnancies were included, which might induce a bias, since little information is known concerning the reason for non-inclusion at the 16th week of pregnancy. More importantly, there was a difference in timing of the examination of the children (7 days for the control children and a median of 38 days in the ICSI children) and in the fact that the examiners were different for both groups and not blinded. Also, the time period of the examination was different and much later in the ICSI than in the control group. The study design made it impossible to adjust in the first publication from this group[17]. In a subsequent study the same authors compared the ICSI data to another prospective birth registry and were able to perform adjustment for different variables, showing that parental background played a role in the increase of congenital malformations in ICSI[37].

Intracytoplasmic sperm injection compared to *in vitro* fertilization

Major malformations in ICSI compared to IVF were studied in a prospective study on 2995 IVF and 2889 ICSI children (liveborn and stillborn) by Bonduelle and colleagues[19]. No difference in malformation rate was found between ICSI and IVF children, with 3.4% major malformation in ICSI and 3.8% in IVF. When the total malformation rate was considered, including terminations for fetal anomaly and stillbirths, similar results were obtained, with 4.2% total major malformations in ICSI and 4.7% in IVF. In this study most of the conditions needed for an ideal prospective study protocol were fulfilled. The authors tried to avoid observation bias by using the same pediatricians blinded for the type of treatment with additional expertise in genetic assessment and examining ICSI and IVF children in the same way and in the same conditions. However, a number of (minor) malformations were detected through more intensive

screening by ultrasound in the neonatal period in ICSI as well as in IVF children. There was also a different time period in which IVF and ICSI children were examined, possibly leading to a bias of finding more anomalies in the ICSI group. No adjustment or matching was done in this study, but the ICSI and IVF groups were similar for different sociodemographic and medical background parameters, owing to the selection of consecutive cohorts of ICSI and IVF pregnancies from the same hospital.

Malformations in different organ systems

Differences in frequency of malformations per organ system were reported by several authors in IVF as well as in ICSI. All these reports were not consistent, apart from the fact that if a difference was found it was always more in the ART group than in the control group. An increase of urogenital malformations after ICSI was reported in several studies[6,16,17], but also in IVF and not in ICSI[7]. Comparison of all urogenital malformations after ICSI compared to IVF by Bonduelle and co-workers led to the conclusion that no difference could be demonstrated in 2840 liveborn ICSI children compared to 2955 IVF children[19]. Information on the urogenital status of the parents is lacking in all these studies (apart from the fact that ICSI is often associated with male factor infertility) and this parental genetic background could be the key factor responsible for this relatively small increase of urogenital malformations.

Intracytoplasmic sperm injection in relation to sperm quality and sperm source

There is increasing evidence that in severe oligo- and azoospermic patients with severe testicular failure a higher chromosomal aneuploidy rate is present in their sperm. Several studies support an association between certain types of morphological aberrations and sperm aneuploidy or between abnormal motility and sperm chromosome aneuploidy. There are therefore reasons to expect more chromosomal anomalies in children born after ICSI from fathers with severe testicular failure. In the series of 1586 prenatal tests described by Bonduelle and co-workers[38], statistically more chromosomal anomalies (2.1%) were found in fetuses when spermatozoa from men with low sperm counts ($< 20.10^6$/ml) were used in comparison to 1.6% chromosomal anomalies when spermatozoa with higher concentrations were used. However, this difference was not reflected in a higher percentage of congenital anomalies in the children born from fathers with more abnormal sperm parameters (including children with chromosomal anomalies presenting congenital malformations as well as children with morphological anomalies and normal chromosomes). No statistical difference was observed on the basis of sperm concentration (3.8%, $n = 1301$ if sperm count was $< 5.10^6$/ml and 2.8%, $n = 1635$ if sperm count was $\geq 5.10^6$/ml), morphology and motility or when spermatozoa from other sources than the ejaculate were used (Table 3). These data were also confirmed by a few other studies analyzing the possible relationship between congenital malformations and sperm parameters as well as sperm source[15,19,39]. Vernaeve and associates also looked into the subgroup of children born after the use of non-obstructive testicular sperm and found no statistical differences from those born from obstructive testicular sperm. However, all these results have to be considered with caution, since in all studies the numbers of children born after the use of sperm from other sources than the ejaculate were still very limited.

Rare imprinting disorders

Genomic imprinting is the exclusive expression of a gene from only one of the parental alleles. Many imprinted genes play a key role in embryonic development and fetal growth. Imprinted genes are functionally haploid and may therefore be more likely to induce disease when subjected to mutations or to epimutations, if these occur during the early exposure of gametes and embryo to artificial conditions (culture media, altered hormonal environment before and during implantation, etc.).

The imprinting process itself may be disturbed by *in vitro* culture (by disturbing methylation) leading to aberrantly imprinted genes. Loss of function of imprinted genes can have severe consequences, as it can lead to a number of syndromes such as Beckwith–Wiedemann syndrome, Angelman syndrome or Prader–Willi syndrome, which result from mutation, inactivation or gain of function of 'imprinting genes'.

Two children with Angelman syndrome (a neurogenetic disorder) due to a sporadic imprinting defect have been reported to date after use of the ICSI procedure[40]. The lack of an imprinting center mutation and the detection of a mosaic methylation pattern in one of the two patients make an inherited defect unlikely and point to an epigenetic post-

Table 3   Malformations after intracytoplasmic sperm injection (ICSI) with epididymal, testicular and ejaculated spermatozoa in the literature

| Authors | Malformations in ICSI liveborn children after use of sperm from different sources | | | Statistics |
	Epididymal	*Testicular*	*Ejaculated*	*Statistics*
Bonduelle *et al.*, 2002[38]	$n = 105$ (3.8%)	$n = 251$ (2.4%)	$n = 2477$ (3.4%)	NS
Ludwig *et al.*, 2002[17]	$n = 26$ (3.8%)	$n = 229$ (9.1%)	$n = 2994$ (8.4%)	NS
Vernaeve *et al.*, 2003[39]		obstructive $n = 193$ (2.1%) non-obstructive $n = 58$ (3.7%)		NS

zygotic defect leading to erroneous imprinting of the maternal chromosome 15. In a small case–control series of ART offspring after cryo-preservation, a single case of Beckwith–Wiedemann syndrome (a human overgrowth syndrome) was reported among 91 cases[41]. One case was reported in a study by Olivennes and colleagues on ART children[42], where no further genetic origin (*de novo* or inherited) could be determined. A recent article by DeBaun and co-workers reports evidence that ART is associated with Beckwith–Wiedemann syndrome on the basis of a higher frequency of history of ART in a Beckwith–Wiedemann syndrome registry than in the general population[43]. A total of seven children with Beckwith–Wiedemann syndrome were born after ART, of whom four were born after ICSI with ejaculated sperm and one after ICSI with testicular spermatozoa. Molecular studies indicated that five of the six children studied had specific epigenetic alterations associated with Beckwith–Wiedemann syndrome. A recent letter by Maher and colleagues[44] describes six more patients (three after ICSI and three after IVF) in a Beckwith–Wiedemann syndrome register in the UK, representing a three-fold increase in the expected number of patients with this syndrome.

Recently, Moll and co-workers found that a higher relative risk (from 4.9 to 7.2) for retinoblastoma, another disease related to imprinting, was associated with IVF in The Netherlands, based on a register of retinoblastoma patients[45]. On the basis of all these findings, sufficient evidence exists to suggest that some aspects of the ICSI procedure may increase the frequency of epigenetic anomalies leading to congenital malformation syndromes. As all imprinting disorders are rare disorders (Beckwith–Wiedemann syndrome affects approximately 1/15 000 newborns, Angelman syndrome affects approximately 1/30 000 newborns, Prader–Willi syndrome affects 1/15 000, retinoblastoma 1/17 000) a large sample size is needed to detect minor increases. Given the known association between Beckwith–Wiedemann syndrome, cancer and an increased frequency of H19 methylation abnormalities, we can postulate that ART is associated with embryonic cancers of childhood where methylation abnormalities have been implicated. Since the incidence of cancer in children with Beckwith–Wiedemann syndrome aged less than 4

years is 0.02 per 110 patient years, these problems would be expected from the moment the patient groups become sufficiently large and when follow-up is beyond the neonatal period (approximately 1/1000 at the age of 5 years).

From all these data we can conclude that there is evidence an increased risk of imprinting disorders in ICSI children and that childhood cancers might be associated with this, but only a few observations in the literature provide data on possible frequencies of these events. Only a systematic survey aimed at those syndromes/diseases which have a known, defined phenotype linked to imprinted genes may clarify whether epigenetic anomalies play a role in ICSI (and IVF) more often than in the general population. In both reports on the Angelman syndrome and on the Beckwith–Wiedemann syndrome, it is the maternal allele that is affected (unmethylated). This makes it unlikely that the problem is related to sperm differentiation and more likely that ICSI or some other aspects of the ART used disturbs methylation in the maternal genome or early embryo. Further biological studies are required in order to understand the pathogenesis of these events and to investigate whether precautions can be taken to prevent their occurrence.

CONCLUSIONS

Most of the recent IVF and ICSI studies indicate that there is a slightly higher risk of congenital malformations in the ART population in comparison with a control group of the general population. This risk seems to be related to the parental background, to influencing factors such as a higher maternal age, a lower parity, a longer period of infertility prior to conception and maternal pre-existing disease. The more influencing factors the studies are controlled for, the lower the residual risk of major malformations in the children. However, none of the studies performed an extensive analysis of the parental genetic background, expressed as, for example, numbers of miscarriages, malformations in the parents or in previous children and first-degree relatives and genetic underlying diseases in the parents. There is more evidence that all these influencing factors determine the differences found in the literature between ICSI, IVF and the naturally conceived children, than are determined by the procedures themselves. Parents should be told that a possible effect of the ART techniques cannot be excluded, but that it is probably far less important than the underlying sociodemographic, medical and genetic parental background. If a major malformation is estimated (following a certain definition and methodology) to be present in approximately 2.5% of the newborns, then in ICSI or IVF children a risk of 3.5% is to be given. Moreover, there could be a very low risk of rare diseases related to imprinting disorders that has to be further elucidated. Extensive counseling and searching for individual risk factors can help to modify the individual risk for each couple. More research is also needed in order to evaluate the importance of the different influencing factors.

ACKNOWLEDGEMENTS

Vera Van Beneden for helping with the references and Julie Deconinck for reviewing the manuscript are kindly acknowledged.

REFERENCES

1. Cohen J, Mayaux MJ, Guihard-Moscarao L. Pregnancy outcomes after *in vitro* fertilisation. A collaborative study on 2342 pregnancies. *Ann NY Acad Sci* 1988;541:1–6

2. National Perinatal Statistics Unit and Fertility Society of Australia. *IVF and GIFT Pregnancies: Australia and New Zealand, 1987*. Sidney: Sidney National Perinatal Statistics Unit, 1988

3. Beral V, Doyle P. Report of the MRC Working Party on Children Conceived by *In Vitro* Fertilization. Births in Great Britain resulting from assisted conception, 1978–87. *Br Med J* 1990;300:1229–33

4. Lancaster PAL. Congenital malformations after *in vitro* fertilization. *Lancet* 1987;1392:3

5. Bergh T, Ericson A, Hillensjo T, *et al*. Deliveries and children born after *in-vitro* fertilisation in Sweden 1982–95: a retrospective cohort study. *Lancet* 1999;354:1579–85

6. Ericson A, Källén B. Congenital malformations in infants born after IVF: a population based study. *Hum Reprod* 2001;16:504–9

7. Hansen M, Kurinczuk JJ, Bower C, Webb S. The risk of major birth defects after intracytoplasmic sperm injection and *in vitro* fertilization. *N Engl J Med* 2002;345:725–30

8. Palermo GP, Joris H, Devroey P, Van Steirteghem AC. Pregnancies after intracytoplasmic sperm injection of single spermatozoon into an oocyte. *Lancet* 1992;340:17–18

9. Van Steirteghem A, Liu J, Joris H, *et al*. Higher success rate by intracytoplasmic sperm injection than by subzonal insemination. Report of a second series of 300 consecutive treatment cycles. *Hum Reprod* 1993;8:1055–60

10. Bonduelle M, Camus M, De Vos A, *et al*. Seven years of intracytoplasmic sperm injection and follow-up of 1987 subsequent children. *Hum Reprod* 1999;14:243–64

11. Bonduelle M, Legein J, Buysse A, *et al*. Prospective follow-up study of 423 children born after intracytoplasmic sperm injection. *Hum Reprod* 1996;11:1558–64

12. Kurinczuk JJ, Bower C. Birth defects conceived by intracytoplasmic injection: an alternative interpretation. *Br Med J* 1997;7118:1260–65;discussion 1265–6

13. ESHRE Task Force on Intracytoplasmic Sperm Injection. European Society for Human Reproduction and Embryology. Assisted reproduction by intracytoplasmic sperm injection: a survey on the clinical experience in 1994 and the children born after ICSI, carried out until 31 December 1993. *Hum Reprod* 1998;13:1737–46

14. Loft A, Petersen K, Erb K, *et al*. A Danish national cohort of 730 infants born after

intracytoplasmic sperm injection (ICSI) 1994–1997. *Hum Reprod* 1999;14:2143–8

15. Wennerholm UB, Bergh C, Hamberger L, *et al*. Obstetric outcome of pregnancies following ICSI, classified according to sperm origin and quality. *Hum Reprod* 2000;15:1189–94

16. Wennerholm UB, Bergh C, Hamberger L, *et al*. Incidence of congenital malformations in children born after ICSI. *Hum Reprod* 2000;15:944-8

17. Ludwig M, Katalinic A. Malformation rate in fetuses and children conceived after intracytoplasmic sperm injection (ICSI): results of a prospective cohort study. *Reprod BioMed Online* 2002;5:171–8

18. Young LE, Fernandes K, Mc Evoy TG, *et al*. Epigenetic change in IGF2R is associated with fetal overgrowth after sheep embryo culture. *Nature Genet* 2001;27:153–4

19. Bonduelle M, Liebaers I, Deketelaere V, *et al*. Neonatal data on a cohort of 2889 infants born after intracytoplasmic sperm injection (ICSI) (1991–1999) and of 2995 infants born after *in vitro* fertilization (IVF) (1983–1999). *Hum Reprod* 2002;17:671–94

20. Sakkas D, Moffatt O, Manicardi GC, *et al*. Nature of DNA damage in ejaculated human spermatozoa and the possible involvement of apoptosis. *Biol Reprod* 2002;66:1061–7

21. Van Dyck Q, Lanzendorf S, Kolm P, *et al*. Incidence of aneuploid spermatozoa from subfertile men: selected with motility versus hemizona-bound. *Hum Reprod* 2000;15:1529–36

22. Engel W, Murphy D, Schmid M. Are there genetic risks associated with microassisted reproduction? *Hum Reprod* 1996;11:2359–70

23. St John JC. The transmission of mitochondrial DNA following assisted reproductive techniques. *Theriogenology* 2002;57:109-23

24. Marchington DR, Scott Brown MS, Lamb VK, *et al*. No evidence for paternal mtDNA transmission to offspring or extra-embryonic tissues after ICSI. *Mol Hum Reprod* 2002;11:1046–9

25. Simpson JL. Registration of congenital anomalies in ART populations: pitfalls. *Hum Reprod* 1996;11:4

26. Meschede D, Lemcke B, Behre HM, *et al*. Non-reproductive heritable disorders in infertile couples and their first degree relatives. *Hum Reprod* 2000;15:1609–12

27. Mills JL, Simpson JL, Rhoads GG, *et al*. Risk of neural tube defects in relation to maternal fertility and fertility drug use. *Lancet* 1990;336:103–4

28. Palermo G, Colombero L, Schattman G, *et al*. Evolution of pregnancies and initial follow-up of newborns delivered after intracytoplasmic sperm injection. *J Am Med Assoc* 1996;276:1893–7

29. *Manual of the International Statistical Classification of Diseases, Injuries and Causes of Death (ICD). Based on the 10th Revision Conference.* Geneva: World Health Organisation, 1992

30. EUROCAT Report 7. *15 Years of Surveillance of Congenital Anomalies in Europe 1980–1994.* Brussels: Eurocat Central Registry, Institute of Hygiene and Epidemiology Brussels, 1997

31. Leppig KA, Werler MM, Cann CI, *et al*. Predictive value of minor anomalies, association with major anomalies. *J Pediatr* 1987;110:531–7

32. Myrianthopoulos NC, Chung CS. Congenital malformations in singletons: epidemiological survey. Report from the Collaborative Perinatal project. *Birth Defects Orig Artic Ser* 1974;10:1–58

33. Aase JM. *Diagnostic Dysmorphology*. New York: Textbook Plenum Medical Book Company, 1990

34. Aylward P, Hatcher R, Stripp B, *et al.* Who goes and who stays: subject loss in a multicenter, longitudinal follow-up study. *J Dev Behav Pediatr* 1985;6:3–8

35. Westergaard H, Tranberg B, Johansen AM, *et al.* Danish National *In-Vitro* Fertilization Registry 1994 and 1995: a controlled study of births, malformations and cytogenetic findings. *Hum Reprod* 1999;14:1896–902

36. Anthony S, Buitendijk SE, Dorrepaal CA, *et al.* Congenital malformations in 4224 children conceived after IVF. *Hum Reprod* 2002;17:2089–95

37. Ludwig *et al.*, 2003; in press

38. Bonduelle M, Van Assche E, Joris H, *et al.* Prenatal testing in ICSI pregnancies: incidence of chromosomal anomalies in 1,586 karyotypes and relation to sperm parameters. *Hum Reprod* 2002;17:2600–14

39. Vernaeve V, Bonduelle M, Tournaye H, *et al.* Pregnancy outcome and neonatal data of children born after ICSI using testicular sperm in obstructive and non-obstructive azoospermia. *Hum Reprod* 2003;18:1–5

40. Cox GF, Burger J, Lip V, *et al.* Intracytoplasmic sperm injection may increase the risk of imprinting defects. *Am J Hum Genet* 2002;71:162–4

41. Sutcliffe AG, D'Souza SW, Cadman J, *et al.* Outcome in children from cryopreserved embryos. *Arch Dis Child* 1995;72:290–3

42. Olivennes F, Mannaerts B, Struijs M, *et al.* Perinatal outcome of pregnancy after GnRH antagonist (ganirelix) treatment during ovarian stimulation for conventional IVF or ICSI: a preliminary report. *Hum Reprod* 2001;16:1588–91

43. DeBaun MR, Niemitz EL, Feinberg AP. Association of *in vitro* fertilization with Beckwith–Wiedemann syndrome and epigenetic alterations of LIT1 and H19. *Am J Hum Genet* 2003;72:156–60

44. Maher ER, Brueton LA, Bowdin SC, *et al.* Beckwith–Wiedemann syndrome and assisted reproduction technology (ART). *J Med Genet* 2003;40:62–4

45. Moll AC, Imhof SM, Cruysberg JR, *et al.* Incidence of retinoblastoma in children born after *in-vitro* fertilisation. *Lancet* 2003;361:273–4

21

Miscellaneous risks and complications

P. De Sutter

INTRODUCTION

Assisted reproductive technologies (ART) such as *in vitro* fertilization (IVF) and intracytoplasmic sperm injection (ICSI) are not at all free of risks. This chapter will not deal with the problem of multiple pregnancies, nor with the ovarian hyperstimulation syndrome (OHSS) and its specific complications. These two major problems related to ART are dealt with extensively elsewhere in this volume. This chapter will discuss miscellaneous risks and complications of ART, those that occur less frequently but may be as severe or even more severe than the two other mentioned complications.

Venn and colleagues have recently screened a large cohort of IVF patients for mortality in a large national registry and compared them with control patients[1]. They found that IVF patients were less likely to die than expected (OR 0.58; 95% CI 0.48–0.69) and they attributed this to a 'healthy patient effect', meaning that the unhealthiest women in the population are deterred from pregnancy and infertility treatment. Also, the socioeconomic status of women undergoing IVF may be higher than average. Whatever the bias, when one looks at the data from this Australian study in 29 700 IVF patients, it does not seem that IVF contains a direct threat to life.

OVERVIEW OF MISCELLANEOUS RISKS AND COMPLICATIONS

Table 1 shows an overview of various large studies published in the literature on risks and complications of ART[2–6]. The values are remarkably consis-

Table 1   Literature data on complication rates after assisted reproductive technologies

Author	Baber et al. (1988)[2]	Bergh and Lundkvist (1992)[3]	Roest et al. (1996)[4]	Serour et al. (1998)[5]	Govaerts et al. (1998)[6]
Number of cycles	600	10 125	2495	3500	1500
OHSS + hospitalization (%)	—	0.7	0.7	1.7	1.8
Serious bleeding (%)	1.3	0.7	—	0.1	0.2
Adnexal torsion (%)	—	—	0.1	—	0.1
Postoperative infection (%)	0.5	0.3	0.3	0.3	0.4
Total (%)	1.8	1.7	1.1	2.1	2.5

tent, and the average complication rate as calculated from these five studies is 1.8% (321/18 220), including hospitalizations from OHSS. If this complication is omitted, the incidence of miscellaneous complications related to ART becomes 0.8% (147/18 220). In none of these series were casualties directly related to the stimulation, nor to the IVF procedure itself, reported. In the series of Serour and co-workers, in 3500 cycles one mortality case was reported following hepatorenal failure in a patient with OHSS[5]. Although mortality is of course the most severe of all possible complications, and probably rare and even more rarely reported, other complications do occur as a result of ART. In general, one may distinguish between the risks related to the ovarian stimulation, the egg retrieval, or the pregnancy itself. Although severe complications are relatively uncommon, they may be potentially life threatening.

RISKS RELATED TO THE OVARIAN STIMULATION

Thrombosis

OHSS is by far the most important risk of ART stimulation, being responsible for a 1% hospitalization rate. OHSS and its possible lethal thrombotic complications will not be discussed further here (see Chapters 12 and 13). However, thrombotic complications related to ovarian stimulation have been described in the absence of OHSS.

Ludwig and associates recently described a patient with activated protein C (APC) resistance who developed deep calf vein thrombosis on the 8th day of human menopausal gonadotropin (hMG) administration[7]. Another patient with antithrombin III deficiency developed a massive deep vein thrombosis as a result of ovarian stimulation for ART[8]. Thrombosis is always the result of hypercoagulability and/or defective anticoagulant mechanisms. Rising estradiol levels may lead to increased liver fibrinogen synthesis and thus to a thrombophilic predisposition in all stimulated women[9]. If a patient has APC resistance or antithrombin III deficiency, she has an increased thrombotic risk. Also, the usage of a high-dose oral contraceptive pill prior to the stimulation cycle, in order to synchro-

nize the treatment, may be a risk factor in such patients. Proper family and personal history taking and, in selected cases, heparin prophylaxis may prevent thrombotic events in such patients who are known to be at risk. One should not forget that the risk continues to be increased during pregnancy as well, and some cases have been reported of thrombotic events during the first trimester of an ART pregnancy[10,11].

Seligsohn and Lubetsky have recently reviewed all inherited causes for thrombophilia and they advise screening all women pursuing treatment for infertility if they have a personal or family history of venous thrombosis[12]. They also propose screening if the women have had three unexplained miscarriages in the past, abruptio placentae, stillbirth, recurrent fetal growth restriction or possibly pre-eclampsia.

Inadvertent exposure to gonadotropin releasing hormone agonists

The introduction of gonadotropin releasing hormone (GnRH) analogs has revolutionized the practice of ART. The use of GnRH analogs has significantly decreased cancellation rates and increased ART efficiency. Most programs use the long protocol and start administering the analog prior to the start of gonadotropin injections, during the midluteal phase of the previous cycle. The result of this practice is that inadvertent exposure of a spontaneously occurring early pregnancy to the analog may take place. GnRH analogs usually have a long half-life and may thus be present in the circulation at the time of early organ formation. In monkeys no teratogenic effects were observed when a single bolus injection of the analog was administered to pregnant mothers[13]. After continuous GnRH analog exposure for a long time, testes of male infants were significantly lighter in the monkey.

Since the start of the use of GnRH analogs, many authors have reported on the outcome of such spontaneous pregnancies[14–17]. Plateau and associates reviewed a total of 453 pregnancies and 383 liveborn babies from the literature[18]. There were in total eight congenital abnormalities (2.1%), which is not different from the rate in the general population. Lahat and colleagues, on the other hand, found neurodevelopmental abnormalities at school age in four out of six children born after GnRH analog administration in early pregnancy[19]. Although these data were not completely convincing, it is clear that the discussion is not yet closed and that more long-term data have to be collected[20]. Administration of the analog while the women is on an oral contraceptive pill, the use of a short GnRH agonist protocol, and finally avoiding the agonist completely or using a GnRH antagonist circumvents this risk.

COMPLICATIONS FOLLOWING OOCYTE RETRIEVAL

These complications mainly follow from puncturing a blood vessel, from traumatizing an anatomically related structure (bowel, ureter) or from introducing an infection into the peritoneal cavity. Bleeding and infections both occur in < 1% of all ultrasound-guided oocyte retrievals (Table 1). Dicker and colleagues reported a total of 14 out of 3656 (0.4%) patients presenting with an acute abdomen after transvaginal oocyte puncture, due to pelvic infection or bleeding[21].

Bennett and co-workers reviewed 2670 ultrasound-directed transvaginal follicle puncture procedures and they reported 8.6% of cases of vaginal hemorrhage, with significant blood loss (> 100 ml) in 0.8%[22]. In two cases (0.1%) they recorded retroperitoneal bleeding from the ovary and in one case this necessitated an emergency laparotomy. In one case an iliac vessel was punctured but the resulting pelvic hematoma settled without intervention. Azem and co-workers reported a case of massive retroperitoneal bleeding from the sacral vein, necessitating an emergency laparotomy[23]. To reduce the risks of hemorrhage at the time of oocyte retrieval, Serour and colleagues advised limiting vaginal punctures to two, visualizing the peripheral follicles with ultrasound in a cross section before the puncture and using color Doppler if available[5]. The vaginal blood loss 24 h after complicated ultrasound-guided transvaginal oocyte pick-up was calculated by Dessole and co-workers to be around 230 ml[24]. These authors described a drop in hematocrit of up to 5% or of hemoglobin of 1.6 g% as normal. They concluded that if the blood loss is estimated to be normal, according to their calculation method, any postoperative acute abdomen must be infectious in origin.

In another series, postoperative pelvic infection occurred in 0.6% of cases, half of which were severe, with the formation of a pelvic abscess[22]. Although in this series there was no increased risk for infection in patients with severe pelvic damage resulting from endometriosis or previous pelvic inflammatory disease (PID), the authors advised avoidance of puncturing endometriomas, pseudocysts or hydrosalpinges during egg collection procedures. They did not recommend routine use of antibiotic prophylaxis during transvaginal oocyte retrieval, although other authors do[21,25].

Ovarian abscesses following oocyte retrieval usually contain a mixture of bacteria. Although *Escherichia coli*, *Bacillus fragilis* or enterococcus may be found, often cultures remain negative. Sometimes abscesses are asymptomatic and remain unrecognized or are diagnosed only during pregnancy or at the time of Cesarean section[26]. Well known is the risk of abscess formation by accidental puncture of an endometriotic cyst. Younis and associates described three patients in whom acute PID occurred 3–6 weeks after oocyte retrieval[27]. In all three cases it was thought that inoculation of the endometrioma occurred at the time of the pick-up, and that the delay between infection and symptoms was due to the slow growth of the bacteria in the blood cyst. These authors cautioned against the aspiration of endometriotic cysts at the time of oocyte collection.

They also pointed out that antibiotic prophylaxis may not be effective in these patients because of the pseudocapsule surrounding the endometrioma, so that antibiotics may not reach the inoculum. Since abscesses after transabdominal puncture have never been described, it may be safer to perform a laparoscopic pick-up in patients with severe endometriosis, to avoid transvaginal inoculation. Another dramatic case of a pelvic abscess following ART was described in which rupture of the abscess occurred at the end of the second trimester of a twin pregnancy, with loss of the pregnancy and fetal death as a result[28].

To avoid the risk of infection, some authors have studied the use of vaginal disinfection prior to transvaginal oocyte puncture. Van Os and co-workers demonstrated, in a prospective randomized trial, that vaginal disinfection with povidone iodine (Betadine®) decreased pregnancy rates (17.2% versus 30.3% clinical pregnancies per embryo transfer), probably because of an embryotoxic effect[29,30]. Disinfection of the vagina therefore does not seem advisable.

A few case reports have been written on rare infectious complications following transvaginal oocyte retrieval. One paper has described an accidental puncturing of the appendix at the time of oocyte pick-up, followed by clinical appendicitis leading to surgery[31]. At inspection of the appendix the puncturing holes could even be recognized! Another case mentions a pyosalpinx developing after oocyte pick-up in a woman with tubal facor infertility undergoing ART. The woman presented with fever and abdominal pain a day after embryo transfer and was treated conservatively with antibiotics[32]. These authors pointed out that this complication resulted from activation of a quiescent tubal infection, bowel puncture, or inoculation with vaginal flora during pick-up or during transfer. It is perhaps wise to avoid aspirating obvious hydrosalpinges at the time of pick-up or to administer prophylactic antibiotics to patients with postinfectious tubal infertility. It has been shown that it is advantageous to IVF outcome to remove the hydrosalpinges before starting IVF, but this is another topic. Also, after embryo transfer without previous oocyte retrieval, as in oocyte donation or frozen/thawed cycles, pelvic infection has been described, although it is an extremely rare event[33].

Besides infections and bleeding, very few other complications have been described in the literature after transvaginal ultrasound-guided oocyte retrievals. One patient presented bradycardia and bradypnea after the pick-up as a possible toxic effect of paracervical mepivacaine[34]. Another woman developed vertebral osteomyelitis after puncturing of a vertebra by the needle tip and contamination from the vagina[35]. Recently a case of ureteral obstruction was published following transvaginal egg retrieval[36]. Another patient developed neurological signs in the left leg following compression of the lumbosacral plexus by a hematoma in the obturator space[37]. These are all unique case reports.

SPECIFIC PREGNANCY COMPLICATIONS AFTER ART

Ectopic pregnancy

Up to 4% of all IVF pregnancies are ectopic[38]. Ectopic pregnancies especially occur in patients with tubal disease. Strandell and colleagues performed a stepwise logistic regression analysis to identify risk factors for ectopic pregnancy after ART and they found that a previous myomectomy, besides tubal damage, was also a risk factor for ectopic pregnancy[38]. These authors suggested that changes in uterine contractility may contribute to the risk for ectopic implantation in patients who had had previous uterine surgery. Another risk factor for ectopic pregnancy seems to be the difficulty of the transfer. Difficult transfer may provoke more uterine contractions, which may increase the chance for an embryo to relocate into the tube. Lesny and co-workers reported an OR for ectopic pregnancy of 3.91 (95% CI 1.49–10.23) for difficult transfers compared with easy transfers, but there could have been a bias, in that difficult transfers may be related to post-infectious sequelae[39]. Interestingly, the increased risk after difficult transfers only held for day-2 transfers, but not for day-3 transfers. The authors explained their findings by the fact that junctional zone contractions may be less pronounced on day 3, because of the 'soothing' effect of progesterone on uterine contractility.

Heterotopic pregnancy

Typically for IVF are heterotopic pregnancies, which present an even higher risk because of the danger of not being recognized early[40]. A relatively recent review mentions the same risk factors as for ectopic pregnancy (especially tubal disease) in conjunction with a high number of transferred embryos[41]. Although two embryos could in theory suffice to lead to a heterotopic pregnancy, the more embryos that are transferred, the higher the risk[42]. The risk is estimated to be as high as 1–3% of all ART gestations, but one may hope that this rate will drop in parallel with a drop in the number of transferred embryos. In the above-mentioned review, in 88.2% of cases the intrauterine pregnancy was combined with a tubal pregnancy, in 6.3% with a cornual, in

2.7% with an abdominal, in 1.8% with a cervical and in 0.9% with an ovarian pregnancy. This last implantation site has recently been correlated with the transfer of blastocysts, but the pathophysiological link between both is unclear[43].

Because of the vital intrauterine pregnancy, diagnosis of a heterotopic pregnancy is often delayed and patients usually present with symptoms of abdominal pain, vaginal bleeding and often shock, because of rupture of the ectopic pregnancy[44]. One report describes a case in which the first symptom was rectal bleeding because of erosion of the intestinal wall by an abdominal pregnancy[45]. Ultrasound and monitoring of human chorionic gonadotropin (hCG) do not help to diagnose a heterotopic pregnancy; in almost all instances diagnosis is suspected only when symptoms occur. However, in this series no mortality was recorded and 72.5% of the involved pregnancies ended with the birth of a live baby. These authors advocate surgery to remove the ectopic pregnancy and do not favor methotrexate or potassium chloride injection in the ectopic gestational sac under ultrasound guidance, as described by Guirgis[46].

Interstitial pregnancy

The cornual or interstitial pregnancy is quite common following ART. Such ectopic localization, occurring alone or combined with an intrauterine gestational sac, represents about 2–6% of all ectopic localizations[41]. The diagnosis is difficult, and often delayed. A cornual implantation may lead to loss of the pregnancy and, on rare occasions, even to hysterectomy because of uterine rupture, hemorrhage and shock. Interstitial pregnancies typically occur in patients having undergone salpingectomy[47,48]. They necessitate a high index of suspicion and close follow-up to avoid obstetric catastrophes[49,50]. Even in the absence of a cornual pregnancy, salpingectomy itself represents a risk factor for rupturing of the uterus in an ongoing intrauterine pregnancy in the second or third trimester.[51]

Bilateral ectopic pregnancy

Bilateral ectopic pregnancies have been reported but remain an extremely rare event, even after ART. They are more easily diagnosed than heterotopic pregnancies, but sometimes in two steps, leading to two interventions[52]. The lesson here is always to inspect the whole abdomen and pelvis, especially the contralateral tube, when performing laparoscopy for an ectopic pregnancy[53]. 'Look beyond the most obvious diagnosis and always expect the unexpected' – this is also the adage of a case report describing a simultaneous rupturing of a tubal pregnancy together with acute appendicitis in a patient who furthermore had an ongoing intrauterine twin pregnancy[54]. Another extraordinary case was described by Ludwig and co-workers[55]. They reported a patient with an ovarian abscess after ovarian puncture of a cyst, followed by a heterotopic triplet pregnancy (one tubal and two intrauterine) after transfer of three embryos.

Adnexal torsion

Another complication that occurs in pregnancies after hormonal hyperstimulation is adnexal torsion. In the series of Roest and associates the incidence was around 0.1%[4]. Kemmann and colleagues reviewed 1303 women who had a total of 6919 gonadotropin-induced cycles[56]. Four women developed adnexal torsion, all of whom were pregnant, representing an incidence of 1 in 162 pregnancies. In patients developing OHSS, however, the incidence of adnexal torsion seems to be much higher. Mashiach and co-workers reported an overall incidence of adnexal torsion of 7.5% in patients with OHSS[57]. Torsion of a stimulated ovary can be managed by laparoscopic untwisting, even when the ovary seems to have become ischemic. Long-term follow-up of patients after laparoscopic detorsion of an apparently non-viable ovary has revealed a normal ovarian appearance at subsequent surgery, with normal function[58]. Before detorsion, it may be necessary to aspirate as much fluid as possible, which allows safe rotation of the ovary without any damage. Another approach may be transvaginal aspiration of the cysts to relieve the tension on the ovarian pedicle. The outcome of these procedures is usually excellent, and normally the pregnancy remains unaffected[59,60].

Maternal mortality

If the IVF pregnancy is ongoing, maternal mortality still is twice as high as in the general population (25.7/100 000 as compared to 10.9/100 000)[1]. This is probably a consequence mainly of the high incidence of multiple pregnancies and of other patient-related obstetric risk factors, such as age. Complications of ART pregnancies in the second and third trimesters are, however, beyond the scope of this overview.

REFERENCES

1. Venn A, Hemminki E, Watson L, *et al.* Mortality in a cohort of IVF patients. *Hum Reprod* 2001;16:2691–6

2. Baber R, Porter R, Picker R, *et al.* Transvaginal ultrasound directed oocyte collection for *in vitro* fertilization: successes and complications. *J Ultrasound Med* 1988;7:377–9

3. Bergh T, Lundkvist O. Clinical complications during *in-vitro* fertilization treatment. *Hum Reprod* 1992;7:625–6

4. Roest J, Mous H, Zeilmaker G, *et al.* The incidence of major clinical complications in a Dutch transport IVF programme. *Hum Reprod Update* 1996;2:345–53

5. Serour GI, Aboulghar M, Mansour R, *et al.* Complications of medically assisted conception in 3,500 cycles. *Fertil Steril* 1998;70:638–42

6. Govaerts I, Devreker F, Delbaere A, *et al.* Short-term medical complications of 1500 oocyte retrievals for *in vitro* fertilization and embryo transfer. *Eur J Obstet Gynecol Reprod Biol* 1998;77: 239–43

7. Ludwig M, Felberbaum RE, Diedrich K. Deep vein thrombosis during administration of hMG for ovarian stimulation. *Arch Gynecol Obstet* 1999;263:139–41

8. Kligman I, Noyes N, Benavida CA, Rosenwaks Z. Massive deep vein thrombosis in a patient with antithrombin III deficiency undergoing ovarian stimulation for *in vitro* fertilization. *Fertil Steril* 1995;63:673–6

9. Harnett MJ, Bhavani-Shankar K, Datta S, Tsen LC. *In vitro* fertilization-induced alterations in coagulation and fibrinolysis as measured by thromboelastography. *Anesth Analg* 2002;95:1063–6

10. Belaen B, Geerinckx K, Vergauwe P, Thys J. Internal jugular vein thrombosis after ovarian stimulation. *Hum Reprod* 2001;16:510–12

11. Arya R, Shehata HA, Patel R, *et al.* Internal jugular vein thrombosis after assisted conception therapy. *Br J Haematol* 2001;115:153–5

12. Seligsohn U, Lubetsky A. Genetic susceptibility to venous thrombosis. *N Engl J Med* 2001;344:1222–31

13. Sopelak VM, Hodgen GD. Infusion of gonadotropin-releasing hormone agonist during pregnancy: maternal and fetal responses in primates. *Am J Obstet Gynecol* 1987;156:755–60

14. Shulman A, Shilon M, Bahary C, *et al.* Inadvertent exposure of early pregnancy to gonadotropin releasing hormone analogue. *J Assist Reprod Genet* 1993;10:387–91

15. Abu-Heija AT, Fleming R, Yates RW, Coutts JR. Pregnancy outcome following exposure to gonadotropin-releasing hormone analogue during early pregnancy: comparisons in patients with normal or elevated luteinizing hormone. *Hum Reprod* 1995;10:3317–19

16. Elefant E, Biour B, Blumberg-Tick B, *et al.* Administration of a gonadotropin-releasing hormone agonist during pregnancy: follow-up of 28 pregnancies exposed to triptoreline. *Fertil Steril* 1995;63:1111–13

17. Taskin O, Gokdeniz R, Atmaca R, Burak F. Normal pregnancy outcome after inadvertent exposure to long-acting gonadotrophin-releasing hormone agonist in early pregnancy. *Hum Reprod* 1999;14:1368–71

18. Platteau P, Gabbe M, Famelos M, *et al.* Should we still advise infertile couples to use (barrier) contraception before IVF down-regulation? *Fertil Steril* 2000;74:655–9

19. Lahat E, Raziel A, Friedler S, *et al.* Long-term follow-up of children born after inadvertent administration of a gonadotrophin-releasing hormone agonist in early pregnancy. *Hum Reprod* 1999;14:2656–60

20. Platteau P, Vandervorst M, Devroey P. Long-term follow-up of children born after inadvertent administration of a gonadotrophin-releasing hormone agonist in early pregnancy [letter]. *Hum Reprod* 2000;15:1421

21. Dicker D, Ashkenazi J, Feldberg D, *et al.* Severe abdominal complications after transvaginal ultrasonographically guided retrieval of oocytes for *in vitro* fertilization and embryo transfer. *Fertil Steril* 1993;59:1313–15

22. Bennett SJ, Waterstone JJ, Cheng WC, Parsons J. Complications of transvaginal ultrasound-directed follicle aspiration: a review of 2670 consecutive procedures. *J Assist Reprod Genet* 1993;10:72–7

23. Azem F, Wolf Y, Botchan A, *et al.* Massive retroperitoneal bleeding: a complication of transvaginal ultrasonography-guided oocyte retrieval for *in vitro* fertilization–embryo transfer. *Fertil Steril* 2000;74:405–6

24. Dessole S, Rubattu G, Ambrosini G, *et al.* Blood loss following noncomplicated transvaginal oocyte retrieval for *in vitro* fertilization. *Fertil Steril* 2001;76:205–6

25. Meldrum DR. Antibiotics for vaginal oocyte aspiration. *J In Vitro Fert Embryo Transf* 1989;6:1–2

26. Zweemer RP, Scheele F, Verheijen RHM, *et al.* Ovarian abscess during pregnancy mimicking a leiomyoma of the uterus: a complication of transvaginal ultrasound-guided oocyte aspiration. *J Assist Reprod Genet* 1996;13:81–5

27. Younis JS, Ezra Y, Laufer N, Ohel G. Late manifestation of pelvic abscess following oocyte retrieval, for *in vitro* fertilization, in patients with severe endometriosis and ovarian endometriomata. *J Assist Reprod Genet* 1997;14:343–6

28. Den Boon J, Kimmel CEJM, Nagel HTC, van Roosmalen J. Pelvic abscess in the second half of pregnancy after oocyte retrieval for *in-vitro* fertilization. *Hum Reprod* 1999;14:2402–3

29. Van Os HC, Roozenburg BJ, Janssen-Caspers HAB, *et al.* Vaginal disinfection with povidon iodine and the outcome of *in-vitro* fertilization. *Hum Reprod* 1992;7:349–50

30. Gembruch U, Diedrich K, Al-Hasani S, *et al.* Die transvaginale, sonographisch gesteuerte Follikelpunction. *Geburtshilfe Frauenheilkd* 1988;48:617–24

31. Van Hoorde GJJ, Verhoeff A, Zeilmaker GH. Perforated appendicitis following transvaginal oocyte retrieval for *in-vitro* fertilization and embryo transfer. *Hum Reprod* 1992;7:850–1

32. Peters AJ, Hecht B, Durinzi K, *et al.* Salpingitis or oophoritis: what causes fever following oocyte aspiration and embryo transfer? *Obstet Gynecol* 1993;81:876–7

33. Friedler S, Ben-Shachar I, Abramov Y, *et al.* Ruptured tubo-ovarian abscess complicating transcervical cryopreserved embryo transfer. *Fertil Steril* 1996;65:1065–6

34. Ayestaran C, Matorras R, Gomez S, *et al.* Severe bradycardia and bradypnea following vaginal oocyte retrieval: a possible toxic effect of paracervical mepivacaine. *Eur J Obstet Gynecol Reprod Biol* 2000;91:71–3

35. Almog B, Rimon E, Yovel I, *et al.* Vertebral osteomyelitis: a rare complication of transvaginal ultrasound-guided oocyte retrieval. *Fertil Steril* 2000;73:1250–2

36. Miller PB, Price T, Nichols JE Jr, Hill L. Acute ureteral obstruction following transvaginal oocyte retrieval for IVF. *Hum Reprod* 2002;17:137–8

37. Van Eenige MM, Scheele F, Van Haaften M, *et al.* A case of neurological complication after transvaginal oocyte retrieval. *J Assist Reprod Genet* 1997;14:21–2

38. Strandell A, Thorburn J, Hamberger L. Risk factors for ectopic pregnancy in assisted reproduction. *Fertil Steril* 1999;71:282–6

39. Lesny P, Killick SR, Robinson J, Maguiness SD. Transcervical embryo transfer as a risk factor for ectopic pregnancy. *Fertil Steril* 1999;72:305–9

40. Tal J, Haddad S, Gordon N, Timor-Tritsch I. Heterotopic pregnancy after ovulation induction and assisted reproductive technologies: a literature review from 1971 to 1993. *Fertil Steril* 1996;66:1–12

41. Rojansky N, Schenker JG. Heterotopic pregnancy and assisted reproduction – an update. *J Assist Reprod Genet* 1996;13:594–601

42. Tummon IS, Whitmore NA, Daniel SA, *et al.* Transferring more embryos increases risk of heterotopic pregnancy. *Fertil Steril* 1994;61:1065–7

43. Oliveira FG, Abdelmassih V, Costa ALE, *et al.* Rare association of ovarian implantation site for patients with heterotopic and with primary ectopic pregnancies after ICSI and blastocyst transfer. *Hum Reprod* 2001;16:2227–9

44. Oliveira FG, Abdelmassih V, Abdelmassih Oliveira S, *et al.* Heterotopic triplet pregnancy: report and video of a case of a ruptured tubal implantation with living embryo concurrent with an intrauterine twin gestation. *Reprod Biomed Online* 2002;5:313–16

45. Fisch B, Powsner E, Heller L, *et al.* Heterotopic abdominal pregnancy following *in-vitro* fertilization/embryo transfer presenting as a massive lower gastrointestinal bleeding. *Hum Reprod* 1995;10:681–2

46. Guirgis RR. Simultaneous intrauterine and ectopic pregnancies following *in-vitro* fertilization and gamete intra-Fallopian transfer. A review of nine cases. *Hum Reprod* 1990;5:484–6

47. Chen CD, Chen SU, Chao KH, *et al.* Cornual pregnancy after IVF-ET. A report of three cases. *J Reprod Med* 1998;43:393–6

48. Dumesic DA, Damario MA, Session DR. Interstitial heterotopic pregnancy in a woman conceiving by *in vitro* fertilization after bilateral salpingectomy. *Mayo Clin Proc* 2001;76:90–2

49. Arbab F, Boulieu D, Bied V, *et al.* Uterine rupture in first or second trimester of pregnancy after *in vitro* fertilization and embryo transfer. *Hum Reprod* 1996;11:1120–2

50. Sills ES, Perloe M, Kaplan CR, *et al.* Uncomplicated pregnancy and normal singleton delivery after surgical excision of heterotopic (cornual) pregnancy following *in vitro* fertilization/embryo transfer. *Arch Gynecol Obstet* 2002;266:181–4

51. Inovay J, Marton T, Urbancsek J, *et al.* Spontaneous bilateral cornual uterine dehiscence early in the second trimester after bilateral laparoscopic salpingectomy and *in-vitro* fertilization. *Hum Reprod* 1999;14:2471–3

52. Sherman SJ, Werner M, Husain M. Bilateral ectopic gestations. *Int J Gynaecol Obstet* 1991;35:255–7

53. Klipstein S, Oskowitz SP. Bilateral ectopic pregnancy after transfer of two embryos. *Fertil Steril* 2000;74:887–8

54. Barnett A, Chipchase J, Hewitt J. Simultaneous rupturing heterotopic pregnancy and acute appendicitis in an *in-vitro*

fertilization twin pregnancy. *Hum Reprod* 1998;14:850–1

55. Ludwig M, Felberbaum RE, Bauer O, Diedrich K. Ovarian abscess and heterotopic triplet pregnancy: two complications after IVF in one patient. *Arch Gynecol Obstet* 1999;263:25–8

56. Kemmann E, Ghazi DM, Corsan GH. Adnexal torsion in menotropin-induced pregnancies. *Obstet Gynecol* 1990;76:403–6

57. Mashiach S, Goldenberg M, Bider D, *et al.* Adnexal torsion of hyperstimulated ovaries in pregnancies after gonadotropin therapy. *Fertil Steril* 1990;53:76–80

58. Ben-Rafael Z, Bider D, Mashiach S. Laparoscopic unwinding of twisted ischemic hemorrhagic adnexa after *in vitro* fertilization. *Fertil Steril* 1990;53:569–71

59. Pinto AB, Ratts VS, Williams DB, *et al.* Reduction of ovarian torsion 1 week after embryo transfer in a patient with bilateral hyperstimulated ovaries. *Fertil Steril* 2001;76: 403–6

60. Gorkemli H, Camus M, Clasen K. Adnexal torsion after gonadotrophin ovulation induction for IVF or ICSI and its conservative treatment. *Arch Gynecol Obstet* 2002;267:4–6

22

Psychological complications of assisted reproductive technologies

J. Boivin and J. Takefman

INTRODUCTION

The psychological and emotional aspects of using assisted reproductive technologies (ART), particularly *in vitro* fertilization (IVF), have been intensely studied since the first successes were recorded in the late 1970s and early 1980s. From a psychological perspective, the main complication arising from ART treatment is deterioration in life quality. The aim of this chapter is to summarize research from a variety of studies examining the effect of ART treatment on psychosocial well-being as well as the effect of psychosocial factors on ART progress and outcome.

ART psychology studies can be grouped broadly into three types. The very first studies sought to examine the psychological profiles of couples about to undergo ART. It was proposed that those using ART might be at high risk for further distress, because IVF was their final medical option, following many years of failure with traditional efforts. These studies helped to isolate risk factors that identified people who would be likely to react poorly to the treatment process and helped to develop pretreatment psychological screening processes. A second body of research investigated the emotional, physical and interpersonal reactions occurring during the ART procedure and after a failed ART cycle. The findings from these studies were important in showing that ART presented patients with unique psychological challenges and that reactions varied greatly over the course of this protracted treatment. However, unexpectedly, these studies demonstrated that ART was not exponentially more

stressful than other infertility treatments, in spite of the fact that these technologies are more complex. A final set of studies investigated the relationship between emotional reactions and the probability of pregnancy with IVF. These studies were important in showing that psychological factors were associated with the progress and outcome of ART treatments.

Before reviewing these three classes of studies it is important to point out their methodological limitations. First, most use only heterosexual couples in their sample. Second, IVF is the primary ART examined. Finally, the effects measured are of short duration following an ART cycle, as opposed to long-term follow-up.

PRE-TREATMENT PSYCHOSOCIAL PROFILING AND SCREENING

As was the case for the initial studies on infertility, initial studies on psychological aspects of ART investigated the psychological status of people about to begin IVF. Interest in this issue was based on the assumption that those embarking on ART treatment would be significantly distressed because of years of unsuccessful medical treatment, lack of other options to become parents and the demanding nature of IVF. Psychological screening and assessment prior to IVF was carried out in depth, with the main aims of such assessment being to evaluate individuals' capacity for parenthood and to identify those at risk for severe psychological distress during IVF.

Evaluating the capacity for parenthood

With respect to identifying couples for whom treatment might be contraindicated, fertility clinics generally operate with the belief that their role is not to decide who has access to treatment ('gatekeepers') but simply to provide fertility services for those who have barriers to conception. The ethical issues inherent in this position cannot be dealt with here. However, survey-type studies have shown that individual fertility clinics generally operate with some policies about who has access to treatment.

Leiblum and Williams carried out a survey with randomly selected members of a large fertility medical association in the USA[1]. The aim of the study was to identify whether fertility clinics had formal policies about excluding patients for treatment and to describe the common criteria that were used to do so. Although half the clinics did not acknowledge any official exclusion policy, all relied on an informal policy to select suitable candidates for treatment. Moreover, two-thirds of the clinics were more likely to apply exclusion criteria when the treatment involved donor gametes than when treatment was with the couple's own gametes. As for the most common exclusion variables, 50% or more of clinics refused treatment in couples where there was active substance abuse, current physical abuse, severe marital strife, the presence of a major personality disorder or severe intellectual impairment and in cases where it was apparent that one spouse was being coerced by the other to undergo treatment. The fact that most policies were unofficial, and that more stringent criteria were applied when donor gametes were used, highlights the fact that most clinics assume the 'gatekeeping' function only reluctantly and only when they may have some responsibility towards a third party (i.e. the donor of the gametes).

Overall, it is fair to conclude that the percentage of couples refused treatment is quite low. One author reported that of 100 patients seeking treatment with donor insemination only 2% were refused treatment, whereas another reported a 3% refusal rate in their sample of 835 couples[2,3]. Factors which influenced the decision about access to treatment in these studies were severe psychological disturbances (i.e. psychosis), severe marital discord

and coercion of one spouse by the other to undergo treatment. A percentage of couples in both these studies (about 20%) were conditionally accepted for treatment pending further psychological counseling. The factors that contributed to this counseling recommendation were ambivalence about using treatment in one or both spouses and stress management. It should be noted that the one exception to this low refusal rate is the case of single women who seek fertility treatment because they do not have a suitable partner. In this subpopulation, rejection rates are closer to 50%, mainly based on impoverished social relationships and psychological disturbance[4]. It is noteworthy that the above-mentioned studies were conducted almost a decade ago. With more couples from all walks of life now accessing fertility services, rejection rates may be rising.

Risk factors for *in vitro* fertilization

Studies on the psychological status of people about to begin IVF have revealed two important findings for those concerned with potential complications of ART. First, people about to begin IVF are psychologically normal; and second, people at risk for high distress can be identified prior to the start of treatment.

Results from survey studies show that couples about to begin ART are not more likely to experience greater anxiety, depression, psychiatric symptomatology, marital dissatisfaction or sexual dysfunction than other infertile or fertile couples. Using various methods to define highly distressed patients, only about 15–20% of all patients are identified, which is consistent with epidemiological surveys of depression in the general population[5]. Furthermore, the same percentage is reported for any infertile population demonstrating that people who choose to undergo ART are not at greater psychological risk than infertile individuals in general.

In light of these findings the principal function of pre-IVF psychological assessment is to identify individuals at risk for high distress during the procedure or following a treatment failure. Studies have identified some personal and social risk factors[6]. The personal risk factors include pre-existing psychopathology (e.g. personality disorder, depression), never having conceived in the past, being a woman, viewing parenting as a central life goal and the use of certain coping strategies (e.g. avoidance, wishful thinking). The social risk factors associated with high distress include a poor marital relationship and an impoverished social network. Excluding the variables related to parenting, these factors are well-known predictors of poor coping for any life crisis.

While these factors can individually predict high distress during IVF it is often a combination of factors that make the distress overwhelming. For example, being anxious before IVF will obviously make treatment more difficult but, combined with an unsupportive partner or social network, treatment can become unmanageable. Conversely, the risk posed by some factors, for example anxiety, may be mitigated by the presence of buffers such as a strong marital relationship and/or good social support.

Identifying people with high distress

Research studies have employed different methods to identify patients experiencing high distress. Some research identifies people based on exceptionally high scores on standardized inventories of psychiatric and psychological adjustment. Other research uses psychiatric diagnostic criteria (e.g. the Diagnostic and Statistical Manual (DSM-IV) in interviews, while self-reports of subjective distress are the basis of identification in other studies. Another method is to monitor people seeking psychological help from mental health professionals working with fertility clinics under the assumption that highly distressed patients will seek the help they need. As the take-up rate for counseling is similar to the incidence of high distress determined by other methods, this may be a reasonable assumption to make.

Although these methods are adequate, there is some indication in the research literature that infertility-specific measurement tools may be better at detecting high distress because they include items that are more representative of problems experienced by infertile people. In recent years a few infertility-specific measurement tools have been developed[7]. These tap into the need for parenthood, guilt, blame, negative self-image, infertility-specific negative affect and concerns related to social, marital and sexual domains. In addition, a new international measure of quality of life among infer-

tile people (FertiQoL) is now being developed that should not only identify those at risk for high distress during treatment, but also allow comparisons to be made among patients from different cultural groups and using different languages. Together, standardized and infertility-specific measurement tools should identify highly distressed patients.

Summary

Although there was concern about the psychological status of people about to begin ART treatment when these treatments first became available, it is now recognized that the rate of psychopathology in this population is more or less the same as that reported for all infertile patients and compared to the population in general. However, IVF is a demanding treatment and certain pre-treatment characteristics may identify those who are likely to experience difficulty during treatment and/or treatment failure. Once this subgroup is identified they can be offered psychoeducational interventions with the aim of ensuring that they are able to continue their pregnancy attempts while maintaining a reasonable quality of life.

EMOTIONAL, PHYSICAL, INTERPERSONAL AND GENDER-SPECIFIC REACTIONS DURING AND AFTER IVF

Emotional reactions

For the majority of couples, the main psychological repercussions of ART treatment will arise during treatment or when the outcome of treatment is known. Although negative reactions are considered appropriate, given this demanding treatment process and high rates of failure, they negatively impact on quality of life and therefore may be considered complications.

Psychological research has shown that reactions to IVF, for both men and women, are dependent on the stage of treatment and, as one might expect, its success or failure. Emotional reactions, especially anxiety and distress, increase just before each stage of IVF (e.g. stimulation, retrieval) and subsequently decrease to pre-treatment levels once the stage has been successfully completed[8,9]. The fluctuating nature of distress has been attributed to anticipatory anxiety with regard to the outcome of each stage. For example, couples worry about whether the woman will have a good response to superovulation medications, whether eggs will be retrieved and then fertilized and whether embryos will implant. These experimental findings measuring distress are consistent with couples' self-reports of mood during the IVF cycle. That is, mood alternates between elation and sadness, confidence and worry, and frustration and relief, depending on whether treatment is progressing well or not. Women's vigilance for any physical signs of pregnancy/lack of pregnancy during the implantation period may similarly cause cycles of hope or despair, depending on whether they feel pregnant or not at any given moment.

Some information is available on reactions when stages are unsuccessful and treatment must be abandoned. Reading found that patients whose treatment was cancelled mid-cycle, owing to a lack of oocytes or fertilization, experienced more anxiety compared to that of women who had had a failed pregnancy test[10]. Our own studies found that women who had less than the maximum number of embryos transferred experienced significantly more distress than those who had the maximum of three transferred[11]. The findings of severe levels of distress among women who experience a premature cancellation are clinically important, because such women are less likely to receive the same support as women who learn that treatment has been unsuccessful at the time of the negative pregnancy test.

Together these results suggest that it is not the intrusive or straining nature of the medical procedures per se that are stressful for couples, but the uncertainty and unpredictability at each stage of IVF. Some authors have suggested that uncertainty is one of the most difficult dimensions of life events because the coping strategies for anticipating an event's occurrence (pregnancy) are incompatible with those of an event's non-occurrence (lack of pregnancy)[12]. The necessity of considering both courses of action can thus lead to confusion, fear and excessive worrying or rumination[12]. This state of conflict is observed in couples undergoing IVF, especially during the 2-week waiting period. Many couples deal with uncertainty by developing the belief that one outcome is more likely than the other. Some might express their pessimism by offer-

ing different reasons for trying IVF even when they believe it will not be successful (e.g. 'get it out of my system', 'for peace of mind'). Others will express their optimism by identifying some factor that makes success more likely (e.g. proper diet, superstitious thoughts) even if the factor in question is not related to IVF success.

As would be expected, a negative pregnancy test is accompanied by feelings of distress, anxiety and hopelessness. The extent of distress in response to a negative pregnancy test, compared to other stages, confirms that what is hardest about IVF is its failure. A variety of reactions have been reported after treatment failure, including an acute period of depression, high anxiety and even suicidal ideation[13-15]. For most patients acute distress usually subsides within 3–4 weeks. However, for those who have made a final attempt or exhibit pre-existing psychological disorders, distress may persist for a longer period of time, with some studies reporting difficulties up to 18 months after treatment failure[15].

Physical reactions

One of the main sources of information concerning physical reactions to IVF is a controlled, prospective study in which women were asked to rate their reactions to IVF on a daily basis. Ratings were made for one IVF cycle and one menstrual cycle without fertility treatment[9]. Most physical changes were dependent on the stage of treatment, as was the case for emotional reactions, and most represented negative changes from usual levels of functioning.

The main physical complaints reflect the side-effects of drug therapy used during IVF. In particular, these include the experience of breast tenderness, ovarian pain, abdominal discomfort and bloating, which increases in concert with rising estradiol levels caused by ovarian stimulation[9]. However, an equally important symptom reported by women is low energy[9]. The need to schedule and manage both the practical demands of treatment (injections, scans, visits to the clinic) and those of daily life during the active stages of IVF often lead to significant fatigue as well as difficulty concentrating on work and social activities[9]. As would be expected, fatigue is greatest during the active stages of treatment (e.g. ovarian stimulation, retrieval and transfer) and lower during stages where the practical demands of treatment are lower (e.g. gonadal suppression, waiting period). Moreover, fatigue is greater among women than men, as the latter are less likely to attend the clinic as frequently and undergo as many procedures[16].

Marital functioning

Changes in the relationship between partners are also dependent on the stage. Past work would predict that marital functioning would deteriorate during IVF because of limited sources of social support (couples are reluctant to talk to others about their infertility) and because of the strain caused by the emotional and physical demands of IVF. However, daily monitoring of data has shown improved rather than declining functioning compared to pre-treatment, especially at the time of retrieval and embryo transfer[13]. During these stages, heightened feelings of closeness and intimacy are most often reported. We additionally showed that couples mainly coped in a positive way with the demands and outcome of treatment, for example through discussion and greater emotional involvement[16].

Convincing and consistent findings have been reported on the negative impact infertility in general has on a couple's sexual relationship, in terms of both sexual self-image and functioning. However, since ART practically requires no additional sexual demands on a couple compared to traditional therapies, it is widely accepted that sexual functioning is not further complicated by participation in ART *per se*. One exception is the additional stress put on the male partner to produce a semen specimen. Given the increased emotional and financial expense of IVF compared to, for example, artificial insemination (AI), the former procedure has been studied in terms of the impact of male performance anxiety on semen quality. These data are reviewed in a later section.

Gender differences

Overall, there is much evidence to show that women react more intensely to IVF than men. Research has shown that prior to treatment women compared to men report more anxiety and depression, less life satisfaction, lower self-esteem and greater anticipatory stress. A retrospective study showed that men and women also differ in terms of their recall of the stress of IVF post-treatment. The extent of distress reported after a treatment failure also appears to be greater for women than for men. It was shown that 25% of women had mild to moderate depression 3 weeks after a failed IVF cycle, while this level of depressive symptomatology was less common among men (12%)[14]. It has been reported that 13% of the women but none of the men in their sample of 86 patients acknowledged some thoughts of suicide after their failed IVF cycle[15]. Some authors have found that gender differences in depression persisted for up to 6 months after the failed IVF cycle[17]. Other findings have shown that men are less interested in psychosocial interventions, less likely to participate in them and, when they do participate, tend to do so for shorter periods of time than women[18].

That such gender differences exist among infertile couples is not surprising, given that they are also well-established in the general population. Indeed, negative affective states tend to be more prevalent in women, regardless of the way in which mood is assessed and expressed[5]. Some reasons for this gender difference include women's ability to express their emotions more openly than men and the finding that typical, self-report instruments are in synchrony with women's and not men's manner of emotional expression[16]. In terms of infertility-related distress, the gender difference can be explained on the basis of social and biological theories that propose mothering to be a more integral part of women's identity and/or physiological needs (e.g. maternal instinct) than fathering. Finally, others suggest that, because women undergo all the physical procedures in IVF, their higher rate of depression could be due to the effects of injections, hormones, etc.[19].

While gender differences are expected and routinely observed, a more surprising finding from detailed analysis of past findings and more recent studies is that in many ways men and women have *consistent* reactions to infertility treatments[16]. Although women rate each stage of IVF as more stressful than do men, couples' relative rankings of each stage show that both recall the 2-week implantation period and the negative pregnancy test as the most stressful stages of IVF[15]. Similarly, although women score higher on measures of distress, both before and after IVF, comparisons between these two assessment times show that men also experience a significant increase in depressive symptoms, anxiety and a variety of other negative emotional reactions when treatment fails[13,14,17]. In support of these findings, a recent prospective study confirmed that men and women exhibit a similar response pattern. For example, both husbands and wives responded to oocyte retrieval and transfer with increased optimism and feelings of emotional closeness with their partners, while for both, the pregnancy test was accompanied by feelings of acute distress and social isolation[16]. Finally, despite their general lack of interest in psychosocial interventions, men benefit from participation as much as do women. However, they report different reasons for improved well-being. Women report that the primary benefit from such interventions is the normalizing effect it has, whereas men report the educational component to be the most beneficial.

Summary

Overall, these findings highlight the emotional challenges IVF places on a significant proportion of infertile couples. Depression and anxiety are the most often recorded psychological disturbances. Research has ascertained that negative reactions are stage-dependent, however, with the greatest difficulties experienced when treatment is canceled prematurely or is unsuccessful. The IVF characteristics that appear the most difficult to cope with are its uncertainty and unpredictability, rather than its high technical demands. Estrogen-dependent symptoms (e.g. breast tenderness) and fatigue are the most frequently reported physical effects of ART. Surprisingly, a couple's interpersonal relationship improves as they proceed through the IVF process. The most illuminating aspect of gender differences in reactions to IVF is that the response pattern of men and women is for the most part consistent as they proceed through IVF, even though women experience reactions more intensely. Together, this group of findings allows clinicians to anticipate typical reactions, when they occur, to what extent and as experienced by whom, so that intervention programs to alleviate such problems can be better tailored to the ART context and thereby presumably be more effective.

IMPACT OF PSYCHOLOGICAL FACTORS ON IVF PROGRESS AND OUTCOME

Given that IVF is associated with such varying emotions, one might reasonably question whether such negative reactions could interfere with the progress of treatment or impact on the probability of conception. While the literature on this topic is extensive for distress as a cause of infertility, it remains relatively sparse with regard to distress as a cause of ART treatment failure, although exceptions occur[20]. Furthermore, most studies are restricted to the possible impact of women's distress on outcome. The research focus on women is long-standing and has been attributed to a number of factors. These include, for example, the fact that women are generally more willing to participate in such research, that the greater treatment demands on women compared to men make them more stressed during treatment, and the belief that the female reproductive system is more vulnerable to such effects[19]. Therefore, the following section will focus primarily on women. In addition, the paradigms used to test the hypothesis that psychological factors are linked to reproductive function vary considerably in experimental rigor, making it difficult to draw firm conclusions about this association. Nevertheless, evidence-based data present some intriguing findings and promising avenues for further research, and will be presented for consideration as a potential complication in ART treatments.

Treatment studies

In this type of prospective design, emotional distress is assessed alongside biological variables at several time points during the actual IVF cycle. The main finding from this type of design is that women who eventually achieve a pregnancy tend to report less stress during treatment than those who are unsuccessful[8]. However, from this correlational design it would not be possible to determine whether higher stress was the cause of the imminent treatment failure or whether awareness of imminent treatment failure was the cause of higher stress. Specifically, feedback provided by medical staff during treatment concerning a woman's response to pharmacological interventions could increase stress level, especially when treatment was not going as well as expected ('negative feedback hypothesis')[11].

Therefore, while studies using this type of design can provide valuable information about stress reactions during treatment, the methodology cannot differentiate whether stress is a cause or a consequence of (imminent) IVF outcome.

Pre-treatment-to-treatment studies

In this type of prospective study, psychological assessments carried out some months prior to the start of IVF are correlated with the biological response during treatment and/or the pregnancy rate on that or a subsequent cycle. The relationship between distress and IVF outcome is determined either by subsequently comparing pregnant and non-pregnant women on these pre-treatment scores or by using pre-treatment scores as predictors of later pregnancy using logistic regression.

Findings from these studies are mixed. In general the between-groups analyses fail to reveal differences between subsequently pregnant and non-pregnant women on standardized measures of mood (e.g. depression, anxiety, distress) or expectations for success. However, analyses that correlate the pre-treatment psychological profile with the biological response to IVF (e.g. number of oocytes) or treatment outcome, converge in showing a moderate positive association. Specifically, those who characteristically respond to stressful situations with anxiety, worry, tension and/or depression tend to have a more unfavorable response to IVF[20].

A few studies have used a similar paradigm to investigate stress effects on semen quality. This type of design compares ejaculates produced at a relatively high stress period during ART treatment (retrieval) to those produced in a relatively less stressful context some months prior to treatment[21]. The need to provide a sperm sample by masturbation on the day of retrieval is psychologically stressful for men, as the sample must be produced in the clinic, for immediate treatment, while the partner and staff are waiting and with the knowledge that failure to do so will terminate the treatment attempt for the couple. Several studies using this pre-treatment-to-treatment paradigm have indeed found that sperm quality (e.g. volume, concentration, motility) is poorer in the treatment ejaculate compared to the pre-treatment sample, with the per cent change in quality ranging from 10 to 40% depending on the study[21]. However, there is

significant intraindividual variation in semen quality and one cannot be sure from these studies whether changes were due to treatment stress or to random fluctuation in semen quality. It has been argued that, as decrements in sperm quality were up to eight times more frequent than increments in these pre-treatment-to-treatment paradigms, it was likely that effects were due to stress[21].

Mediating pathways

Different hypotheses have been offered to explain how negative personality characteristics and stress might impact on reproductive health. Some hypotheses concern indirect effects via lifestyle choices associated with high stress (e.g. smoking or alcohol use). Others concern personality factors (e.g. defeatism, ambivalence about parenthood) which might reduce the likelihood of patients persisting with treatment and thus succeeding. However, the main hypotheses concern the interaction between the hormonal system which regulates the stress response and that which regulates reproductive functioning. Whilst such interactions have proved pivotal in explaining stress effects in non-human mammals, their application in humans undergoing ART treatment has proved more problematic.

Animal studies would suggest that the final neuroendocrine event causing stress-induced disruptions to reproductive function in untreated women is inhibition of the hypothalamic gonadotropin releasing hormone (GnRH) pulse generator and slowing of luteinizing hormone (LH) pulse frequency[22]. Inhibition of GnRH is ultimately caused by an increase in corticotropin releasing hormone (CRH), which reflects the increased activity of the hypothalamic–pituitary–adrenal axis during stress[22]. Additionally, research with non-human mammals has shown that implantation can be compromised by stress-induced disruption in the estradiol : progesterone ratio during the luteal phase. Although these possibilities offer a reasonable theoretical framework for how stress might affect pregnancy outcome, medication administered during ART blocks or by-passes these natural processes. Consequently, the applicability of such findings in treated women is questionable, unless future research can demonstrate that stress reduces the effectiveness or somehow compromises the actions of such medication.

The biological pathways offered to explain stress effects on semen quality have also drawn from animal studies and have targeted psychoneuroendocrinological interactions. In particular, reductions in LH and testosterone, which over time would negatively affect the 72-day sperm developmental process, have been proposed. As was concluded for stress effects in women, further research would be needed to elucidate both the nature of stress effects on semen quality and the biological pathways that could mediate these effects in men.

Summary

Prospective studies in women and men do indeed provide converging evidence of a correlation between stress and biological parameters important for ART success. However, some data come from designs that cannot clearly demonstrate a causal link between these variables. Moreover, hypotheses offered to explain stress effects at a biological level are conceptually problematic. In the case of women, the pharmacology of ART treatment is powerful and seemingly difficult to by-pass, especially given the magnitude of stress or psychological disturbance reported. In the case of men, the most reliable effects on semen quality come from acute stress paradigms, making such findings difficult to integrate with the 72-day spermatogenic cycle. Despite these thorny issues, the stress–reproduction link does have a basis in the context of ART, and is therefore worthy of further research attention.

CONCLUSION

As was stated at the outset of this chapter, the main complication for patients undergoing ART is reduced quality of life, which is reflected by increased psychological distress and emotionality, compromised physical health and difficulty coping with treatment failure. The one exception to the general trend of deterioration in quality of life is the couple relationship, which does not appear to weaken during this process. However, one must consider that, given the inherent demands IVF places on a couple in terms of financial expense, disruption to work and lifestyle, physical side-effects

and the roller-coaster of emotions, it is surprising that the majority of patients endure this procedure with only transient and manageable disturbances to life quality. Nevertheless, it is our duty as practitioners and service providers constantly to strive to improve conditions surrounding ART. The psychological literature has given us much information in this regard. We are now able to screen out those who are not appropriate candidates for such treatment, to anticipate the different reactions of males and females, to predict the various stages of IVF that will generate the most difficulties and to identify those who are at greater risk for emotional upheaval. Thankfully, there exists at our disposal a variety of psychoeducational tools to help couples navigate their way through the obstacles of ART. It behoves us to make use of these tools. This body of research also offers a hint of evidence to suggest that, if we reduce the stress associated with ART, we might also succeed in improving pregnancy rates, our ultimate goal.

REFERENCES

1. Leiblum SR, Williams E. Screening in and out of the new reproductive options: who decides and why. *J Psychosom Obstet Gynaecol* 1993;14:37

2. Humphrey M, Humphrey H, Ainsworth-Smith I. Screening for parenthood by donor insemination. *Soc Sci Med* 1991;32:273–8

3. Micioni G, Jeker L, Zeeb M, Campana A. Doubtful and negative psychological indications for AID: a study of 835 couples – treatment outcome in couples with doubtful indication. *J Psychosom Obstet Gynaecol* 1987;6:89

4. Baetens P, Ponjaert-Kristoffersen I, Devroey P, Van Steirteghem A. Artificial insemination by donor: an alternative for single women. *Hum Reprod* 1995;10:1537

5. Ohayon MM, Priest RG, Guilleminoult C, Caulet M. The prevalence of depressive disor-

ders in the United Kingdom. *Biol Psychiat* 1999;45:300

6. Boivin J, Kentenich H. *ESHRE Monographs: Guidelines for Counselling in Infertility*. London: Oxford University Press, 2002:9–10

7. Newton CR, Sherrard W, Glavac I. The Fertility Problem Inventory: measuring perceived infertility distress. *Fertil Steril* 1999;72:54–62

8. Demyttenaere K, Nijs P, Evers-Kiebooms G, Koninckx P. Coping and the ineffectiveness of coping influence the outcome of *in vitro* fertilisation through stress responses. *Psychoneuroendocrinology* 1992;19:655

9. Boivin J, Takefman J. The impact of the *in vitro* fertilization–embryo transfer (IVF-ET) process on emotional, physical and relational variables. *Hum Reprod* 1996;11:903

10. Reading AE. Psychological preparation for surgery: patient recall of information. *J Psychosom Res* 1981;25:57

11. Boivin J, Takefman JE. Stress levels across stages of *in vitro* fertilization in subsequently pregnant and nonpregnant women. *Fertil Steril* 1995;64:802

12. Lazarus RS, Folkman S. *Stress, Appraisal, and Coping*. New York: Springer, 1984:81–91

13. Leiblum SR, Kemmann E, Lane MK. The psychological concomitants of *in vitro* fertilization. *J Psychosom Obstet Gynaecol* 1987;6:165

14. Newton CR, Hearn MT, Yuzpe AA. Psychological assessment and follow-up after *in vitro* fertilization: assessing the impact of failure. *Fertil Steril* 1990;54:879

15. Baram D, Tourtelot E, Muechler E, Huang KE. Psychological adjustment following unsuccessful *in vitro* fertilization. *J Psychosom Obstet Gynaecol* 1988;9:181

16. Boivin J, Andersson L, Shoog-Svanberg A, *et al.* Psychological reactions during *in vitro* fertilisation (IVF): similar response pattern in husbands and wives. *Hum Reprod* 1998;13: 3262

17. Slade P, Emery J, Lieberman BA. A prospective, longitudinal study of emotions and relationships in *in-vitro* fertilization treatment. *Hum Reprod* 1997;12:183

18. Boivin J. A review of psychosocial interventions for infertility. *Soc Sci Med* 2003;57: 2325–41

19. Berg BJ, Wilson JF, Weingartner PJ. Psychological sequelae of infertility treatment: the role of gender and sex-role identification. *Soc Sci Med* 1991;33:1071

20. Eugster A, Vingerhoets AJJM. Psychological aspects of *in vitro* fertilisation: a review. *Soc Sci Med* 1999;48:575

21. Harrison RF, Callan VJ, Hennessey JF. Stress and semen quality in an *in vitro* fertilization programme. *Fertil Steril* 1987;48:633

22. Ferin M. Clinical review 105: stress and the reproductive cycle. *J Clin Endocrinol Metab* 1999;84:1768

23

Philosophical and ethical considerations regarding assisted reproductive technologies

G. Pennings

INTRODUCTION

Medically assisted reproduction has shown an exponential growth, as has the number of children born. Currently, 1–3% of all children are born after medical assistance in Europe. Moreover, the treatment options are steadily expanding. More and more patients can be helped with technically more and more complicated solutions. Since the early start with *in vitro* fertilization (IVF), a spectrum of ethical problems has been generated by this technology. Some of these problems, such as the moral status of the embryo, have received an inordinate amount of attention while others, such as justice in the distribution of and access to treatment, have been largely ignored. In this contribution, two ubiquitous elements in the evaluation of ART are analyzed: the responsibility of the physician and the welfare of the child. A large part will be focused on where these elements overlap, e.g. the physician's responsibility for the well-being of the future offspring.

THE WELFARE OF THE CHILD

The 'welfare of the child' is a very useful concept in a discussion: everyone agrees that it should be taken into account but no one knows exactly what it means. The concept is sufficiently broad and vague to allow everyone to appeal to it in all kinds of circumstance. Whatever the reason for one being

opposed to certain interventions, the argument that the well-being of the future child is jeopardized always puts the speaker in a strong position. Nevertheless, the importance of the right to reproduce, as part of a person's autonomy, places the burden of proof on the one who proposes to restrict another's reproductive plan on the basis of the threat to the welfare of the future child.

The first problem that needs to be addressed is the calculation of the life quality of a person. The debate within the field of genetics and prenatal diagnosis about the quality of life of those born with certain disabilities clearly illustrates the difficulties in measuring the concept. However, even if we were able to calculate the total happiness or well-being of a future person, we would still have to decide how a certain amount should be evaluated. Suppose we determine that the life quality of a certain future person will be 75 quality-adjusted life years (QALY), is 75 QALY sufficient, since the child will have a reasonably happy life, or insufficient, because the parents could have a child with 95 QALY, or too low but acceptable, since the parents could not have had a child without the defect? Without entering deeply into the discussion, three standards for the evaluation of welfare can be found in the literature on medically assisted reproduction. The strictest standard is the 'maximal welfare' standard, according to which no medical assistance should be provided when there are indications that the life conditions of the future child will not be optimal. On the other side of the balance, there is the 'wrongful life' or 'worse than death' standard. Medical assistance to reproduction is unacceptable only if the life quality of the child is so low that it would have been better if the child had never been born. Practitioners frequently appeal to this standard when stating that without the medical intervention the child would not exist at all. This is a complicated philosophical topic, because it depends on whether bringing a person into existence is a benefit for that person. If it is, and the child has a life worth living, then the net result of the infertility treatment is positive. In my opinion, this reasoning is based on the mistaken assumption that the situation when a person exists can be compared to the situation where one has to decide whether to bring a person into existence or not. Once a person exists, his life should be very bad before he can return to a state of non-existence (death); when we have to decide whether to create a person, we should be able to offer him more than a life just worth living. Both standards mentioned above lead to a number of highly counterintuitive judgements regarding acceptable reproduction. The intermediate position, the 'reasonable welfare' standard, avoids such judgements and puts into balance both the right to reproduce of the parents and the right to a decent life of the child[1]. Responsible parenthood implies that couples should avoid having children if there is a foreseeable high risk that the future child will have a serious disease, disability or handicap. Predictably, the focus of this discussion shifts to the meaning of a 'serious' disease and a 'high' risk. In a more positive way, the same standard can be expressed as 'the child should have a reasonable chance of having a reasonably happy life'[2]. Although different definitions can be found about what constitutes a 'decent' or 'reasonable' welfare level, the common core of most definitions is that a person has a decent quality of life when he or she has the abilities and opportunities to realise those dimensions and life plans that in general make human life valuable. This leaves a large gray zone of borderline cases in which conflicts may arise between the different parties involved.

The third problem, besides the difficulty of calculating the life quality and the choice of the evaluation standard, is the presence of other values that influence the decision-making process. In other words, not all actions are exclusively directed at the welfare of the future child. Two such intervening values will be analyzed in what follows: the genetic link and the success rate of infertility treatment.

The value of the genetic link

From the early start of infertility treatment, the rationality of the wish to have genetically related children was questioned. According to some philosophers, the desire is irrational, since there is no real difference between rearing one's own child and rearing that of another person. If there is a difference, it is fully belief-dependent, i.e. if in reality the child has no genetic link but the parent believes that it has, he will experience the same satisfaction. Many men have raised children in the erroneous belief that the child was their genetic offspring when it was not and they did not even notice. This type of reasoning, however, takes dubious short-cuts by ignoring more abstract reasons for wanting genetically related children. It is important in this context to separate goals that can be realized only by having genetically related children from goals that can be realized by having children. The wish to experience pregnancy and childbirth, for instance, would not count, because it could equally well be fulfilled after oocyte donation. Moreover, we are not looking for the reasons people actually give for having genetically related children (some of these may be selfish or based on wrong assumptions), but for reasons that could justify the desire for genetically related children[2]. Some goals, such as the wish for a certain form of immortality, the wish to participate in the creation of a person or the wish to incarnate the love between partners, can be fully realized only when there is a genetic relationship. The genetic link is not exclusively valued because it will lead to qualitatively different experiences as a parent. If this were the case, then the rationality of the desire could indeed be doubted. However, if the value and rationality of these other goals is accepted, the real existence of a genetic link is crucial. In a theory which gives priority to wish fulfilment rather than wish satisfaction, it could be argued that those who have these goals are harmed when they are falsely made to believe that they have a genetic link with their children.

New techniques

Progress in medicine implies a certain degree of risk taking. However, steps can be taken to reduce the risks. First, standard measures of safety and precaution should precede the application of a technique. Second, long-term follow-up studies to verify the outcome should be planned. When new treatment methods are proposed, we will always be confronted with the tricky transition from the research phase to the first (pre-)clinical trial. The application of the new techniques in assisted reproductive technologies has been criticized because many procedures have been performed in the absence of any basic research to evaluate either the efficacy or the potential risks[3]. A carefully monitored and limited experiment with a thorough examination of the children does not remove the risks completely, but presents the best compromise between reticence and recklessness. Even for the mainstream techniques, such as 'classical' IVF, it is important to set up large-scale studies to check the physical and psychological development of those who are born as a result. It is disconcerting to read in a consensus statement published in 2003 that 'so far little attention has been paid to the safety of ART, i.e. to its adverse effects and complications'[4].

The whole field of medically assisted reproduction started as an enterprise to give people a genetically related child. While initially the interventions were focused on bypassing tubal obstruction or disease, they increasingly contained some kind of manipulation of the gametes. Intracytoplasmic sperm injection (ICSI) is probably the best known example of such manipulation, with the intention to remedy incompetent or 'bad' sperm. A small but significantly increased rate of *de novo* chromosomal anomalies and inherited malformations in children born after ICSI compared to the general population has been demonstrated[5]. The counterpart for the 'bad' oocyte is ooplasm or germinal vesicle transfer to repair oocytes or to compensate for mitochondrial defects[6]. A small part of the cytoplasm of a donor oocyte is injected into the cytoplasm of the recipient oocyte. The number of offspring in humans after cytoplasmic transfer is very limited (approximately 30) at present, but there are already indications (e.g. increased incidence of Turner's syndrome) that this method, too, might generate

risks for the health of the children. Moreover, the long-term consequences of a number of other findings, such as mitochondrial heteroplasmy in the children, are unknown. Some defects can be heritable and may be transmitted to the next generations. In the past few years, experiments have been started on haploidization or 'semi-cloning' for individuals with a total lack of competent gametes. In haploidization, the nucleus of a somatic cell from one of the parents is transferred into an enucleated oocyte. The oocyte can bring this diploid cell nucleus to undergo reduction division resulting in a pseudo-polar body and a pronucleus that can be fertilized with the gamete of the other parent[7]. This technology is explicitly promoted as an ethically more acceptable way than full cloning for enabling people to experience genetic parenthood. Haploidization has not yet led to pregnancies in humans, but animal data point at abnormalities in the development of the embryos. 'Full' cloning would have been the last step, were it not for legal prohibition. The ban on human reproductive cloning, beside concerns about uniqueness and rights to individuality, is to a large extent based on the risks for the future offspring.

The steps outlined above constitute a logical evolution as long as genetic parenthood is the primary goal. Since every step is but a small addition to the previous one, there is no clear-cut point at which a new cost–benefit analysis or means–end balance has to be made. In fact, the present controversy about human cloning may be a consequence of making too big a leap from existing techniques. When haploidization is applied (supposing it will ever work), the gap becomes much smaller and cloning can be fitted more easily into the classical justification of helping people to have genetically related children. Moreover, when the media hype has died down and the rogues have disappeared from the cloning scene, we will be left with couples for whom there is no other way of having a child that is genetically related to one of them[8]. This justification differs only gradually from that used to apply ICSI, cytoplasmic transfer or haploidization.

Acceptable risk

Although the genetic link is important to obtain the more symbolic goals of parenthood, its value should not be overestimated. This link counts for something and it compensates for a certain degree of additional risk taken for the health of the children. The question now becomes how the threshold of acceptability is determined. What, for instance, is the acceptable risk when the child might have a disease such as cystic fibrosis or Huntington's disease? One way to determine a threshold is by comparing different situations which involve reproductive risk taking. These situations can be compared from several points of view, such as severity, probability, and efforts needed to diminish or eliminate the risk. Two points are important for this strategy. First, the base rate of major malformations in the general population is 3–5%. Every child has a 3–5% chance of having a serious disease or handicap. There is no such thing as risk-free reproduction. Apparently, when little can be done about it (or when the reduction of the probability would require a disproportionate effort of testing and screening), this chance is considered acceptable. Second, the issue of acceptable risk in the context of medically assisted reproduction is mainly about risk added to the base rate either because of specific characteristics of the parents or because of the technique employed. This additional risk must in most cases be balanced against the desire for genetically related offspring.

The judgement about the acceptability of a risk for a disease in the method described above is not justified on its own, but is justified by being fitted into a set of judgements regarding the acceptability of other diseases. In other words, when we want to argue that a 10% chance of HIV infection is ethically unacceptable, we have to take into account our judgement regarding a 25% chance of cystic fibrosis, a 3% chance of chromosomal abnormality, etc. This 'coherentist' position differs from the traditional ways of justification, because we tend to raise the question of acceptability for specific diseases and risk situations. This strategy does not avoid interpersonal disagreement but at least it strives for a coherent position on all diseases and handicaps.

In the matrix for the classification of diseases, four options exist on the dimensions 'severity' and 'probability': low–low, low–high, high–low and high–high. The choice will be especially difficult for the intermediate positions. Infertility treatment for HIV-positive persons is an example of a severe lethal disease with a low probability. HIV-positive men

increasingly request artificial insemination with washed sperm in order to reduce the risk of infection of their partners and thus indirectly of their offspring. Current data pertaining to a few thousand cases of insemination with washed sperm and several hundred births have not shown a single seroconversion. This permits the conclusion that the risk of infection, when all precautions are taken, is very small. Demanding the use of donor sperm for such a minor risk requires a complete denial of the value of the genetic link.

The inverse is the combination of a relatively minor disadvantage with a high probability. This is the case in ICSI for men with microdeletions on the Y chromosome. The male children resulting from this treatment are likely also to be infertile. They will have to go through the same process as their father if they want to build a family themselves. Although there is disagreement on whether it is ethically acceptable for parents (and more specifically for the father) to burden their child with this ordeal, the disease is only moderately serious in the sense that the main consequence, i.e. infertility, can be circumvented by technology. However, a recent study also showed that couples in which the man had an abnormal karyotype did not refrain from ICSI treatment despite an increased risk of having a chromosomally abnormal child[9]. Given the severity of some of these abnormalities, one may start wondering whether the wish for a genetic child by the parents has outweighed the disadvantages for an affected child.

The existence of alternatives

A very important element in the evaluation of the decisions regarding responsible (assisted) reproduction is the existence of alternatives. However, we are so caught in the mold of genetic parenthood that the use of donor gametes is frequently not even considered as an alternative, either by those requesting help or by the providers of these services. Only when all possibilities of reaching this goal are exhausted, is donor material proposed. The French CECOS Genetics Advisory Board, for instance, only allows the use of donor sperm as an alternative when the genetic condition is serious, the risk of transmission is very high and the illness is not detectable prenatally[10]. Ignoring this option alters the problem situation completely. Harris, for instance, has repeatedly argued that, when people can have only a disabled child, it is morally better to have it than having no child at all (at least as long as the child will have a worthwhile life)[11]. However, donor gametes will, in almost all cases (genetic as well as infectious diseases), fully eliminate the risk for the offspring. The choice is not between having a disabled child or no child, but between taking a high or increased risk of having a genetically related but disabled child and a healthy but not genetically related child. This perspective gives rather a different view on the parental choice.

A broader framework

The greatest challenge for the future of medically assisted reproduction is to construct a framework in which the desire to have genetically related children can be placed. We will be able to prevent this wish from becoming absolute only if we manage to build a broader structure that incorporates theories of parenthood, genetic relationships and identity. This framework will have to incorporate other values that should be balanced against the satisfaction derived from having genetically related children. It should also include the investment and effort made by the people involved and by society in general to fulfil the desire. After the initial acceptance of the techniques, the discussion on the health economics of medically assisted reproduction was referred to the sidelines. However, the importance of infertility as a need or desire should be compared to other needs and desires in order to establish the part of the health-care budget that should be accorded to this treatment. The existence of a strong wish to have a genetically related child does not mean that every possible tool should be used to realize this wish.

The present remark is not a disguised attempt to stop medicine from developing new methods to treat infertility but intends to stimulate a critical analysis of the efforts. This exercise should be taken up at regular intervals to prevent doctors from becoming caught in the stream they themselves have created and to induce others simply to follow new developments. Apparently, such an analysis is not considered unfeasible for other desires. The wish to have a child of a particular sex for social reasons by means of preimplantation genetic diagnosis is rejected because, amongst other reasons, the goal is not in proportion to the investment physi-

cians and society have to make[12]. Why could the same balance not be made for the treatment methods used to fulfil the desire to have a child of one's own?

THE RESPONSIBILITY OF THE PHYSICIAN

People frequently reproach physicians for performing risky techniques or offering infertility treatment to controversial groups of patients. Nevertheless, little has been written on the moral responsibility of the physician in the context of assisted reproduction. Partially this is due to the peculiar nature of responsibility. Does the physician's responsibility differ from the responsibility of the intentional parents? Can they both carry full responsibility for the outcome? To a large extent, the answer to these questions will indicate who has the authority to decide about certain aspects of the treatment.

The basic scheme underlying the patient–physician relationship in the context of medically assisted reproduction is one of principal and collaborator (or accomplice). The intentional parents are the principals, because they take the initiative for the project and because they will raise the child. Fertile people carry the full responsibility themselves. When they experience difficulties in becoming pregnant, they can appeal to others for assistance in realizing the project. The other can be a surrogate, a gamete donor or a doctor. These persons have to decide whether or not to participate in the parental project. The doctor helps by providing information, performing diagnostic tests and actions. Since he contributes to the treatment as a causal agent, he is accountable for the result. The doctor must make a normative judgement about the correctness of his actions. Since his decision to collaborate is voluntary and deliberate, he engages himself as a moral agent and thus blocks the possibility of hiding behind the requesting parents. In other words, he cannot reduce himself to an instrument or a 'technical agent' who merely executes the parents' wishes. A 'technical agent' would be responsible only for the skill, proficiency and technique with which his interventions are performed, but not for the value choices that are made[13]. Precisely this personal moral responsibility gives the physician the right to appeal to conscientious objections. If the parents only were accountable for the outcome, the physician's personal moral standards could never be infringed by his or her participation.

The structure 'principal–accomplice' also implies that the fundamental ethical decision rests on the project of the intentional parents. If their plan is morally acceptable, permissible or good, the physician should be allowed to collaborate. He cannot be blamed for participating in an acceptable project. This position implicitly denies that the physician would be bound by a higher standard than the principals. Some authors have argued that physicians, owing to the deontological code of their profession, have a commitment to try to maximize well-being (and/or minimize harm)[14]. For these authors, the parents are allowed to accept a higher risk for the health of the future child than the doctor. However, I fail to see why this would be the case. Both the parents and the fertility specialist should refrain from action leading to reproduction when there is a high risk that the child will be seriously harmed. The main problem is that parents, physicians and society do not always agree on the evaluation of a parental project.

Physician's responsibility for multiple gestations

Risk for the welfare of the offspring is one factor amongst many in the decision-making process in assisted reproduction. Risk minimization is not the sole important criterion by which to evaluate a treatment. The risk will always be weighed against the efforts that have to be made to decrease the risk. In the case of medically assisted reproduction, the increase of risk is justified by the heightened success rate. However, the urge and pressure to increase success rates have resulted in a deviation from the original goal, i.e. the birth of healthy singletons. It is a well-established fact that multiple pregnancies generate a highly increased risk of obstetric complications, perinatal mortality, congenital malformations, maternal and fetal mortality and long-term social, psychological and financial difficulties. These negative effects have until now been accepted as the price to be paid for an increased pregnancy rate.

The responsibility of the physician for a multiple pregnancy deserves a thorough analysis. The Practice Committee of the American Society for Reproductive Medicine stated that a multiple gestation is an unintended result of assisted reproduction[15]. However, this statement is false for those physicians who still believe that twins are a good, or at least an acceptable outcome. But let us, for the sake of argument, accept that, in the overwhelming majority of cases, the doctor does not directly intend to create a multiple pregnancy. His immediate reason for replacing several embryos is to increase the chance of a pregnancy. Nevertheless, people can be blamed not only for what they intend to bring about but also for what they intentionally bring about, i.e. for the consequences of which the doctor is morally certain will occur. When he knows or is able to foresee that in a number of cases his actions will lead to adverse results, he is morally responsible and accountable to those who suffer the harm[16].

The fact that multiple gestations are iatrogenic is sometimes mentioned as an aggravating characteristic. However, in itself this is not true. This impression is due to the fact that the danger is induced by the physician's actions. In a way, he initiates and generates the risk. The general justification for causing harm or taking risks is the good that results from the same act. In this case, the physician knows that, by replacing several embryos, he is causing harm by creating multiples, but he judges that the good (more births of children with reasonably happy lives) resulting from the increased pregnancy rate outweighs the harm of multiple gestations. This is a dubious statement as it stands, but even more problematic is that a number of other conditions also apply to this justification. First, there should exist no alternative that brings about a better balance between harm and benefit; and second, there should be no acceptable way to diminish the harm. Precisely on these points the justification fails. The unfavorable results should occur as an inevitable or unexpected side-effect of the treatment. This would apply only if women could not become pregnant, not even of a singleton, *unless* two or more embryos were replaced. The most damaging fact about multiple pregnancies is that they are to a large extent neither unexpected nor inevitable.

In balancing the benefits and disadvantages, there is a general misrepresentation of the different options: implicitly the message is given that it is either a multiple pregnancy or no pregnancy at all. In reality, the choice is between having multiples now and having a singleton later. Most women who become pregnant of multiples would have become pregnant of a singleton if they had undergone more cycles. Obviously, it is impossible to predict with certainty whether a woman who has three or more embryos replaced and becomes pregnant of triplets would have become pregnant in a subsequent cycle if only one embryo had been replaced. Nevertheless, a number of elements (embryo and patient characteristics) are known to affect the pregnancy rate. Sufficient data have been collected in recent years to estimate the risk of ending with a multiple gestation when a certain number of embryos with certain morphological characteristics are replaced[17]. The question then becomes whether a physician who takes a high risk of creating multiples is guilty of negligence or recklessness. Risk taking is condemned as reckless when the person is aware of an unjustified risk but still proceeds. As noted above, risk is a combination of seriousness and probability of harm. If we take into account the possibility of preventing the harm by replacing one embryo during more cycles, then the cost (in terms of money, psychological distress, etc.) of this strategy is easily outweighed by the harmful consequences of a multiple pregnancy rate of approximately 25%.

The acceptance of the negative effects of multiple pregnancies, demonstrated by the reluctance of practitioners to take drastic measures to reduce the multiple gestation rate, shows a striking inconsistency in the application of the 'welfare of the child' criterion. Postmenopausal pregnancies are rejected because the obstetric and health risks for mother and child are too high. Lesbians are denied access to infertility treatment because of the expectation that their children would suffer detrimental psychological consequences of growing up in a fatherless family. All these (frequently putative) consequences pale into insignificance when compared with the effects of multiple pregnancies. The selective use of the 'welfare of the child' standard demonstrates that its use frequently hides moral prejudices. It expresses the belief that children should be born in 'normal' families, i.e. families composed of young heterosexual married or stable parents with their genetically related children.

Sharing responsibility: who decides?

More and more, the need to provide patients with full information on the risks and benefits is stressed. The preference of infertile patients for replacing several embryos and the fact that they welcome twins are explained by inadequate counseling and incomplete information about the psychological, physical and financial challenges of having multiples. If the patients knew better, they would choose differently. In a similar vein, pleas are made in favor of providing more complete information on the risks involved in ART in general and ICSI more specifically[18]. It is beyond doubt that this is a laudable proposal: autonomous and rational decision making by patients presupposes adequate information and counseling. Nevertheless, other messages might also (even if not intended) underlie such initiatives. First, it is up to the patient to decide what should be done; and second, when full information is provided, the physician's responsibility for the choice (and outcome) is diminished.

Applied to the question of how many embryos to replace, some practitioners adopt the position that the physician's role should be restricted to informing the patients about the possible risks and benefits. The candidate parents should make the final decision on the basis of that information. There are, however, strong arguments to oppose this position. First of all, the autonomous and rational character of the decision by the candidate parents can be doubted. A number of findings from surveys among fertility patients raise doubt about the patients' competence: women with children are significantly more negative towards having multiples than childless women (which indicates an underestimation of the difficulties of raising children) and a large majority of infertility patients would elect to have quadruplets rather than forfeit the opportunity to have biological children. These findings strongly suggest that the desire to have children dominates and distorts the way infertile individuals look at the situation. Second, as emphasized earlier, the physician cannot reduce himself to a 'technical agent' whose job it is to realize the patients' wishes. As a free and autonomous agent who collaborates in the reproductive project of the candidate parents, the physician remains accountable. In fact, this can be made clear by imagining 'extreme' circumstances. Suppose a 32-year-old woman and her partner are relatively poor and can pay for only one IVF cycle. After being informed of the chance of pregnancy and the multiple pregnancy rate, they ask for four embryos to be replaced. The couple argues that, given their financial situation, the success rate is very important. Moreover, it is unlikely that the woman will have quadruplets. They also indicate that they do not intend to have a reduction if a multiple gestation is detected, because a multiple will give them a complete family at once. Is it acceptable for the physician, possibly after informing them again about all possible risks and scenarios, to replace four embryos? If so, then what about replacing six embryos?

Leaving the decision completely to the patients is simply untenable. I believe that the doctor should err on the safe side and should opt for single- or double-embryo transfer, depending on the characteristics of both the embryo(s) and of the woman. Ultimately, given the questions about the competence of infertile people to make a rational decision regarding this point and given the physician's obligation to avoid causing harm to the patients and their possible offspring, it is the fertility specialist who should decide how many embryos to transfer (unless the patient wants fewer). Increased patient participation in the medical decision process cannot serve as a factor to discharge the physician from his duty to make clinical management decisions based on objective knowledge[19]. The physician's attitude can be both paternalistically and non-paternalistically motivated. He can rightly argue that it is better for the intentional parents not to have multiples. Parents are better off with a healthy singleton. But even when every form of paternalistic behavior is rejected, there still remains the direct responsibility of the physician for the well-being of the future offspring.

An interesting point when considering the personal accountability of the physician is whether it is acceptable that the collaborator imposes conditions. Conditional infertility treatment makes sense within the principal–collaborator framework. A physician who judges that the risk taken by the intentional parents falls outside the reasonable risk range can introduce conditions to reduce the risk. He could, for instance, agree to participate in the reproductive project of an HIV-positive man on the

condition that donor sperm were used. Most fertility centers will demand prenatal or preimplantation genetic diagnosis for couples with a high risk of cystic fibrosis, or screening of the female partner of men who need ICSI for congenital bilateral absence of the vas deferens. Similarly, prenatal diagnosis followed by a termination of pregnancy could be a condition before ICSI treatment is started in men with chromosomal abnormalities. This implies that the procreative liberty of the couple is restricted to a certain extent. In theory, patients are free to accept the conditions or not, but in practice, the circumstances are rarely so simple. Therefore, such measures should be imposed only when the physician or the fertility center is convinced that unconditional collaboration is unacceptable. Nevertheless, especially when the measure would lead to a drastic reduction of risk, the physician has the right to lay down conditions. If he were obliged to comply with every request patients proposed, he could not be liable for the outcome. It is precisely because his collaboration is free and deliberate that he is morally accountable. To stipulate risk-reducing actions should not be seen as an infringement of the patient's autonomy but as a way to enable the physician to justify his participation.

The contribution of society

The physician's responsibility cannot be isolated from the social context in which he functions. The physician is not acting within a social vacuum. His rights and duties towards society in general are increasingly recognized. Several steps can be taken in the management of the health-care system to decrease the number of multiple gestations. This presupposes that the causes of the current practice are identified. On the positive side, incentives can be given to clinics that manage to hold down the percentage of multiples. This financial benefit might counteract the profit motive that drives directors, boards and fertility specialists to maximize the success rate. Statistics become publicity if the intake of patients is determined by the success rate (especially when published in IVF league tables). Commercialization of IVF has been identified as an important cause of the present transfer policy. In addition, reimbursement for a reasonable number of cycles might mitigate the pressure exerted by patients on their doctors to replace more embryos.

A recent study in Denmark showed that one-quarter of women who initially disagreed would accept single-embryo transfer if they were offered more than the three reimbursed treatments they received at the time[20]. For a considerable number of countries, three reimbursed cycles would already be a major improvement compared to the present situation. If such positive measures would remain ineffective, there is still the possibility of coercion by law, as in Sweden and the UK, where a maximum limit for the number of transferred embryos is determined. Heavy fines for clinics and physicians with higher-order multiples or with a disproportionally elevated number of multiple gestations is also an option. This could help to compensate for the additional cost of every multiple pregnancy for the health-care budget.

CONCLUSION

The quest for new ways to initiate a pregnancy has resulted in a set of techniques that encompass a more or less invasive manipulation of the embryo or the gametes. Most of these methods generate known and unknown risks for the health of the offspring. It is vital for the further development of ART that a framework be constructed to prevent the wish for genetically related children becoming absolute. A debate should be started within society to determine how much effort the community should invest in the realization of this wish and how much risk for the child intentional parents should be allowed to assume in order to fulfil this wish.

Although the welfare of the child is frequently presented as the fundamental criterion for the moral evaluation of infertility treatment, the analysis of clinical practice shows that other criteria intervene. Two other considerations make clinical practice deviate from maximizing the health and general well-being of the child in the strict sense, i.e. the genetic link and the pregnancy rate in ART.

REFERENCES

1. Pennings G. Measuring the welfare of the child: in search of the appropriate evaluation criterion. *Hum Reprod* 1999;14:1146–50

2. Strong C. Overview: a framework for reproductive ethics. In Dickenson DL, ed. *Ethical Issues in Maternal–Fetal Medicine*. Cambridge: Cambridge University Press, 2002:17–35

3. Hawes SM, Sapienza C, Latham KE. Ooplasmic donation in humans: the potential for epigenic modifications. *Hum Reprod* 2002;17:850–2

4. Land JA, Evers JLM. Risks and complications in assisted reproduction techniques: report of an ESHRE consensus meeting. *Hum Reprod* 2003;18:455–7

5. Bonduelle ML. ICSI-related risk for the children. PhD thesis, Brussels Free University, Brussels, 2003

6. Barritt JA, Willadsen S, Bremer C, Cohen J. Cytoplasmic transfer in assisted reproduction. *Hum Reprod Update* 2001;7:428–35

7. Tesarik J. Reproductive semi-cloning respecting biparental embryo origin: embryos from syngamy between a gamete and a haploidized somatic cell. *Hum Reprod* 2002;17:1933–7

8. Bonnicksen AL. Procreation by cloning: crafting anticipatory guidelines. *J Law Med Ethics* 1997;25:273–82

9. Giltay JC, Kastrop PMM, Tuerlings JHAM, *et al.* Subfertile men with constitutive chromosome abnormalities do not refrain from intracytoplasmic sperm injection treatment: a follow-up study of 75 Dutch patients. *Hum Reprod* 1999;14:318–20

10. Novaes SB. Making decisions about someone else's offspring. Geneticists and reproductive technology. In Fortun M, Mendelsohn E, eds. *The Practices of Human Genetics*. Dordrecht: Kluwer Academic, 1999:169–84

11. Harris J. *Wonderwoman and Superman: the Ethics of Human Biotechnology*. Oxford: Oxford University Press, 1992

12. Pennings G. Personal desires of patients and social obligations of geneticists: applying preimplantation genetic diagnosis for non-medical sex selection. *Prenat Diagn* 2002;22: 1123–9

13. Blustein J. Doing what the patient orders: maintaining integrity in the doctor–patient relationship. *Bioethics* 1993;7:289–314

14. Savulescu J. Should doctors intentionally do less than the best? *J Med Ethics* 1999;25: 121–6

15. American Society for Reproductive Medicine. *Guidelines on Number of Embryos Transferred.* A Practice Committee Report. Birmingham, AL: American Society for Reproductive Medicine, 1998

16. Dworkin G. Intention, foreseeability, and responsibility. In Schoeman F, ed. *Responsibility, Character, and the Emotions: New Essays in Moral Psychology.* Cambridge: Cambridge University Press, 1987:338–45

17. Gerris J, Van Royen E. Avoiding multiple pregnancies in ART: a plea for single embryo transfer. *Hum Reprod* 2000;15:1884–8

18. Kurinczuk JJ. Safety issues in assisted reproductive technology. From theory to reality – just what are the data telling us about ICSI offspring health and future fertility and should we be concerned? *Hum Reprod* 2003;18: 925–31

19. Brinsden P. Controlling the high order multiple birth rate: the European perspective. *Reprod BioMed Online* 2003;6:339–44

20. Pinborg A, Loft A, Schmidt L, Nyboe Andersen A. Attitudes of IVF/IVSI-twin mothers towards twins and single embryos transfer. *Hum Reprod* 2003;18:621–7

Appendix

CLASSIFICATION OF OVARIAN HYPERSTIMULATION SYNDROME

The classification of OHSS has evolved with time, owing to changes in diagnostic methods and also in stimulation aims. Initially, only essays of urinary estrogens were available to evaluate the stimulation during controlled ovarian stimulation, which aimed at obtaining a natural conception, and to elicit maturation of as few follicles as possible to avoid multiple pregnancy.

On this basis, Rabau[1] proposed in 1967 a first classification of OHSS cases, which was later modified by Schenker and Weinstein in 1978. A simplified classification consisting of three grades has been proposed by the World Health Organization (WHO).

The classification by Schenker and Weinstein was mostly used until Golan and colleagues[2] proposed a new system in 1989:

(1) *Mild OHSS:*

Grade 1 Only laboratory evidence of OHSS exists: total urinary estrogens above 150 μg/24 h and pregnanediol excretion above 10 mg/24 h

Grade 2 Grade 1 features plus enlargement of the ovaries but less than 5 cm

(2) *Moderate OHSS:*

Grade 3 Features of mild OHSS plus abdominal distention

Grade 4 Features of grade 3 plus nausea, vomiting and/or diarrhea (less frequently). Ovarian enlargement between 5 and 12 cm

(3) *Severe OHSS:*

Grade 5 Features of moderate OHSS plus ascites and/or hydrothorax

Grade 6 All of the above plus a change in blood volume and increased blood viscosity due to hemoconcentration, resulting in reduced renal perfusion complicated by anuria and renal failure

WHO classification (1973):

(1) *Degree I (mild):* Grades 1 and 2 (Schenker and Weinstein)

(2) *Degree II (moderate):* Ovarian cysts and digestive symptoms

(3) *Degree III (severe):* Large cysts and ascites or hydrothorax

The situation is currently quite different, since serum levels of estradiol and progesterone are available, as is measurement of follicle size and number by using vaginal sonography. The latter technique is also able to diagnose ascites before the appearance of clinical symptoms. On the other hand, many ovulation inductions are carried out with the aim of obtaining a supraphysiological number of oocytes in the context of IVF. Therefore, the mild OHSS grade, according to the criteria of Rabau and of the WHO, has become a situation that is part of almost every stimulation cycle in IVF. Consequently, in the absence of symptoms, it cannot be considered as a true complication. Moreover, ovarian size was one of the major criteria in the previous classifications. Unfortunately, it is no longer useful in IVF. Indeed, oocyte collection and follicular aspiration induce early iatrogenic intrafollicular hemorrhage, thus modifying ovarian size.

Currently, the Golan classification based on clinical signs seems to be more appropriate, and in accordance with new treatment and investigation methods:

(1) *Mild OHSS:*

Grade 1 Abdominal distention and discomfort

Grade 2 Features of grade 1 plus nausea, vomiting and/or diarrhea. Ovaries are enlarged to a size of 5–12 cm

(2) *Moderate OHSS:*

Grade 3 Features of grade 2 plus ultrasonic evidence of ascites

(3) *Severe OHSS:*

Grade 4 Features of moderate OHSS plus clinical evidence of ascites and/or hydrothorax or dyspnea

Grade 5 All of the above plus change in blood volume, increased blood viscosity due to hemoconcentration, coagulation abnormalities, and diminished renal perfusion and function

Finally, Navot and colleagues made a distinction between the severe form and a life-threatening form of OHSS[3]. The latter is characterized by one of the following criteria: ARDS, tense ascites with or without hydrothorax, severe hemoconcentration (hematocrit > 55%) and very high leukocytosis (> 25 000), oliguria, creatinine level of > 1.6 mg/ml, creatinine clearance of < 50 ml/min, renal failure and thromboembolic phenomena.

Lyons and co-workers separated OHSS into early and late occurrences[4]. Onset of OHSS follows two different patterns: early OHSS occurs 3–7 days after hCG administration, whereas late OHSS, which is most often severe, occurs 12–17 or more days after hCG injection.

Early OHSS is an acute effect, owing to exogenous hCG, administered 35 h before oocyte retrieval, and can occur in patients who do not become pregnant. Spontaneous resolution occurs when the exogenous hCG concentrations fall, probably resulting in reduced production of unknown substance(s) which induce OHSS.

Late OHSS is induced by endogenous hCG from the implanting pregnancy. It is seen only in patients who become pregnant, more often with two or more gestational sacs. This form is known to subside rapidly after spontaneous or therapeutic abortion. In the initial publication by Lyons's group, no patient with early OHSS developed late relapse and no patient with late OHSS had demonstrated early OHSS.

Early and late forms are characterized by different risk factors. Lyons and colleagues applied a step-wise multiple logistic regression to find factors that might predict early or late onset of OHSS[4]. Estradiol and oocytes collected were identified as statistical predictors for the early form, and only the number of gestational sacs, the serum hCG level and serum progesterone level on days 11–13, after hCG administration, were identified as statistical predictors for the late form. Estradiol levels on the day of hCG administration, the slope of the estradiol curve prior to hCG administration, the number of oocytes collected and serum estradiol and progesterone levels 7–8 days after hCG administration were all non-predictive of late-onset OHSS[4]. These results were confirmed by Mathur and colleagues in a series of 48 cases[5]. Lyons and co-workers emphasized that it was essential to separate early- and late-onset forms, since they depend on different predictive factors, and because, by analyzing them together, some predictive factors of either form may remain unidentified.

However, among the small series of Lyons and co-workers ($n = 10$), mixed forms (early onset, with prolongation for long periods) were not described. These mixed forms are due to stimulation by exogenous hCG first and then by endogenous hCG, when the patient becomes pregnant, rendering the distinction between early- and late-onset theoretical. Indeed, some authors consider that there are not two separated entities, but rather two phases of a self-limiting condition. These phases coincide with the initial preovulatory hCG level and the second rise in hCG due to the pregnancy[6].

In conclusion, OHSS can be subdivided into an early form that is less severe, occurs more often in younger women and is more dependent on stimulation conditions. When these patients do not become pregnant, spontaneous resolution of OHSS ensues. The late form is often severe. Estradiol levels that are reached during stimulation are less elevated and the OHSS develops during pregnancy. If early pregnancy is arrested, the OHSS problem resolves itself rapidly.

Whether the onset of OHSS is either early or late, its degree of gravity needs to be evaluated by established criteria. We believe that the Golan classification (1989) should be preferred, since it is better adapted to modern infertility treatment and management.

REFERENCES

1. Rabau E, David A, Serr DM. Mashiach S, Lunenfeld B. Human menopausal gonadotrophins for anovulation and sterility. Results of 7 years of treatment. *Am J Obstet Gynecol* 1967;98:92–8

2. Golan A, Ron-el R, Herman A, Soffer Y, Weinraub Z, Caspi E. Ovarian hyperstimulation syndrome: an update review. *Obstet Gynecol Surv* 1989;44:430–40

3. Navot D, Bergh PA, Laufer N. Ovarian hyperstimulation syndrome in novel reproductive technologies: prevention and treatment. *Fertil Steril* 1992;58:249–61

4. Lyons CA, Wheeler CA, Frishman GN, Hackett RJ, Seifer DB, Haning RV Jr. Early and late presentation of the ovarian hyperstimulation syndrome: two distinct entities with different risk factors. *Hum Reprod* 1994;9:792–9

5. Mathur RS, Akande AV, Keay SD, Hunt LP, Jenkins JM. Distinction between early and late ovarian hyperstimulation syndrome. *Fertil Steril* 2000;73:901–7

6. Murdoch AP, Evbuomwan I. Severe complications of ovarian hyperstimulation syndrome are preventable. *Hum Reprod* 1999;14:2922–3

Index